Faulkner & Gray's
Medical Outcomes and Practice Guidelines Library
Volume 4

Patient-Focused Care in the Hospital:

Restructuring and Redesign Methods To Achieve Better Outcomes

Carolyn E. Aydin, PhD
Linda Burnes Bolton, DrPH, RN, FAAN
Scott Weingarten, MD, MPH

F&G

Patient-Focused Care in the Hospital

Faulkner & Gray, Inc.
Eleven Penn Plaza
New York NY 10001

ISBN: 1-881393-45-3

Published by Faulkner & Gray's
Healthcare Information Center
11 Penn Plaza
New York NY 10001

Spencer Vibbert, Sponsoring Editor
James DeAngelis, Project Editor
Nancy Frohlich, Production Manager

PRINTED IN THE UNITED STATES OF AMERICA

Table of Contents

The Editors

Carolyn E. Aydin, PhD, is assistant administrator for nursing research at Cedars-Sinai Medical Center and assistant clinical professor at the University of California-Los Angeles, School of Nursing. She has more than twenty years experience in evaluating the impacts of health care innovations.

Linda Burnes Bolton, DrPH, RN, FAAN, is director of nursing research and development and surgical nursing at Cedars-Sinai Medical Center; assistant clinical professor at the University of California-Los Angeles, School of Nursing; and a Fellow in the American Academy of Nursing. In addition, Dr. Burnes Bolton is president of the National Black Nurses Association and is a member of the Advisory Council for the Agency for Health Care Policy and Research.

Scott Weingarten, MD, MPH, is director of health services research for the Cedars-Sinai Health System; and assistant professor, University of California-Los Angeles, School of Medicine. A nationally recognized authority on guideline development, Dr. Weingarten is currently vice chair of clinical guidelines for the American College of Physician Executives.

Acknowledgements

The Editors would like to acknowledge the work of the executive leadership of Cedars-Sinai Medical Center, particularly Gerry Popolow, RN, project director, and the hundreds of Cedars-Sinai employees who spent numerous hours each week for two years or more to make the projects described in this book a reality. Patient-focused care was a group effort in which individuals from throughout the entire organization truly learned to work together in teams.

Forward

Changes in America's health care system have, in recent years, been nothing short of breathtaking. Advances in fundamental biology and human genetics, which have led to rapid development of new health care technologies and the increasing enrollment in group health and managed care delivery systems, are only two examples of changes that have profoundly affected health care in the 1990s. Neither of these could have been anticipated fifteen years ago.

A more recent development—identified by the phrase "patient-focused care"—may lack the drama of new scientific discovery, or the attention given to changing economic relationships within the health care industry. But its impact on America's health care system is certain to be highly significant.

Patient-focused care, with its emphasis on meeting the overall needs and preferences of the patient rather than a more narrow focus on treating specific diseases or medical conditions, is a perspective that offers enormous potential for increasing patient satisfaction, facilitating continuity of care and improving quality of care. Indeed, this represents a major conceptual breakthrough in health services research and practice.

The move toward patient-centered care will require a host of changes. Some of these may be relatively minor and, for the most part, easily accomplished. Others will require major shifts in mind-sets and attitudes and will involve fundamental alterations in how caregivers interact with patients and how they spend their time.

Some changes on the path to patient-focused care will require little or no expense. Others may be quite costly, perhaps involving architectural redesign or remodeling of health care facilities to better accommodate the needs and preferences of patients.

Several seemingly unrelated developments that are now gaining respectability and influence in health care are, indeed, quite consistent with a move toward patient-focused care. For example, increasing attention to the role of patient preferences in clinical decision-making reflects a fundamental change in the way health care professionals have learned to approach the development of science-based clinical practice guidelines. Today, guidelines increasingly stress the importance of patient preferences in determining what treatment option to pursue (including decisions to rely on "watchful waiting," or not to treat at all). By explaining the options and trade-offs among possible treatments, the practitioner's role is vital in arriving at a patient-focused decision. But the final, best decision is the patient's alone.

In the area of outcomes research, we are also learning more about the need to base evaluations of medical effectiveness on patients' perceptions of their health status and function, especially in the light of often less-than-definitive "clinical" evidence. For example, analyses of quality and satisfaction now often include utility measures designed to gauge patient satisfaction with specific treatment outcomes. Such measures are an important factor in evaluating the outcomes of alternative clinical treatments. For patient-focused care to work, consumers must have access to good information about their health care and health care options. This is also a critical area where health services research can contribute to a better health care system.

Consumer information needs to be accessible and understandable so consumers can use it to make better choices about their own health care. This will include consumer satisfaction surveys; good "measures" for determining what constitutes quality in health care; and "report cards" which consumers can use to make comparisons among health care plans. Research is currently underway on such topics as how well consumers understand their health care plans and quality indicators and the extent to which they find these indicators useful in making health care choices.

The concept of patient-focused care will occupy an increasingly important place in America's future health care system. Additional research is needed to fully define the benefits of patient-focused care in real-life clinical settings, and there remains much to be learned about the practical aspects of implementation. Patient-Focused Care in the Hospital provides timely and useful information and is a significant contribution to this end.

Clifton R. Gaus, ScD
Administrator
Agency for Health Care Policy and Research

Chapter 1

Patient-Focused Care, Clinical Practice Guidelines, And Outcomes Research: Essential Links in a Changing Health Care Environment

Carolyn E. Aydin, PhD
Linda Burnes Bolton, DrPH, RN, FAAN
Scott Weingarten, MD, MPH

The driving forces affecting health care systems have escalated over the last five years, with regulatory and market driven demands compelling hospitals and health care systems to lower costs and design systems which will enable them to compete on the basis of quality outcomes. In this context, Dr. Kenneth Shine, President of the Institute of Medicine, has challenged health institutions to constantly modify and reassess quality of care approaches as a part of their public and societal commitment.[1] The goal of these change efforts is to sustain quality while undergoing organizational redesign to reduce costs. One of the many challenges facing these organizations, however, is the development of valid, responsive, and reliable evaluation and monitoring systems to determine the effects of changes in structure and processes on clinical and organizational outcomes.[2] Health care institutions need to be able to answer basic questions of what works and at what costs. How much data should be collected, how is quality measured, and what is the relationship between quality monitoring and organizational design?

While quality is often translated into outcomes monitoring, outcomes may not comprehensively or completely measure organizational effectiveness.[3,4] Donabedian acknowledged this paradox in 1966 in attempting to comprehensively measure quality, and recommended the structure-process-outcome framework which is widely used today.[5] This volume returns to Donabedian's basic structure-process-outcome framework and provides the reader with case studies of work in progress which link efforts to redesign orga-

CAROLYN E. AYDIN, PHD—Assistant Administrator for Nursing Research, Cedars-Sinai Medical Center and Research Institute; Assistant Clinical Professor, University of California-Los Angeles, School of Nursing.

LINDA BURNES BOLTON, DRPH, RN, FAAN—Director, Nursing Research and Development, Director, Surgical Nursing, Cedars-Sinai Medical Center and Research Institute; Assistant Clinical Professor, University of California-Los Angeles, School of Nursing; and Associate Professor, California State University, Los Angeles.

SCOTT WEINGARTEN, MD, MPH—Director, Health Services Research, Cedars-Sinai Health Care System and Research Institute; Assistant Professor, University of California-Los Angeles, School of Medicine.

nizational structures, retool organizational processes of care, and implement medical guidelines and clinical pathways to observable outcomes at both the patient and organizational levels. The need for comprehensive data to evaluate performance and enhance health provider capacity and clinical decisionmaking is imperative to achieving better patient outcomes.

The outcomes research reported here evaluates the effects of structural and process changes on organizational quality and effectiveness. We have delineated and evaluated structures and processes at the clinical and organizational levels simultaneously. Work redesign, clinical guidelines and pathways, and resource management organizational change efforts are examined for their effectiveness in achieving patient and institutional outcomes. The individual chapters also provide readers with detailed information on the processes undertaken to bring about predetermined clinical and organizational outcomes. This work is representative of the national effort to deliver quality health care in the midst of continuous change related to market and economic forces. As such, we report on processes implemented and on their effects, while simultaneously recommending additional refinements and improvements in structures and processes.

Our experience in assessing the costs and benefits of clinical processes and organizational structural changes is shared in hope that others may benefit. This experience is particularly valuable to other institutions because our efforts were undertaken in the "real world" context of an institution faced with the need to respond to the changing health care environment in order to survive and prosper. The projects described in this book have had little or no extramural funding, nor were they conducted as pilot or demonstration projects without concern for cost constraints. We have employed the continuum of health services research tools, including measures of customer satisfaction, patient functional status, cost benefit care model analysis, decision analysis, physician satisfaction, and patient caregiver interpersonal and teamwork analysis. The products of this multidisciplinary initiative, along with the forward by Dr. Clifford Gaus of the Agency for Health Care Policy and Research and the work of our guest authors Dr. Robert Kaplan and Dr. Peter Rosen, contribute data which will hopefully help us to design effective outcomes monitoring systems that are useful to health providers, payers, and consumers.

The following sections provide detailed background information on the health care initiatives underlying the institutional change efforts described in this book. The evaluation of the impacts of these and other change efforts on the delivery of health care forms the core of the relative new discipline of applied health services research. The first section below describes the patient-focused care (PFC) movement in American hospitals to redesign the delivery of patient care, followed by background information on clinical practice guidelines and pathways. The discussion of PFC also includes an overview of recent market and regulatory forces that constitute the driving forces for all of these change efforts.

Patient-Focused Care: The American Expression

Patient-Focused Care (PFC) can be broadly defined as "the redesign of patient care so that hospital resources and personnel are organized around patients rather than around various specialized departments."[6] PFC is one of a number of initiatives currently being adopted by hospitals in response to pressures to become more responsive to patient needs while providing cost-effective care. PFC is unique, however, in that it involves a fundamental rethinking of hospital structures and processes. While other initiatives such as total quality management (TQM) and continuous quality improvement (CQI) attempt to maximize the performance of structures and processes already in place, PFC works backward from the desired end product, or patient outcome, to redesign the entire system.[7]

Organizational and Economic Factors Stimulate Change

Rethinking the Structure of Hospitals. Faced with the demand from patients, physicians, and third-party payers for cost-effective services, hospital administrators have begun to realize that traditional organizational structures may no longer be viable.[8,9] In fact, the structure of the modern American hospital still reflects the organizational needs of the early twentieth century. At that time, physicians wanted easy access to hospitals equipped with facilities such as clinical laboratories to meet their needs, but did not want to become hospital employees themselves.[10] In order to ensure that their needs were met, the American College of Surgeons established standards for certification that required hospitals to have a laboratory with a physician, perferably a pathologist, in charge. Clinical pathologists then began a program for certifying laboratory personnel with various levels of education so that tests could be performed by specialists who were not physicians, with physicians interpreting the results of their tests. Over time, additional provider groups carved out other discrete portions of the care process (e.g., respiratory therapy, physical therapy, and others), creating new departments as well as new state regulations to define the licensure required to perform specific tasks.[11] This proliferation of provider groups is underscored by the fact that, by 1987, thirty-five separate health professions and occupations were subject to licensing by one or more states.[12] All of these factors have combined to create a complex health care process delivered by frequently bureaucratic and inefficient organizations whose operations respond to the needs of departments and disciplines rather than patients.[13]

Patient-focused care represents a paradigm shift in which patient care outcomes (i.e., improvements in patient health and well-being, changes in health-related knowledge and behavior, and patient satisfaction[14]) rather than the needs of the organization and its departments provide the starting point from which to examine the structures and processes of care. This paradigm shift is being reinforced and institutionalized by the Joint Commission on Accreditation of Healthcare Organizations' (JCAHO) recent transition from articulating requirements for structures and processes as ends in themselves to relating performance of essential processes to patient outcomes.[15] This approach also echoes the longstanding emphasis of Donabedian and others on the importance of the relationships among structures, processes, and outcomes for the quality of health care.[16]

The current heightened awareness of this new paradigm, however, can also be traced directly to the trends in the economics of health care.

Responding to the New Economics. Despite the need to restructure health care's complex and unwieldy systems, there was little impetus for change over the years that hospitals remained profitable. Before the 1980s, reimbursement was based almost exclusively on hospital costs or charges. Physicians had exclusive control over treatment decisions and the hospital industry benefited financially from increases in the intensity and scope of hospital-based treatment.[17] In fact, in this fee-for-service or cost based system, individual departments such as the laboratory, radiology, respiratory therapy, physical therapy, and others became important revenue or overhead generators for hospitals. Even with the introduction of prospective payment in the 1980s, large numbers of hospitals were able to shift costs between public and private payers, undermining the incentives of prospective payment. Although the mid 1980s were characterized by a shift to shorter lengths of stay and an increase in outpatient treatment, and some hospitals did reduce costs, hospitals with less competition or whose payer mix included a larger proportion of Blue Cross and commercial insurers were still able to shift costs and maintain their financial viability.[18] By the late 1980s, however, some hospitals, faced with a shortage of registered nurses coupled with the need to reduce costs and improve customer service, began to consider a patient-centered framework for restructuring the delivery of care.[19]

By the early 1990s, the payer mix began to shift in many areas of the country. The ever-increasing costs of health care premiums led corporations to look for alternatives to the traditional Blue Cross and commercial insurance plans and to organize efforts to limit the large annual increases in premiums. Marking the beginning of what has been termed the "economic era of competition,"[20] hospitals and group practices began to merge into systems that could compete for managed care contracts. Many of these contracts include capitation and financial risk sharing among providers (i.e., arrangements in which the provider receives a fixed monthly amount per subscriber, whether or not medical care is provided).[21] Competition for these contracts places tremendous pressure on hospitals to deliver high-quality, low-cost services, and hospitals and health systems are being forced to adapt to these pressures by becoming more efficient.[22] In the course of contract negotiations, hospitals may be required to provide information beyond financial data such as practice parameters, quality indicators, and patient satisfaction methodology and results.[23]

Expert opinion on the future is mixed and many regions of the country may not feel the impact of capitation and financial risk-sharing for several years. Preparation for capitation, however, involves the implementation of systems that will enhance both quality and efficiency in the delivery of health care. Cost management in a capitated system requires "reducing both the volume of services and the cost per unit, while maintaining the quality of care and customer satisfaction."[24] Although the early patient-focused care projects existed before cost issues came to the fore, PFC's focus on enhancing service to patients through improvements in the efficiency of hospital systems makes it a potent tool in the search for ways to improve service while reducing costs. The following section provides an overview of patient focused care goals nationwide and evidence of the results of the initiative to date.

Goals of PFC Nationwide

In 1993, the publication *Hospitals* reported on a national survey designed to explore the PFC movement nationwide.[25] At that time, close to half of the 311 CEOs responding to the survey indicated that they were planning or already inplementing PFC programs. Ninety percent of the efforts were less than three years old and experts predicted that most hospitals would implement PFC programs within ten years. When asked about their motivation to embark on PFC projects, 87.6% of respondents saw PFC as the best way to provide high quality patient care, supporting the concept that PFC's primary goal is to enhance service. Lowering expenses, however, was also important to over half (54.5%) of the respondents. Additional reasons for PFC programs included attracting and/or retaining nurses (43.4%), as a survival strategy (37.2%), improving the hospital's reputation (35.9%), meeting payers' demand for cost/quality data (28.3%), and others. The following section describes the underlying themes of the national PFC movement to redesign hospital processes, summarized from responses to the *Hospitals* survey and other sources.

Renegotiating the Care Process. Hospitals can be thought of as "politically negotiated orders"[26] in which the division of patient care tasks is determined by legal requirements and conscious negotiation among subgroups, traditionally without considering the efficiency of the resulting patient care process.[27,28] The PFC design process involves renegotiating this traditional care process to create more efficient systems that focus on the needs of patients rather than on the needs of departments and health care professionals. Accomplishing this goal generally involves redesigning both the structures and processes of the organization to put as many services as close to the patient as possible. Basic tenets include decentralization of services, cross-preparation of employees, work redesign, and physical and geographical reorganization of delivery systems.

With these general goals in mind, the renegotiation process frequently begins with multidisciplinary groups working together to assess potential weaknesses in the structures and processes of care. These work groups may begin by asking a series of questions basic to patient care such as: "(1) *What* is being done to, for, and by the patient? (2) *Why* is it being done? (3) *Who* is doing it? (4) *How* is it being done? (5) *When* is it being done? (6) *Where* is it being done? And (7) *What* is a better way in which it could be done?"[29] This analysis and the subsequent redesign of an institution's systems actually constitutes a renegotiation of the care process itself. The scope of the project may include a single department, the entire institution, or something in between. Projects that begin "with a clean sheet of paper" and focus on business processes as well as the delivery of patient care are sometimes termed "reengineering" rather than PFC projects.[30] Many experts, however, do not see important differences between the various concepts and many PFC projects include the restructuring of admissions, billing, and other business systems.

Although specific redesign strategies vary from hospital to hospital, findings from the *Hospitals'* survey indicate a number of characteristics common to most programs.

Survey findings reveal two predominant themes underpinning most redesign efforts. The most frequent theme reported by survey respondents focuses on *who* cares for the patient. Hospitals report that they are creating caregiver teams to be responsible for most of the care for designated groups of patients. Specific characteristics mentioned by survey respondents that illustrate this theme include an emphasis on caregiver team interrelationships (87.2%), cross-trained staff to create teams of multidisciplinary caregivers (79.8%), shared decisionmaking among physicians, nurses, and allied professionals (65.4%), and a reduced number of caregivers with whom patients have contact (57.9%).

The second theme focuses on the elements of the care process itself and responds to the *what, why, how, when,* and *where* questions listed above. Program characteristics cited by respondents that focus on these aspects of the care process include implementing clinical pathways or protocols (76.7%), starting or strengthening case management (62.4%), developing a continuum of care (61.7%), strengthening the discharge planning process (69.9%), and strengthening patient/family education (69.2%).

The survey also provides information on the extent of individual initiatives and the departments involved in PFC efforts nationwide. Only 34% of the institutions responding planned hospital wide initiatives, while 59% named specific departments. The predominant departments involved included medical/surgical (62%), clinical specialty departments (e.g., orthopedics, cardiology, etc.) (49%), ancillary services (e.g., lab, pharmacy) (32%), and support services (e.g., materials management, housekeeping) (28%). Approximately 74% of the projects addressed decentralizing (or planning to decentralize) services and moving them closer to the patient. Nursing was mentioned by 78% of respondents, followed by housekeeping (67%), lab (65%), pharmacy (63%), respiratory therapy (62%), as well as other services such as admissions, physical therapy, food service, radiology, medical records, rehabilitation, and materials management. Thus these services and departments find themselves part of an effort that results in changes in both the structure and process of departmental operations and services, in effect altering the traditional structure of the hospital and the patient care process.

Outcomes of PFC Nationwide

Implementation Issues. Implementing organizational changes as fundamental as those posed by PFC is seldom an easy process.[31] *Hospitals* survey respondents were questioned about obstacles encountered, while a number of other articles describe issues of cultural change and staff responses to organizational transformation.[32, 33] Obstacles described by survey respondents included perceived threat of job loss (49%), prospect of shared decisionmaking seemed threatening (40%), program's purpose and goals difficult to convey (39%), limitations in information systems (37%) and physical plant (36%), inadequate management skills (33%), and an existing corporate structure not conducive to change (32%). Issues commonly listed by other authors include staff anxiety and resistance to change. Symptoms described include fear, insecurity, and uncertainty; frustration, resentment, and anger; sadness, depression, and guilt; and feelings of unfairness, betrayal, and distrust.[34] Hospitals survey responses showed that top management, nursing executives and managers, and trustees were the most supportive of the change. The middle category included department heads, floor nurses, other health professionals and the medical staff. (Some hospitals cited medical staff resistance as a reason for their decision not to initiate PFC.) Non-clinical staff were rated as least supportive of PFC initiatives. Frequently, additional education, communication, and team building efforts were implemented to help employees deal with change.

Another barrier to PFC implementation was the time and organizational commitment required. In fact, 55% of the *Hospitals* respondents who did not start PFC initiatives said it was because they had "no time to do it right." While 26% of the responding CEOs had essentially delegated the initiative, 38% spent from 10% to 50% of their time directing the initiative. About 74% said they had attended educational programs, while 36% hired consultants to help with PFC implementation. Approximately 36% also talked with other CEOs with existing initiatives.

Evaluation Findings. Patient-focused care goals include improved service, to be reflected in improved customer satisfaction; reduced costs; and equal or better quality of patient care. Outcomes data to date are mixed, however, with few comprehensive studies to substantiate the common belief that the PFC model is effective.[35,36] One study demonstrated success in PFC redesign on a pilot nursing unit, measuring success in terms of patient, staff, and physician satisfaction and proportion of time nurses spent in direct patient care, but cost-benefits could not be demonstrated with only one unit redesigned.[37] Lakeland Regional Medical Center's pioneering project showed a 9.2% reduction in cost per occupied bed after adjusting for differences in the scope of services between the PFC model unit and a traditional general surgical unit.[38] In a different setting, patient-focused re-engineering of women's services showed a 9.8% decrease in cost per case.[39] Another project, operating within a cost neutral model, documented improvements in nursing satisfaction, but no changes in physician satisfaction and mixed results for patient satisfaction.[40] Other projects have published mixed reports of improvements in customer and staff satisfaction, including some indications of cost savings as well.[41, 42, 43, 44]

The measurement of cost and effectiveness of PFC projects is difficult because of the complex organizational context of each aspect of change in the care delivery process. A number of hospitals reported that they did not plan PFC projects because of the lack of hard-core evidence of improvements in patient care and hospital resources. Others reported that they saved money indirectly through reduced turnover, better staffing, higher productivity, and increased patient and physician satisfaction. Areas that needed continuing attention for the early implementers generally concerned communications and finding new means of staff motivation to maintain the project's initial momentum. Physician reactions to the early pilot projects was mixed, with a majority reasonably satisfied and a minority vocal and unhappy with changes in habits and procedures.[45] While proponents believe that PFC is cost-effective, their reasons for embarking on the initiative are focused on service and improving the traditional hospital structure. As one CEO noted, "We did it because it was the correct way to treat people."[46]

The preceding sections have provided a brief overview of the background and characteristics of PFC nationwide, as well as the driving forces for both PFC and other health care reform initiatives such as the implementation of clinical guidelines and pathways. Each of the elements of PFC will be discussed in greater detail in subsequent chapters. The next section gives an overview of health services research and the development and implementation of clinical guidelines and pathways to improve the management of patient care, followed by a description of the organization of this book.

Health Services Research: Evaluating Clinical Practice Guidelines and Pathways†

"Health services research is a global term applied to studies of health care delivery approaches and the systems in which health care is provided. Studies focus on interventions designed to improve the effectiveness, efficiency, and quality of health care services." [47, 48] The evaluation of clinical practice guidelines, as well as the collection and reporting of patient outcomes information and the evaluation of health care delivery innovations such as PFC, are among the many contributions of this relatively new academic discipline.[49] The products of health services research have the potential to enhance patient outcomes and improve patient satisfaction. In addition, many research studies have demonstrated less costly methods of providing medical care. Unfortunately, much of this research, and the millions of dollars it represents, remains secluded in medical journals and is never operationalized by hospitals, health maintenance organizations (HMOs), and other health care systems. This research has enormous potential and may represent a "sleeping giant" in health care and health care reform. It is necessary, however, to cull out those aspects of health services research that have the greatest applicability and potential to benefit patients, hospitals, and health care plans. The greatest challenge is then to apply these principles and this information in the ongoing care of patients. The current movement to develop and implement clinical guidelines and pathways in health care institutions provides one example with the potential to directly benefit patients through the application of health services research.

Clinical Guidelines and Pathways

Clinical practice guidelines have been defined by the Institute of Medicine as "systematically developed statements to assist practitioner and patient decisions about appropriate health care for specific clinical circumstances." [50] The Agency for Health Care Policy and Research (AHCPR), created by Congress in 1989, is the federal government's focal point for general health services research and is required by statute to arrange for the development of clinical practice guidelines.[51] For many years it has been recognized that

† Portions excerpted and adapted with permission from " Applied Health Services Research: Responding to the Changing Health Care Environment," by Scott Weingarten and A. Gary Ellrodt in *Physician Executive*, 21 (4) 1995: 19-20.

there are wide and often unexplainable variations in the provision of medical care by physicians. Practice parameters such as clinical practice guidelines may help physicians in clinical decisionmaking by identifying a range of appropriate strategies for the management of specific clinical conditions or by specifying a range of appropriate uses for specific diagnostic and therapeutic interventions.[52] Guidelines that are based upon solid research and updated continuously can enable physicians to practice evidence-based medicine and compare their own findings with scientific literature. Practice guidelines and expert systems that are based on outcomes research may enable attainment of the goal of providing patients with services that are most likely to improve their outcomes. Guidelines can also be used in medical education to teach new methods of analyzing evidence for new therapies and clinical interventions and by the purchasers of health care to study the appropriate use of medical resources.[53] For all of these purposes, the development of clinical practice guidelines and pathways has become a major activity in health care institutions and other public and private organizations over the last several years.[54, 55]

In addition to focusing efforts on practice guidelines, many institutions are also developing clinical pathways (i.e., structured, multidisciplinary, outcome-based plans of care for specific groups of patients) to support those guidelines.* [56] Clinical pathways supplement guidelines by providing the day-to-day practice protocols that guide the multidisciplinary team caring for those patients. The concept of clinical pathways stems from a nursing case management initiative at Boston's New England Medical Center. According to Zander, the project attempted to answer four questions:

1. What's required by each discipline to bring patients with similar diagnoses to realistic outcomes?
2. What's the best way to produce that work?
3. Who's accountable for those outcomes?
4. How can we restructure care so that this happens more consistently?[57]

Within this model, the pathways themselves provide an abbreviated version of care processes that "articulate crucial incidents, together with the proper interventions, which should take place on a given day of hospitalization to achieve the standard outcomes within the DRG and allotted length of stay." [58] The pathway goes with the patient throughout his or her route through acute care. Although pathways were first designed and initiated by nursing, the identification of patient-centered, measurable outcomes also requires a new level of collaboration with physicians.[59] Today, the most advanced institutions use clinical pathways in conjunction with other multidisciplinary, systemwide changes such as total quality management and patient-focused care.

Implementation of Clinical Guidelines and Pathways

There are a number of important challenges if guidelines and pathways are to accomplish the goals envisioned for them.[60, 61] The introduction and effective use of guidelines

* At Cedars-Sinai Medical Center the name "clinical pathways" has been adopted; other names in use include critical paths, care maps, clinical protocols and many more. See Lumsdon and Hagland, 1993 for comprehensive list of names used.

and pathways represents substantial organizational change. They must be acceptable to physicians and other providers and be subsequently adopted for use in day-to-day practice. These requirements suggest the need for detailed dissemination and implementation strategies. Furthermore, acceptance depends to a large extent on whether physicians have confidence on the process through which the guidelines and pathways were developed.[62] On a day-to-day basis, the implementation of pathways as a clinical tool also depends upon the education and expertise of the nursing staff who are most involved with the patient around the clock. These nurses will need enhanced knowledge, skills, and values. [63] Finally, it is essential that guideline and pathway implementation be linked with other organizational efforts such as work redesign, as well as being incorporated into ongoing quality improvement frameworks. In developing and implementing clinical practice guidelines and pathways and linking them to the institution's resource management program, Cedars-Sinai has recognized the challenges described above. The chapters in the later sections of the book describe some of Cedars-Sinai's responses to these challenges, evaluate their success, and offer suggestions to other institutions embarking on similar projects.

Organization of this Book

This book is organized in four sections. The first section describes the Cedars-Sinai's PFC project in detail, beginning in Chapter 2 with the PFC design principles adopted by Cedars-Sinai, as well as details on the specific service and financial targets and the analytic processes required to define those targets. Chapter 3 describes the overall project organization and strategies used to gain organizational commitment for PFC planning and implementation in an institution with over 6,000 employees. These strategies are followed by details of the analytic tools and methods developed and adapted in collaboration with the health care consulting firm APM (San Francisco) and used to create the pilot orthopedic model and, subsequently, to adapt that model to the other services and patient populations institution-wide. The tools and methods are followed by a detailed description of the orthopedic pilot unit care model development process and final model. The next five chapters cover the patient-focused care models developed for other areas of the institution—including critical care units, the operating room, respiratory therapy and rehabilitation services, and social services and utilization management.

The second section focuses on the hospital-wide organizational systems required to support the patient-focused care models detailed in Section I. The first three chapters include new concepts for documentation, the evolution and adaptation of existing technology to develop systems to support PFC within existing cost constraints, and new models for materials management, transportation, and housekeeping services. Chapter 13 details the extensive education program required to cross prepare caregivers throughout the institution for PFC implementation, while Chapter 14 turns to human resources and team building issues. Finally, Chapter 15 details the comprehensive evaluation methodology developed by a multidisciplinary team to evaluate the impacts of PFC while Chapter 16 provides the results of these evaluation efforts for the pilot unit as well as preliminary results for the housewide project.

Section III moves from the PFC work redesign efforts to Cedars-Sinai's ambitious program to develop clinical practice guidelines and pathways for patient populations throughout the medical center. Chapter 17 provides an introduction to evidence based medicine while Chapter 18 discusses common issues in the development, implementation, and evaluation of clinical practice guidelines, including details on strategies for success and lessons learned. Chapter 19 details the comprehensive, institution-wide project to link the development of clinical practice guidelines with the institution's resource management targets. Chapter 20 concludes the section with a description of the Quality of Well-Being (QWB) Scale, an instrument designed specifically to measure health related quality of life, and its potential uses in today's changing health care environment.

Section IV provides case studies in the areas of practice guidelines, clinical pathways, and outcomes management. Specific topics include outcomes measurement and management in medical rehabilitation, clinical practice guidelines for patients with chest pain, implementation of clinical pathways, the development of specific targets for VBAC in Cedars-Sinai's obstetrical population, cost effective methods of delivering bronchodilators, pharmacy involvement in guideline development, and the development of appropriate patient care monitoring guidelines for patients with epidural or intrathecal morphine for postoperative pain. Taken together, these case studies provide wide-ranging, varied examples of individual projects that institutions can undertake without extramural funding and that can have important implications for clinical outcomes and quality of care as well as reducing costs for the institution. Combined with the patient-focused care project described in the first sections of the book, the intent is to provide guidance and a wide range of examples for both implementation and evaluation strategies to improve patient care and service and reduce costs as health care institutions seek ways to survive and prosper in a changing health care environment.

References

1 Shine K. *America's Health in Transition: Protecting and Improving Quality.* Institute of Medicine, Academy Press: Washington DC, 1994.

2 Bergman R. "The Measuring Stick: Is Health Care Ready for Full-Scale Outcomes Measurement?" *Hospitals and Health Networks* 1993:36-42.

3 Mark B. "The Black Box of Patient Outcomes Research." *Image: The Journal of Nursing Scholarship* 27(1) 1995:42.

4 Taulbee P. "Measuring Quality: A Tricky Task with Costly Implications, Says Eddy." *Report on Medical Guidelines and Outcomes Research.* 4(9) 1993:5-6.

5 Donabedian A. "Evaluating the Quality of Medical Care." *Milbank Memorial Fund Quarterly* 44 Part II 1966:166-196.

6 Sherer JL. "Putting Patients First: Hospitals Work to Define Patient-Centered Care." *Hospitals* 1993:14-18.

7 Wakefield DS, et al. "Understanding Patient-Centered Care in the Context of Total Quality Management and Continuous Quality Improvement." *The Joint Commission Journal on Quality Improvement* 20(3) 1994:152-161.

8 Sherer JL, 1993.

9 Wakefield DS, et al., 1994.

10 Starr PE. *The Social Transformation of American Medicine.* New York, NY: Basic Books, 1982.

11 Wakefield DS, et al., 1994.

12 Jacobson J and JM Buckle. "Regulatory Forces." In *Clinical Practice Improvement: A New Technology for Developing Cost-Effective Quality Health Care,* Horn SD and DSP Hopkins, Eds. New York, NY: Faulkner & Gray, 1994.

13 Sherer JL, 1993.

14 Donabedian A. "Defining and Measuring the Quality of Health Care" in *Assessing Quality Health Care; Perspectives for Clinicians,* Wenzel R, Ed. Baltimore: Williams & Wilkins. 1992:41-64.

15 Joint Commission on Accreditation of Healthcare Organizations. *1995 Accreditation Manual for Hospitals,* Oakbrook Terrace, IL: Joint Commission on Accreditation of Healthcare Organizations, 1994.

16 Donabedian A. "Defining and Measuring the Quality of Health Care" in *Assessing Quality Health Care; Perspectives for Clinicians,* Wenzel R, Ed. Baltimore: Williams & Wilkins. 1992:41-64.

17 Manheim LM and J Feinglass. "Hospital Cost Incentives in a Fragmented Health Care System." *Health Care Management Review* 19(1) 1994:56-63.

18 Manheim LM and J Feinglass, 1994.

19 Robinson NC. "A Patient-Centered Framework for Restructuring Care." *Journal of Nursing Administration* 21(9) 1991:29-34.

20 Johnson RL. "HCMR Perspective: The Economic Era of Health Care." *Health Care Management Review* 19(4) 1994:64-72.

21 Kolb DS and JL Horowitz. "Managing the Transition to Capitation." *Healthcare Financial Management* February 1995:64-69.

22 Hudson T. "Scoping Out 1995: How Experts See the Health Care Year Unfolding." *Hospitals and Health Networks.* January 5, 1995:21-29.

23 Kolb DS and JL Horowitz, 1995.

24 Kolb DS and JL Horowitz, 1995.

25 Sherer JL, 1993.

26 Strauss A, et al. "The Hospital and Its Negotiated Order." In *The Hospital in Modern Society,* E. Freidson, ed. New York, NY: Fre Press, 1963.

27 Meyer JD and B Rowan. "Institutionalized Organizations: Formal Structure as Myth and Ceremony." In *Organizational Environments: Ritual and Rationality,* Meyer JD and WR Scott, eds. Beverly Hills, CA: Sage, 1983.

28 Aydin CE. "Professional Agendas and Computer-Based Patient Records: Negotiating for Control." *Topics in Health Information Management* 15(1) 1994:41-51.

29 Wakefield DS, et al., 1994.

30 Bergman R. "Reengineering Health Care." *Hospitals and Health Networks.* February 5, 1994:28-36.

31 Clarke RW and JG Lee. "Should Your Hospital Implement Patient-Focused Care?" *Health Care Strategic Management* 12(2) 1994:10-12.

32 Sherer JL. "Changing Cultures: Hospital Staffs Get Used to Patient-Centered Care Plans." *Hospitals* 1993:18-19.

33 Triolo PK, PA Allgeier, and CE Schwartz. "Layoff Survivor Sickness: Minimizing the Sequelae of Organizational Transformation." *Journal of Nursing Administration* 25(3) 1995:56-63.

34 Triolo PK, PA Allgeier, and CE Schwartz, 1995.

35 Lathrop JP. *Restructuring Health Care: The Patient Focused Paradigm.* San Francisco, CA: Jossey-Bass Publishers, 1993.

36 Sherer JL, 1993. "Putting Patients First."

37 Moffitt GK, et al. "Patient-Focused Care: Key Principles to Restructuring." *Hospital & Health Services Administration* 38(4) 1993:509-521.

38 Watson PM, DL Shortridge Jr, DT Jones, RT Rees, and JT Stephens. "Operational Restructuring: A Patient-Focused Approach." *Nursing Administration Quarterly* 16(1) 1991:45-52.

39 Bernd DL and MM Reed. "Re-engineering Women's Services." *Healthcare Forum Journal* 37(1) 1994:63-67.

40 Parsons ML and CL Murdaugh. *Patient-centered Care: A Model for Restructuring.* Gaithersberg, MD: Aspen, 1994.

41 Reisinger T. "Provider Profile: Teaming Up for Patient-focused Care." *Health Progress* November 1993:62-67.

42 Farris BJ. "Converting a Unit to Patient-Focused Care." *Health Progress* April 1993:22-25.

43 Murphy R, F Pearlman, C Rea, and L Papazian-Boyce. "Work Redesign: A Return to the Basics." *Nursing Management* 25(2) 1994:37-39.

44 Abts D, M Hofer, and PK Leafgreen. "Redefining Care Delivery: A Modular System." *Nursing Management* 25(2) 1994:40-43,46.

45 Lathrop JP. 1993.

46 Anderson HJ. "New Planning Models: Reasons for Transforming Hospital Go Beyond Financials." *Hospitals* 1993:20-22.

47 Ingersoll GL, N Hoffart, and AW Schultz. "Health Services Research in Nursing: Current Status and Future Directions." *Nursing Economics* 8(4) 1990:317-326.

48 Public Law 100-177. *Public Health Service Amendments of 1987. Title I - Health Research, Technology, Statistics, and Preventive Health Programs.* 1987.

49 Weingarten S and AG Ellrodt. "Applied Health Services Research: Responding to the Changing Health Care Environment." *Physician Executive* 21(4) 1995:19-20.

50 VanAmringe and Shannon, 1992.

51 VanAmringe M and TE Shannon. "Awareness, Assimilation, and Adoption: The Challenge of Effective Dissemination and the First AHCPR-Sponsored Guidelines." *Quality Review Bulletin* 18 1992:397-404.

52 Kibbe DC, AD Kaluzny, and CP McLaughlin. "Integrating Guidelines with Continuous Quality Improvement: Doing the Right Thing the Right Way to Achieve the Right Goals." *The Joint Commission Journal on Quality Improvement* 20(4) 1994:181-191.

53 Kibbe DC, AD Kaluzny, and CP McLaughlin. 1994.

54 Kibbe DC, AD Kaluzny, and CP McLaughlin. 1994.

55 Joint Commission on Accreditation of Healthcare Organizations. "Making Good on the Promise: Disseminating and Implementing Practice Guidelines." Theme issue. *Quality Review Bulletin* 18 1992: 389-492.

56 Zander K, and R McGill. "Critical and Anticipated Recovery Paths: Only the Beginning." *Nursing Management* 25(8) 1994:34-40.

57 Lumsdon K, and M Hagland. "Mapping Care." *Hospitals & Health Networks* 1993:34-40.

58 Guiliano KK, and CE Poirier. "Nursing Case Management: Critical Pathways to Desirable Outcomes." *Nursing Management* 22(3) 1991:52-55.

59 Zander K. "Managed Care Within Acute Care Settings: Design and Implementation Via Nursing Case Management." *Health Care Supervisor* 6(2) 1988:27-43.

60 Kibbe DC, AD Kaluzny, and CP McLaughlin. 1994.

61 Office of Technology Assessment, Congress of the United States. *Identifying Health Technologies that Work: Searching for Evidence.* Washington DC: U.S. Government Printing Office. 1994.

62 Kibbe DC, AD Kaluzny, and CP McLaughlin. 1994.

63 Zander K, and R McGill 1994.

Section I

Patient-Focused Care: Redesigning Patient Care Models To Maintain Satisfaction, Competency, and Quality of Care

This section presents the organization and methodology used by Cedars-Sinai to develop patient-focused care (PFC) models for organization-wide implementation. Chapter 2 discusses how to get the project started, including ways to assess the external and internal environments, establish design principles for the project, and set service and financial targets. Chapter 3 describes the project organization and gives a step-by-step overview of the analytic methods used to develop the PFC patient care models. Chapters 4 through 9 then provide concrete examples of model building (Chapters 4 and 5) and detail the application of patient-focused care principles in areas such as the operating room and clinical departments including respiratory therapy, physical medicine and rehabilitation, and social work and utilization management. Each chapter presents PFC from a different point of view, together creating a picture of the organization-wide PFC effort.

Chapter 2

Getting Started: Assessing the Environment, Defining Design Principles, and Setting Targets

Gerry Popolow, RN, MSN
Jane Ramseyer, RN, MPA
Carolyn E. Aydin, PhD
Linda Burnes Bolton, DrPH, RN, FAAN
Pat Eastman, MHA
Elaine Auerbach, MHA

Chapter 1 provided an overview of the history and characteristics of patient-focused care (PFC) nationwide. This chapter describes the background of patient-focused care at Cedars-Sinai Medical Center and details the assessment, design principle definition, and target setting phases of the project. These sections set the stage for the chapters that follow, but they also focus on the implications of the Cedars-Sinai experience for other institutions embarking on PFC projects. The chapter begins with a description of Cedars-Sinai's participation in the Robert Wood Johnson Foundation/Pew Charitable Trusts "Strengthening Hospital Nursing" project, since many important aspects of that grant were carried over into the PFC design process.

"Strengthening Hospital Nursing" Sets the Stage for PFC

In the late 1980s, Cedars-Sinai Medical Center was similar to many institutions grappling with a nursing shortage and the need to clearly define the role of the registered nurse while improving customer service and reducing in the cost of medical care. At that time

GERRY POPOLOW, RN, MSN—Vice President, Patient Care Services, Cedars-Sinai Medical Center.

JANE RAMSEYER, RN, MPA—Associate Vice President, Patient Care Services, Cedars-Sinai Medical Center.

CAROLYN E. AYDIN, PHD—Assistant Administrator, Nursing Research, Cedars-Sinai Medical Center and Research Institute; Assistant Clinical Professor, University of California-Los Angeles, School of Nursing.

LINDA BURNES BOLTON, DRPH, RN, FAAN—Director, Nursing Research and Development Director, Surgical Nursing, Cedars-Sinai Medical Center and Research Institute; Assistant Clinical Professor, University of California-Los Angeles, School of Nursing; Associate Professor, California State University, Los Angeles.

PAT EASTMAN, MHA—Associate Vice President, Medical Affairs, Cedars-Sinai Medical Center.

ELAINE AUERBACH, MHA—Associate Vice President, Medical Affairs (former), Cedars-Sinai Medical Center.

Cedars-Sinai—a nonprofit, community-based teaching hospital and tertiary care center located in Los Angeles, CA—had close to 1,200 licensed beds and a voluntary medical staff of approximately 2,000 physicians. In August 1989, Cedars-Sinai was one of eighty hospitals nationwide to be awarded a one-year planning grant entitled "Strengthening Hospital Nursing" by The Robert Wood Johnson Foundation and The Pew Charitable Trusts.[1, 2, 3, 4]

The purpose of the grant was to encourage hospitals to develop new models for patient care that would enable them to both meet the challenge of the nursing shortage that existed at that time and to improve service to customers, including patients and their families, physicians, and the community. Although the amount of money was small ($50,000) in proportion to the work required, the foundations used the prestige of the grant and the prospect of a five-year implementation award ($1,000,000) to twenty hospitals to leverage change in the health care industry through the efforts of these eighty pilot projects. The "Strengthening Hospital Nursing" planning year project meant that individuals from disciplines and departments throughout Cedars-Sinai met and began to develop model approaches to the delivery of patient care. The outcomes and lessons learned from this planning year set the stage for the PFC project in years to come. For Cedars-Sinai, the most important aspects of the "Strengthening Hospital Nursing" legacy included the involvement of executive management in planning for organizational change, the establishment of multidisciplinary project teams, early efforts at work redesign, and developing a focus on outcomes. These elements, each of which is discussed in detail below, helped lay the foundation for the PFC project to come.

Involvement of Executive Management

The foundations sponsoring the "Strengthening Hospital Nursing" project used these grant awards as an opportunity to shape the future of health care by requiring that the executive management of each recipient organization be committed to and participate in the project if the institution was to receive the award. This participation that included mandatory attendance by the CEO, vice president for nursing, chief medical officer, a member of the governing board, and a representative from the medical staff at a two-day educational seminar offered at a central location in the United States. The educational seminar was attended by their counterparts from other institutions nationwide receiving the award. The sessions involved the individuals attending in creative discussions on ways to "wipe the slate clean" and use Russell Ackoff's "interactive planning" approach organizational change.[5, 6] While conference attendees did not return with any solutions (several agreed that the process seemed to resemble "Jell-O"), the magnitude of the challenge and the importance of executive management involvement had become clear to the project leaders.

Multidisciplinary Project Teams

Although the project was entitled "Strengthening Hospital Nursing," the awarding foundations made it clear early in the year that this was not a "nursing grant."

Participating institutions were required to form multidisciplinary teams to examine the processes of care in their institutions and make plans for change. Interactive planning emphasizes planning done at all levels of the organization simultaneously and interdependently. At Cedars-Sinai, a number of task forces were formed to examine the admissions process, patient care delivery on nursing units, and the use of ancillary and support services in patient care. Each of these task forces developed preliminary analyses, flow charts, and recommendations for change that were later enlarged upon and implemented by PFC task forces. This phase also provided individuals in the institution with education and experience in working in multidisciplinary groups. This experience proved invaluable during the start-up phase of PFC, a time in which individuals are typically reluctant to abandon their own professional territory to address the issues from an organizational perspective.[7] In addition, the Cedars-Sinai's leaders became adept at leading those same multidisciplinary groups.

Work Redesign

The "Strengthening Hospital Nursing" project also encouraged Cedars-Sinai to make a first attempt at work redesign. One multidisciplinary task force examined patient care tasks on the unit and recommended the use of assistant personnel to work with registered nurses in the delivery of patient care. These assistant personnel, termed medical-surgical technicians (MSTs) or critical care technicians (CCTs), were frequently nursing students or other individuals with patient care experience (e.g., emergency medical technicians) who then attended a Cedars-Sinai educational program to enable them to perform those basic patient care tasks that did not require licensure in the state of California. (See Chapter 13 for details of the MST/CCT program.) The program was implemented in 1991-92 on all nursing units.

Focus on Outcomes

"Strengthening Hospital Nursing" at Cedars-Sinai also included a detailed evaluation component, one that was enlarged upon for the later PFC project. Evaluation questions and outcomes for the assistive personnel project included the following:

1. **Question:** Have technicians been safely integrated into care delivery teams?
   Outcome: Performance checklists, surveys, and quality assurance data indicated that technicians performed tasks with "good" or "excellent" ratings with no untoward events reported as a result of the program.
2. **Question:** Has the program affected RN/LVN job satisfaction?
   Outcome: Longitudinal job satisfaction surveys showed no decrease in the generally high levels of job satisfaction.
3. **Question:** Has the technician program affected patient satisfaction?
   Outcome: Press/Ganey patient survey results showed improvements in items measuring the impact of assistive personnel, including: "Response of nursing to your calls," and "The attention you received from nursing."

4. **Question:** What is the financial impact of the program?
   Outcome: Findings indicated increased nursing hours with decreased and/or controlled costs on nursing units.

The "Strengthening Hospital Nursing" project set the stage for PFC in a number of important ways at Cedars-Sinai and positioned the institution to embark on the more comprehensive PFC project early in 1993. The remaining sections in this chapter describe the essential elements of the assessment, definition of design principles, and target setting phases of PFC using Cedars-Sinai's experience as an example.

Assessing the Need for Change

As the preceding sections have illustrated, many of the elements of PFC at Cedars-Sinai Medical Center had their roots in the "Strengthening Hospital Nursing" project in 1989-90. Despite the institution's history of organizational change projects, however, PFC was a far more comprehensive change effort than any of its forerunners. Rather than attempting to fix parts of the system, PFC creates a new system of patient care. The first step in embarking on such a project requires an assessment of both the internal and external environments of the institution in order to set project goals that will meet the needs of the organization. Before describing the PFC assessment and goal setting methodologies, however, it is important to understand the broad timeline of PFC at Cedars-Sinai, since the external environment underwent a number of changes during the project period. In addition to the environmental changes described in the following sections, competition in the local health care market and shortened lengths of stay required additional downsizing initiatives (accompanied by some layoffs) unrelated to PFC in early 1994 and again in 1995. The average length of stay decreased from 7.5 days in 1993 to 5.6 in 1994. These factors, along with damage to some patient care facilities in the January 1994 Northridge earthquake, led to a reduction in the number of beds. Cedars-Sinai's budgeted average daily census went from 713 in 1993 when PFC planning began, to 585 at the time of housewide PFC implementation in 1994, and further reduced to 533 in July 1995.

Assessing External and Internal Forces for Change

The first step in any change effort is to assess both the external and internal forces driving the need for change and delineate appropriate responses to those forces. External forces might include cost and marketing concerns, competition in the local health care market, or the demand by payers for statistics such as cost per case and lengths of stay, outcome and/or quality indicators, and patient satisfaction data. Internal factors might include issues such as defining the optimal use of resources, redundant and/or needlessly complex systems, lack of communication between caregivers, employee and physician satisfaction, and others. Assessing and defining these issues will shape the goals and solutions developed during the PFC planning process.

External Forces for Change. At Cedars-Sinai, executive management began to consider the need for a more complete restructuring of the care delivery process in 1992, following the implementation of the assistive personnel (MST/CCT) project described above. At that time, competition between hospitals in the Southern California health care market had been increasing for several years. There were excess beds in the market and utilization was decreasing as well. Physicians and managed care providers were uniting for contracting leverage and the pool of available indemnity lives was shrinking. Major competitors were also implementing cost reduction and service improvement initiatives.

Internal Forces for Change. While Cedars-Sinai had an undisputed reputation for delivering quality care, the institution's reputation for service was not as good as employees or patients believed it should be. And while the institution still remained competitive, pressures to reduce the costs of care were also intensifying. Internally, the payer mix was deteriorating while patient acuity was increasing. Communication and collaboration with physician and other disciplines needed improvement, and patients did not perceive themselves as having a role in their own care and recovery.

Responding to the Need for Change. Acknowledging the forces for change described above, Cedars-Sinai's executive leadership examined the experience of other institutions at that time and decided that patient-focused care, with its focus on service improvements, would best meet the challenges facing the institution. A decision was made to work with a consulting firm, APM, and implement patient-focused care, beginning the planning process for the pilot unit in February 1993. Plans also initially called for gradual expansion to additional units. In April 1993, two months into the planning phase for the pilot unit, however, the hospital's census began to drop and cost containment became an issue. The Cedars-Sinai effort shifted from a pilot project with a long timeline to a housewide implementation program with an accelerated schedule and cost reductions as well as service improvements as the dual goals.

Implications for Other Institutions. This shift in the implementation timeline for PFC makes the project particularly significant to the PFC experience nationwide. The original PFC hospitals implemented their projects on pilot units at a time when cost savings were not a high priority. Many of these hospitals were very successful in meeting expectations, but cost reduction was not a goal for many of these projects. They could afford to indulge in the luxury of a long time line, letting attrition and/or re-education take care of any necessary reductions in staff and, to gain the support of the work force, guaranteeing that no employee would be laid off as a result of restructuring.[8] While the Cedars-Sinai project began under these conditions, the accelerated timeline transformed the project into a "real world" test of organizational change in an institution facing all of the constraints of a competitive health care environment. Every proposal for decentralizing services or improving care delivery had to show demonstrable benefits, including cost benefits, in the short term as well as the long term. Furthermore, the housewide nature of the project offered an opportunity to conduct a comprehensive evaluation of both the service and cost impacts of PFC, something not possible at the early PFC institutions where only the pilot units implemented PFC models and hospitals continued to operate under two different care delivery systems.

Defining Design Principles

Following the assessment of the internal and external forces for change, the second step in the PFC process is to define the design principles to guide the change process. These principles are actually general goals that provide a conceptual foundation for the organizational changes to be proposed as well as a basis for evaluating the success of the project. The principles themselves should lead the organization into changes specifically designed to help the institution meet the challenges identified in the assessment phase described above. Defining these design principles is essential because these principles are used time and again during the redesign process to test progress and determine whether a particular solution furthers the agreed upon direction of the project.

Although most PFC projects embrace the same general goals, the specific design principles and the relative importance placed upon each may differ from institution to institution. Working with APM, Cedars-Sinai project leaders adopted three design principles to focus the institution's efforts in improving the quality and efficiency of care delivery and to gauge progress toward the project goals of improved service and reduced cost. These design principles were defined as the following: (1) managed demand, (2) redesigned work, and (3) empowered employees. Each is described in detail below while **Figure 2.1** provides examples of the predicted outcomes stemming from these design principles for patients, physicians, managers, and employees.

Figure 2.1: Design Principles

WHAT DESIGN PRINCIPLES MEAN TO...

PATIENTS	PHYSICIANS	MANAGERS	EMPLOYEES
• Knowing all the members of my care team by name	• Timely turnaround of test results	• Increased patient, physician, and employee satisfaction	• Less time spent on documentation
• Being able to call upon all members of the care team when assistance is needed	• Timely admission process	• Patients of like diagnosis grouped together (easier to train staff and anticipate patients' needs)	• Coordinated schedule of procedures and services
• More time spent with patient care providers	• Increased patient satisfaction	• Fewer census fluctuations (easier to prepare staffing schedule)	• Recognition as part of the patient care team
• Less need to be transported around the Medical Center; less time waiting for procedures	• Highly skilled team of professionals caring for my patients	• Less time spent on documentation	• Increased patient and physician satisfaction
• Improved quality of care and service	• Improved system for scheduling surgeries and procedures	• Coordinated schedule of procedures and services	• Enhanced decision-making authority
• More personalized care and service	• More personalized service for me and my patients.	• Less time waiting to get something accomplished	• Less time scheduling, coordinating, and waiting
		• Enhanced decision-making authority	• More time providing, or supporting, patient care

Managed Demand. Managed demand focuses on ways in which an institution can control and predict the volume of patient care to be delivered on a specific unit or by a specific group of caregivers. Methods to manage demand include grouping patients by clinical similarity to maximize resource consumption of like services, enable customized care and predictable scheduling, designing units to be "full," with less work load fluctuations, and designing clinical pathways to ensure quality and cost-effective care. Institutions, which are able to manage demand, should be able to provide more cost-effective care using care processes tailored to specific groups of patients. Chapter 3 provides details of the analyses that can be used to determine optimal ways to manage demand and reaggregate patients into clinically similar groups for a specific institution.

Redesigned Work. PFC redesigned work refers to patient care processes in which ancillary, administrative, and support services are moved closer to the patient where clinically and economically sensible. Cross-prepared teams provide most of the care for a specified group of patients. Redesigned jobs provide the appropriate employee to take care of the patient at the bedside and the proper skill mix on the unit. Tasks and processes are restructured, unnecessary work is eliminated, and technology is fully utilized. Chapter 3 describes the steps and Chapters 4 and 5 provide detailed examples of the work redesign process and the empowerment of employees through work redesign.

Empowered Employees. In a redesigned work environment with the proper skill mix on the unit, fewer workers interact with any one patient. Additionally, employees are empowered to have the authority, responsibility, and accountability for patient care appropriately aligned with minimal responsibility hand-offs.

Each of these three design principles was used frequently throughout the planning process to gauge progress toward project goals. Examples on changes made in the care delivery process to meet these criteria will be presented in later chapters. Chapter 5, in particular, provides a specific example of the ways in which proposals for critical care models are matched with the design principles (see **Table 5.1**).

Setting Targets

Organizational change is a complex and multidimensional concept. Achieving desired outcomes requires vertical and horizontal planning, communication, and commitment.[9] In setting targets for change efforts, it is critical that their fit within the institution's culture and strategic plan be considered. The outcomes from the design phase should be directly related to the overall business goals. Failure to "plan the plan" can result in loosely formulated goals and targets unrelated to the organization's primary mission. Goals and outcomes of the target setting process for restructuring efforts articulate a means for achieving overall organizational performance goals. They cannot be separated. Service outcomes must be linked to who provides what services. The question should be posed "if we change who provides what services will there be an observed change in the quality of service as observed by the customer?" This principle question links overall institutional goals for customer service with specific restructuring goals. Similarly, financial and clinical outcomes must be linked to reengineering and work redesign and patient outcomes research for both.

Specific, measurable targets provide a way to measure the success of the project objectively. At Cedars-Sinai the initial focus was on service targets. While cost of care was always important, at the time the pilot unit planning began, the goal was to redesign care and remain budget neutral. During the planning period, as competition in the local market intensified and the patient census began to drop, specific financial targets were also set for each clinical area.

Defining Service Targets

Since PFC fundamentally aims to improve service, goals for improving service, or service standards, should be defined early in the planning process. These service standards are then used in the development of PFC care models to help ensure that changes in the delivery of patient care are designed to meet customer service requirements. At Cedars-Sinai, a design team assessed service needs and defined service standards for the project. The service standards design team included individuals from patient care, ancillary, and support departments who came in direct, regular contact with patients and their families, physicians, and employees and who had knowledge about patients'/families' needs, concerns, and issues. Patient and/or family representatives who are willing to be involved in the design process can also make important contributions to understanding patient and family needs. The group's charge was to identify key customer service requirements and recommend measurement strategies and targets. Defining service standards involved the following steps:

1. Reviewing Existing Data: Group members must first review existing information on customer satisfaction (e.g., findings from physician, patient, and staff surveys, interviews, or focus groups, patient complaints, etc.) and determine whether additional data is needed.

2. Brainstorming: At Cedars-Sinai the design team, using the existing data and group members' knowledge of customer service issues, brainstormed a list of approximately seventy-five different service attributes required to meet the needs of patients, physicians, and employees. These included items such as more time spent by the caregiver at the bedside, courteous hospital employees, timeliness in answering call lights, cleanliness of the room, and responsiveness to patient/family and physician requests.

3. Grouping: These seventy-five attributes were then grouped into categories by project staff and revised and approved by the team. Redundant items were eliminated and items addressing similar concepts were grouped into the eight categories detailed in **Table 2.1.** Grouping the items made it easier to address service needs in a systematic manner. The categories and the items within them were later used by the group designing the PFC care model to ensure that the model would meet customer needs. For example, the model needed to include systems that would make it possible to respond to call lights quickly, allow more time for caregivers at the bedside, have staff available to clean rooms in a timely manner, and so forth.

4. Prioritization: The individual attributes were also prioritized according to criteria developed by the team. According to these criteria, those attributes to be included as service targets in the evaluation plan were attributes that were the following:

- Measurable,
- Visible to patients, physicians, and/or employees, and
- Potentially changeable through PFC.

A number of attributes did not meet these requirements and were eliminated from the list.

5. Measurement: The design team also recommended specific measurement strategies for the identified service elements. Team members divided themselves into four subgroups—the physician, patient, employee, and data subgroups. The physician subgroup identified those the key service elements that were relevant to physicians and designated appropriate measurement methods. The group decided that physicians were concerned with seven of the eight key categories detailed in **Table 2.1** (all categories except-patient information/education/communication). They also decided that an adaptation of a previous physician survey with revised response categories and additional questions to measure responsiveness would provide valid and reliable pre-post measurement of service targets from the physicians' perspective.

The patient subgroup made a similar determination, specifying that patients should respond to all categories except "bureaucracy." The group reviewed the ongoing patient surveys and recommended that these be supplemented by patient interviews for more detailed information on specific service issues. The employee and data subgroups conducted similar analyses. Data methodologies recommended using ongoing quality or service measures (e.g., staff satisfaction surveys and reporting systems for surgical site infections, falls, dermal ulcers, etc.) as well as work sampling observation techniques to determine the amount of staff time spent in specific activities, litter counts to evaluate unit cleanliness, and others. These evaluation recommendations were approved by the project task forces and passed on to the PFC Evaluation Team for refinement and incorporation into the comprehensive PFC evaluation plan (see Chapters 15 and 16).

Table 2.1: Service Categories Designated by Services Standards Design Team

1. **Responsiveness** (e.g., call light response time, physician rating of unit responsiveness to their needs)
2. **Interpersonal interactions** (e.g., physician and staff ratings of teamwork on unit.)
3. **Teamwork** (e.g., physician and staff ratings of teamwork on unit)
4. **Coordination of Services** (e.g., number of different faces interacting with unit, number of missed treatments, and amount of staff time spent scheduling and coordinating)
5. **Clinical/Technical Competence** (e.g., skills assessment of all cross-prepared staff)
6. **Bureaucracy** (e.g., physician and employee rating of how well they are informed about important changes in the organization)
7. **Patient Information/Education/Communication** (e.g., patient ratings of how well they are informed about tests and treatments and how well they are prepared for discharge, and amount of time spends documenting)
8. **Environment/Ameninites** (e.g., litter count)

Setting Financial Targets

Along with service targets, setting the financial expectations for any PFC project and communicating those expectations to the project's task forces comprises the other essential element of the target setting process. While the early PFC projects were primarily aimed at improving service, hospitals currently implementing PFC generally expect cost savings as an outcome of the project. Early pilot programs also found it difficult to evaluate cost savings when PFC was implemented only on selected units, since savings are difficult to realize until institutions are able to reduce and/or restructure central departments.[10] Before financial target setting can begin, however, it is essential that project participants accept the need for financial targets and agree upon the principles by which those targets will be set.

Figure 2.2: Financial Target Setting Steps

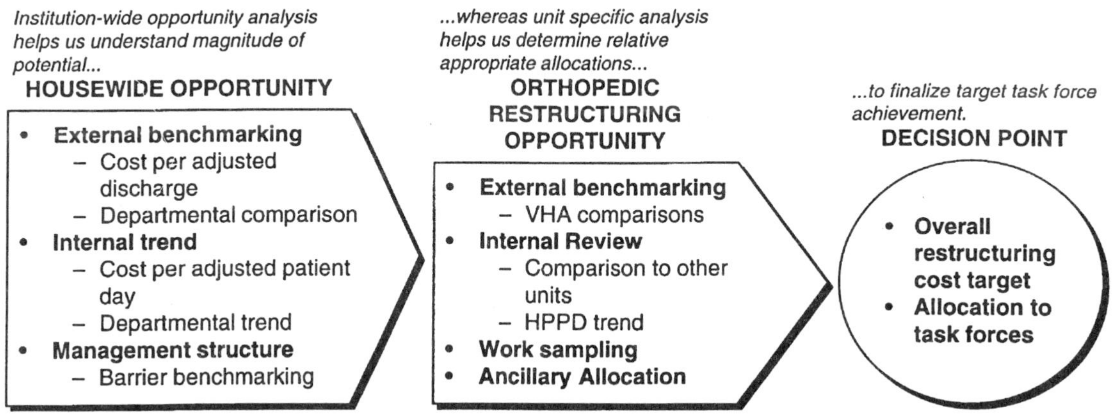

Figure 2.3: External Benchmarking Example

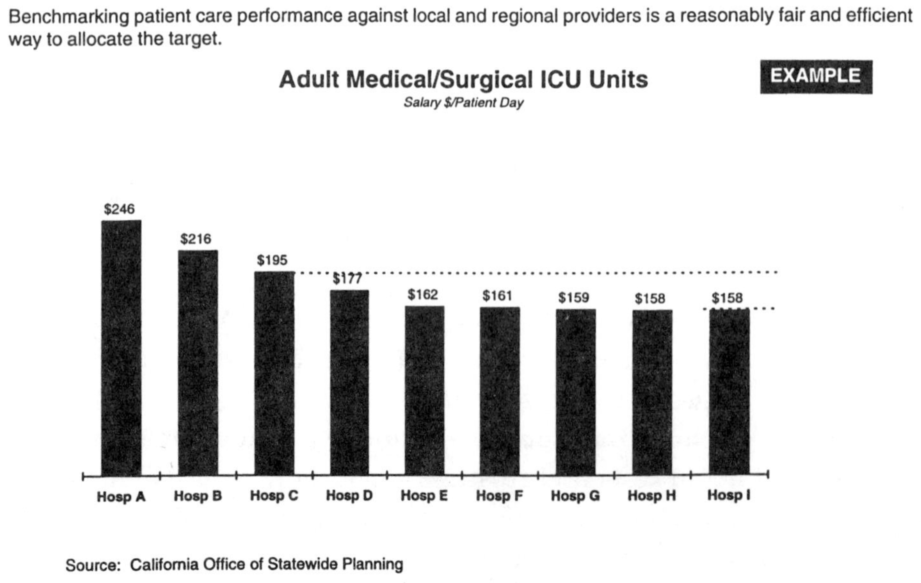

Establishing the Ground Rules. Project participants come to the project with varying levels of knowledge about the forces in health care today. PFC task force leaders and members need to be educated concerning the findings of the assessments of external and internal forces for change such as those described above and in Chapter 1. In addition, Cedars-Sinai defined the following target setting principles:

1. Targets must be consistent with the overall strategic needs of Cedars-Sinai to:
   - Meet the financial need, and
   - Achieve cost competitiveness.
2. Targets must be set fairly (i.e., don't penalize the most efficient performers)
3. Targets must be set efficiently (i.e., invest more time in developing solutions than in perfecting targets).

At Cedars-Sinai each of these principles played an essential role in ensuring managers' acceptance of their allocated targets so that the PFC task forces could move forward to the design phase. Based upon these principles, Cedars-Sinai worked with APM to define a financial target setting methodology that included, among other things, the elements described in the following sections. The data, while carefully researched, were meant to represent the direction and magnitude of the potential cost reduction opportunities only. They were pulled from a variety of sources and considered from a number of different angles to create a valid, composite picture of opportunities available for the institution to reduce costs. Analyses were conducted for both the orthopedic pilot unit and the institution as a whole. **Figure 2.2** provides an example of the steps in the target setting process. Overall, the data generated during this process were intended to provide a basis for reaching consensus on final cost targets. These analyses allowed the institution to make an overall determination of the cost savings required to function in the current and future health care environment and then to delineate that portion of the cost savings that could realistically be assigned to the PFC project.

External Benchmarking. For Cedars-Sinai the specific environmental factors driving the need for cost targets in 1993 included the fact that, in the past, the institution had been able to command a 60% price premium in the marketplace based upon its reputation for premier medical care, a situation that was not likely to continue indefinitely. Major competitor hospitals were undergoing major cost cutting efforts, physicians and managed care providers continued to unite for contracting leverage, and market bed utilization was falling. Conducting a cost opportunity analysis was one way to consider a variety of different comparison approaches for determining the relative magnitude of the cost target. This step involved external benchmarking of the institution's performance against local and regional competitors, both overall and by service (e.g., medical/surgical, intensive care, post-acute care, women's care, psychiatry, etc.). Analyses used publicly available data for other institutions and inflated the data to compare with the most recent Cedars-Sinai data available. **Figure 2.3** provides an example of regional benchmarking of adult medical/surgical intensive care units.

Internal Analyses. In addition to external benchmarking, examination of the internal cost structure and internal benchmarking can also be useful in determining cost targets. **Figure 2.4** provides a sample of the cost structure of a similar medical center while the example in **Figure 2.5** traces the growth in labor costs over a four-year period. Internal benchmarking also provides information useful in establishing the Cedars-Sinai's most efficient performers and allocating the target to different service lines within the institution. **Figure 2.6** compares medical surgical units at Cedars-Sinai revealing that, although orthopedics showed cost savings opportunities when compared externally, it was one of the most efficient units internally. Similar external and internal comparisons for other departments such as the laboratory, imaging, pharmacy, and food and nutrition services can also provide useful information for allocating cost targets.

All of the data were then verified with Cedars-Sinai managers to ensure that they agreed with the information on their relative position in the marketplace. Occasionally addi-

Figure 2.4: Example Medical Center Cost Structure

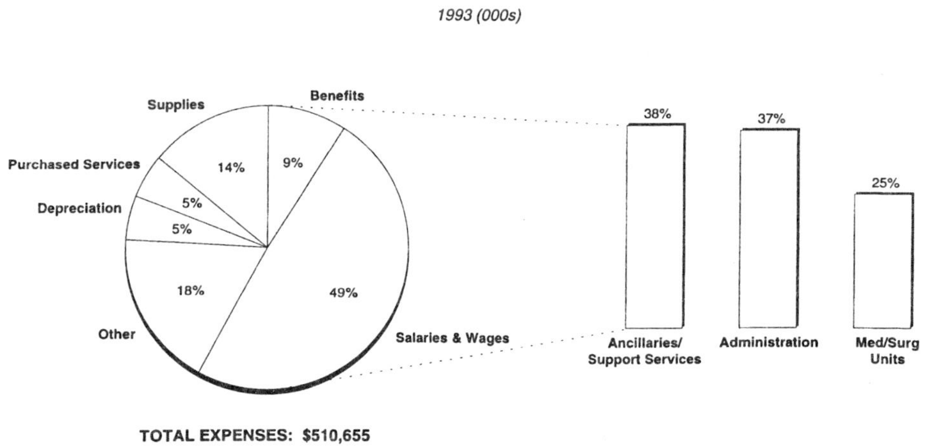

Figure 2.5:Example of Growth in Labor Cost Per Adjusted Patient Day

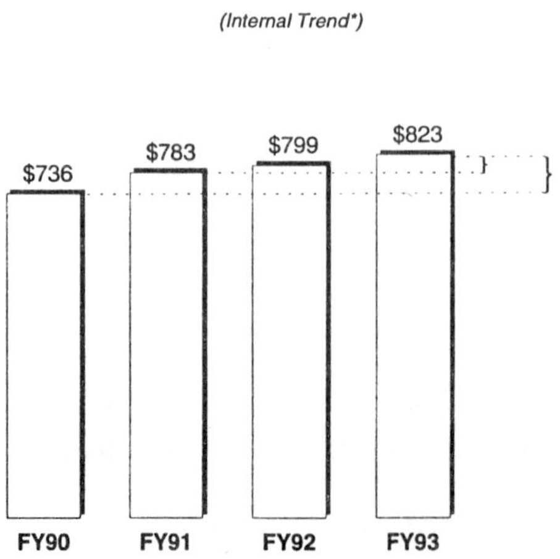

tional benchmark hospitals were added to the analysis if managers were dissatisfied with the comparison hospitals used. The data were then used to arrive at the overall cost target and allocation to task forces. At the time Cedars-Sinai housewide implementation planning began (late fall of 1993) the overall institutional cost savings target was defined as $24 million. This target was divided among a number of different initiatives in the medical center, including PFC and resource management (see Chapter 19). PFC's portion of the target was $5-8 million. **Figure 2.7** details the preliminary allocation of this target to the PFC task forces.

Figure 2.6: Internal Benchmarking Example

A comparison of the Cedars-Sinai med/surg units indicates an opportunity for Orthopedics of $80,000.

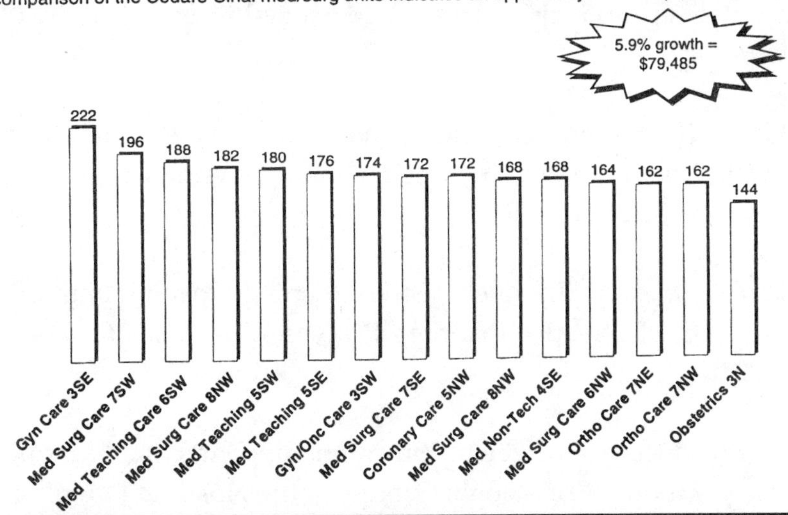

Figure 2.7: Suggested Task Force Targets

Applying the target-setting methodology results in the following targets:

Preliminary
Based on External Benchmarking
12-6-93

Task Force	Total Pt. Care Salaries & Benefits ($000)[1]	Suggested Target ($000)	Target as a Percent of Labor Dollar
Medical	$18,044	$1,479 - 2,367	8.2 - 13.1%
Surgical	$10,626	$831 - 1,330	7.8 - 12.5%
Peds	$8,384	$542 - 867	6.5 - 10.3%
Psych/CCD	$3,570	$123 - 197	3.5 - 5.5%
SNAC/Rehab	$3,711	$284 - 453	7.7 - 12.3%
Women's Care	$12,192	$711 - 1,138	5.8 - 9.3%
Critical Care	$12,743	$1,029 - 1,646	8.1 - 12.9%
Total	**$69,270**	**$5,000 - 8,000**	**7.2 - 11.6%**
As a point of Reference: Ortho	$3,232	$300	9.3%

1 4/1/93 - 9/31/93 YTD*2

Summary

This chapter has provided details on the history of PFC at Cedars-Sinai, including the driving forces for change in the Southern California marketplace. These conditions are being mirrored in varying degrees throughout the United States, and no institution can afford to ignore their implications or the need to examine the cost efficiency of its delivery of patient care. The design principles, as well as the service and financial target setting methodologies can help other institutions lay the groundwork for their own PFC initiatives. While local conditions may differ, setting clear targets that are congruent with the institution's business plan is an essential step in any change effort. The following chapter describes the project organization and methodologies used to plan patient-focused care delivery models specifically designed to meet the institution's service and cost targets.

1 Taft SH and JE Stearns. "Organizational Change Toward a Nursing Agenda: A Framework from the Strengthening Hospital Nursing Program." *Journal of Nursing Administration* 21(2) 1991:12-21.

2 Taft SH, PK Jones, & EL Minch. "Strengthening Hospital Nursing, Part 2: Characteristics of Effective Planning Processes." *Journal of Nursing Administration* 22(6) 1992:

3 Taft SH, PK Jones, & EL Minch. "Strengthening Hospital Nursing, Part III: Differences Among Professional Groups in the Hospital Planning Process." *Journal of Nursing Administration* 22(8) 1992:41-50.

4 Adams RA and AR Rentfro. "Strengthening Hospital Nursing: An Approach to Restructuring Care Delivery." *Journal of Nursing Administration* 21(6) 1991:12-19.

5 Ackoff RL. *Creating The Corporate Future*. New York: Wiley, 1981.

6 Ackoff RL, J Gharajedaghi, & EV Finnel. *A Guide to Controlling Your Corporation's Future*. New York: Wiley, 1984.

7 Burnes Bolton L, et al. "Ten Steps for Managing Organizational Change." *Journal of Nursing Administration* 22(6) 1992:14-20.

8 Lathrop JP. *Restructuring Health Care: The Patient Focused Paradigm*. San Francisco, CA: Jossey-Bass Publishers, 1993.

9 Burnes Bolton L, et al. 1992.

10 Lathrop JP. 1993.

Chapter 3

Tools and Methods for Organizing the Project and Developing the Patient Care Model

Gerry Popolow, RN, MSN
Jane Ramseyer, RN, MPA
Linda Burnes Bolton, DrPH, RN, FAAN
Carolyn E. Aydin, PhD

This chapter describes the Cedars-Sinai patient-focused care (PFC) project organization and the tools and methods required to develop a patient-focused model for delivering patient care. The first sections focus on organizing both the planning and implementation phases of the project. These sections are followed by a step-by-step description of the model building process. Chapters 4 and 5 then provide concrete examples of both the interactive planning process and model building, using detailed descriptions from the pilot orthopedic patient care model and the several critical care models implemented at Cedars-Sinai.

Organizing the Project

A collaborative process is essential for the implementation of a patient-centered health delivery system. Diverse perspectives (ie., the physicians', nurses', administrators', board of directors', physical therapists', educators') must unite, speak, and act with one purpose—to provide quality care efficiently and effectively. This is a formidable task requiring active planning and organization. The theoretical framework for Cedars-Sinai's project structure had its roots in Russell Ackoff's "interactive planning" process in which the entire organization simultaneously engages in planning for change.[1,2] The model employs an open environment in which stakeholders from various subsystems are brought together to create and reengineer systems. This interactive planning frame-

GERRY POPOLOW, RN, MSN—Vice President, Patient Care Services Cedars-Sinai Medical Center.

JANE RAMSEYER, RN, MPA—Associate Vice President, Patient Care Services, Cedars-Sinai Medical Center.

LINDA BURNES BOLTON, DRPH, RN, FAAN—Director, Nursing Research and Development Director, Surgical Nursing Cedars-Sinai Medical Center and Research Institute; Assistant Clinical Professor, University of California-Los Angeles, School of Nursing; Associate Professor; California State University, Los Angeles.

CAROLYN E. AYDIN, PHD— Assistant Administrator for Nursing Research Cedars-Sinai Medical Center and Research Institute, Assistant Clinical Professor, University of California-Los Angeles, School of Nursing.

work was utilized throughout the planning and implementation phases of the project. The following sections describe the structure employed to organize work teams to achieve project goals.

Executive Commitment (Steering Committee)

The Cedars-Sinai project began at the top. The chairman of the board of directors, chief executive officer and president, operational vice president, chief medical officer, members of the voluntary medical staff, chief financial officer, and chief nursing officer were organized as the Steering Committee for the project. The committee was chaired by the organization's president. The Steering Committee had the final approval for the care model designs, financial targets, and timeline for implementation. The Steering Committee met monthly for 60-90 minutes to receive reports from design teams and project management. Eventually, the Steering Committee was co-chaired by the chief medical and nursing officers.

The Steering Committee was chartered following an all-day executive retreat. The retreat was organized by the Project Director, Gerry Popolow, RN, Vice President for Patient Care Services, and the APM consulting group. The purpose of the retreat was to review national, state, and internal data and determine the need to proceed with an organizational restructuring effort. The consulting firm presented data on national efforts to restructure health delivery systems—state benchmarketing data comparing Cedars-Sinai costs per case, length of stay, full-time equivalents, occupied beds, and various clinical outcome measures and internal variation data across clinical service lines. (See Chapter 2 for examples of external and internal benchmarking data used for target setting.) The data and supportive presentations provided the executive leadership with the necessary information to arrive at a consensus for change.

Overall Project Management (Project Team)

Following the executive retreat, the Steering Committee approved the chartering of multidisciplinary work teams and a project management team to begin the restructuring effort. The project management team ("project team") guided day-to-day operations, provided staff resources to task forces, served as liaison between the consultants and work teams, and facilitated task force productivity. The project team consisted of the vice president for patient care services, who chaired the team, project staff members from administration, nursing research and development, and the consultant team. These project team personnel and their activities were absolutely essential to successful project management. The project director, team leadership, and the consultants assured a successful project implementation.

Consultants

The APM consulting firm provided consultation and supportive services throughout the project planning, design, and initial implementation phases. The value of a consulting firm lies in its access to data from previous restructuring efforts, provision of technical support and analytical services, and its lack of stakeholder bias that can limit project designs. However, it is absolutely essential that the project must be overseen and operated by the institution. Consultants work for their clients. They provide advice, data, and experience, which the institutional project management staff can choose to use or disregard as appropriate.

The project director must set the ground rules to govern consultant utilization. Since a variety of consultants and firms provide technical and analytical support for organizational restructuring efforts, it is wise to interview a minimum of three. Leaders from institutions embarking on restructuring efforts should also visit projects supported by these consulting firms to evaluate their work and obtain feedback from other clients before selecting the final consultant candidates.

Key issues, such as communication, technical support, data analysis deliverable, the cost of consultants, the size of the consultant team and its roles and responsibilities, should be negotiated prior to project initiation. Consultant team members and the specific skills they provide should also be negotiated prior to the project and renegotiated during the project as needed. On a day-to-day basis, the project coordinator should work closely with the consultants, ensuring that their efforts are expended in areas most needed by the institution.

One important deliverable in the Cedar-Sinai consultant agreement concerned technology transfer. In addition to the analysts provided by the consulting firm, Cedars-Sinai analysts also provided support for the project. An important aim of the project was to ensure that the institution's own personnel acquired the technical and analytical skills and methods brought to the project by the consultants, enabling the institution to become independent when the need arose for future analytical or restructuring projects or for refining the PFC models.

Project Structure

Patient-focused care at Cedars-Sinai was a two-step process, beginning with the design and implementation of the pilot orthopedic unit and proceeding to housewide implementation. Both steps were completed within a two-year time period. Orthopedic model development was accomplished through the work of four design teams (see **Figure 3.1**). The work of the service standards design team was described in detail in Chapter 2 in the discussion of target setting. Chapter 4 provides details on the work of the other design teams working on the pilot unit care model. **Figure 3.2** illustrates the project structure for the housewide model development and implementation. The housewide task forces were formed immediately following the October 5, 1993 "go-live" date for the pilot unit. The following sections detail the roles and responsibilities of each of the task forces and committees shown in **Figure 3.2.**

Figure 3.1: Design Team Structure for Pilot Unit

DESIGN TEAM	OBJECTIVES
CARE MODEL *(Support Empowered Employees)*	• Options for patient-focused care models • Constraints and vision for care delivery
SERVICE INTEGRATION *(Support Redesigned Work)*	• Strategy to provide ancillary and support services to Orthopedic Unit • Consolidate accountability to unit, improve service responsiveness/continuity of care
PATIENT ORGANIZATION *(Support Managed Demand)*	• Patient grouping strategy to improve resource utilization, increase demand predictability, and minimize patient dispersion by diagnosis and physician
SERVICE STANDARDS *(Support Empowered Employees)*	• Identify and measure performance on service requirements • Recommend targets to Steering Committee

Figure 3.2: Patient-Focused Care Project Organization

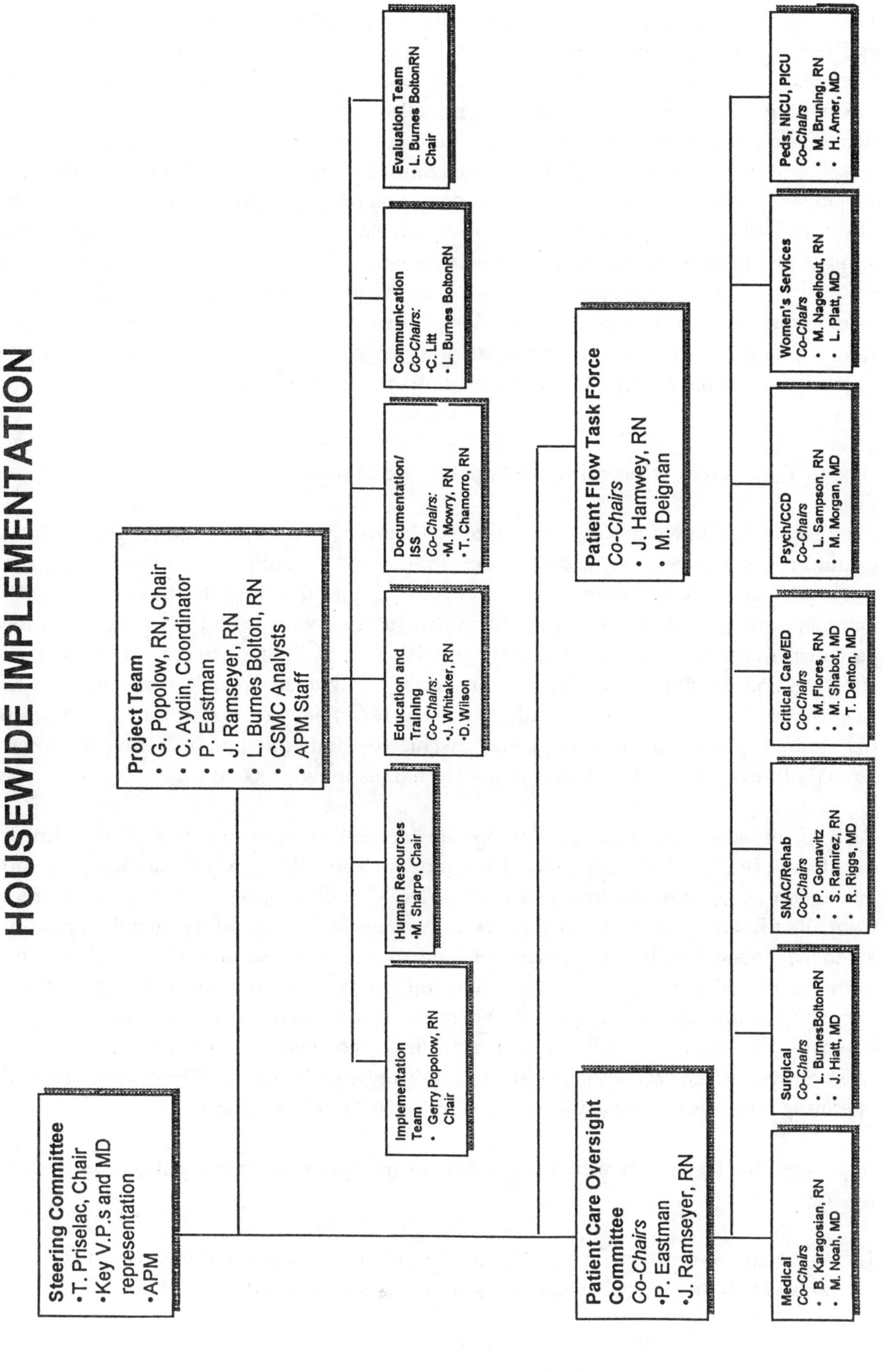

Patient Care Oversight Committee

The Oversight Committee was co-chaired by the associate vice presidents for nursing and medical affairs. This committee was charged with reviewing and approving task force plans for service line restructuring and assuring inter- and intradisciplinary team functioning and compliance with design principles. The Oversight Committee met every two weeks for 90 minutes to receive task force reports and provide feedback from all stakeholder departments. Members of the committee included directors and/or representatives of pathology and laboratory medicine, imaging, pharmacy, food and nutrition, physical medicine and rehabilitative services, social services, utilization management, admissions, finance, transportation, housekeeping, plant operations, information systems services, medical records, quality management, materials management, medical media, volunteer services, human resources, nursing, house officers, voluntary medical staff, nursing research and development, and health services research. The Oversight Committee forum was critical to the generation of ideas across departmental and service lines.

Design Task Forces (Designing the Patient Care Models)

The task forces shown across the bottom of **Figure 3.2** were chartered by the Steering Committee to develop specific care models for defined patient populations. Included in the task force responsibilities were the review of data detailing the following: which patient populations were housed on which patient units; who provided what care for the patients; and what barriers existed to the provision of quality patient care in an efficient, effective, and satisfying manner. The project began with seven task forces—medicine, surgical, pediatric, women's health, critical care/emergency department, sub-acute (rehabilitation and skilled nursing), and psychiatry—and added an operating room services (OR) task force as the others completed the planning process.

Task forces were co-chaired by appropriate medical, nursing, and other department directors. Members included medical and nursing leadership (i.e., clinical directors and managers) from all of the involved units, selected staff members, and representatives from all of the other clinical and support departments (e.g., laboratory, imaging, materials management, environmental services, and so on). Because of the heavy time commitment required to attend multiple meetings, representatives from some of these departments attended meetings only when the agenda involved issues related to their departments. They were always readily available, however, for subgroup meetings to work on specific aspects of the care models. Examples of the work of the critical care and operating room services task forces are included in Chapters 5 and 6.

In general, the task forces were responsible for providing recommendations on the following:

1. Aggregation of patients (i.e., determining which patient populations would be housed together to enable care teams to manage to demand),

2. Defining the specific care processes essential for these patient populations,

3. Determining who was providing care currently and whether the required care process could be implemented by another care team member based on licensure and regulatory standards,

4. Decreasing response and turn around time for key care processes, and

5. Improving operational efficiency.

The model development process is described in greater detail later in this chapter.

Staff Committees

Supporting the work of the task forces were staff committees. These work units provided supportive and technical assistance and evaluative services. They included the groups described below.

Communication Team. The multidisciplinary communication team was chartered by the project team to facilitate communication about the project among stakeholders at all levels of the organization. The team developed a comprehensive communication plan to keep employees, the governing body, medical staff, patients, and the community informed. Tools employed included press releases, newsletters, weekly flyers, and open forum informational sessions. The committee met weekly and was responsible for disseminating communication throughout the internal and external community.

Human Resources. The human resources committee was chaired by the vice president of human resources and consisted of vice presidents from each functional unit—patient care services, support services, and medical affairs—and project management staff. The committee was chartered by the steering committee to develop, implement, and evaluate a human resource management plan to guide the implementation of the patient-focused care models. Committee responsibilities included the development and adaptation of new policies and the creation of new job classes. Chapter 14 describes the membership and work of this group in greater detail.

Education. The Education Task Force was co-chaired by the director of employee development and an education program coordinator from nursing research and development. This committee was chartered by the project team to develop, implement, and evaluate an educational program to cross prepare the work force to provide core processes identified by the task forces. The membership and work of this committee is described in Chapter 13.

Documentation/Information Systems. The Documentation Committee worked closely with each task force to develop appropriate documentation strategies for specific patient population(s). Chapter 10 describes Cedar-Sinai's new documentation system in detail, while related technology enablers are detailed in Chapter 11.

Evaluation Team. The Evaluation Team was chaired by the director of nursing research and development and included members from nursing, information systems services, utilization management, health services research, resource management, physical medicine and rehabilitation, pulmonary services, laboratory services, volunteer services, finance, and the unit manager from the pilot unit. The team was chartered by the Steering Committee to develop and implement an evaluation plan to determine the effectiveness of the patient care models to achieve identified goals. Members of the evaluation team worked with each care model task force to tailor the generic evaluation plan to meet the evaluation needs of that patient population. The specific process and outcomes of the team's work are described in Chapters 15 and 16.

Supportive Services. In addition to the task forces detailed above, smaller work units were deployed by the project team to develop specific implementation plans for the enablers supporting the new patient care models. Each plan included a set of operating assumptions to maximize care team functions and enable the implementation of the models. The work of the specific teams addressing materials management, renovations, and information systems implementation are described in Chapters 11 and 12.

Implementation Team. Subsequent to the approval of task force care models by the Steering Committee, an implementation team was formed to implement the designed models. The implementation team met weekly and was chaired by the project director, the vice president for patient care services. Each patient care unit manager, director, and supportive staff met with project management staff to review plans for model implementation. Unit managers joined the group a few weeks prior to their own unit's implementation date. The education, human resources, communication, and supportive services groups provided updates weekly. Prior to implementation, each patient care model was approved, team job classifications were verified, individuals were cross prepared, and stakeholders (employees, medical, and administrative staff) reviewed the comprehensive communication plan. The implementation team provided an essential forum to consider the immediate implementation issues facing each unit as their implementation dates approached. As issues, concerns, and questions about tasks to be completed were brought up, unit managers were able to get immediate answers to their questions, since representatives of all of the appropriate task forces were present. The "go live" timeline extended over a six month period beginning with surgical units in April-May 1994, followed by medicine and the other service lines. Implementation of all areas was complete by the end of September 1994.

Patient Flow Task Force. This group was charged by the project team to deliver the "best practice" structure for patient admissions and placement. The team was guided by the design principle of managing to demand in their deliberations. Specific recommendations for actual patient aggregation were made by the individual care model task forces. Patient flow task force recommendations for an improved admissions process required physical renovations and re-programming of existing information systems and are being implemented in late 1995.

Aggregating Patients and Developing the Patient Care Model

Most institutions embarking on PFC projects employ similar analytical methods to design patient care models within the patient-focused care paradigm. The concepts behind these analytical frameworks were reviewed in Chapter 1 and are also described in detail by Lathrop.[3] Cedars-Sinai worked with APM to develop a design process based upon the PFC conceptual framework that would meet the specific needs of the institution. As mentioned above, PFC at Cedars-Sinai was sequential, beginning with the pilot unit and moving on to housewide implementation. While both the pilot unit and housewide implementation task forces used the same methods, the housewide task forces were able to build upon the work of the pilot unit in designing their patient care models.

The primary task force deliverables included (1) a reaggregation plan for patient care units and (2) care models with positions, job descriptions, staffing plans, and cost analyses for each unit. In analyzing their processes, the task forces created flow charts and brainstormed new ways to perform tasks that were overly complex (see **Figure 3.3** for an example). They also used work sampling data (see Chapters 15 and 16) to define nonvalue-added activities specific to individual units. They worked with the committees described above to design a new documentation system, identify technology and other enablers to improve problem areas, determine the most common DRGs and make recommendations for the development of clinical guidelines and pathways, and develop service line specific evaluation plans. All of these areas are described in greater detail in other chapters.

This chapter focuses specifically on the steps required to identify appropriate patient aggregation and develop unit-specific care models. As each task force was chartered, however, APM and project staff members also worked with task force co-chairs to develop appropriate background information to present to the task force members, as well as ground rules to help set the tone for the restructuring process. Each task force was given a financial target to meet through cost savings realized from their efforts in all of the areas described above, and time was spent at the initial task force meetings making sure that all members understood the target and agreed that it was fair. It was at this point that some additional benchmarking hospitals were added to help clarify the targets for task force members. **Figure 3.4** details the restructuring ground rules underlying the process while the preliminary financial targets for each task force are detailed in Chapter 2. Chapter 5 provides a participants' description of the work processes used by the critical care task force.

Figure 3.3: Sample Flow Chart

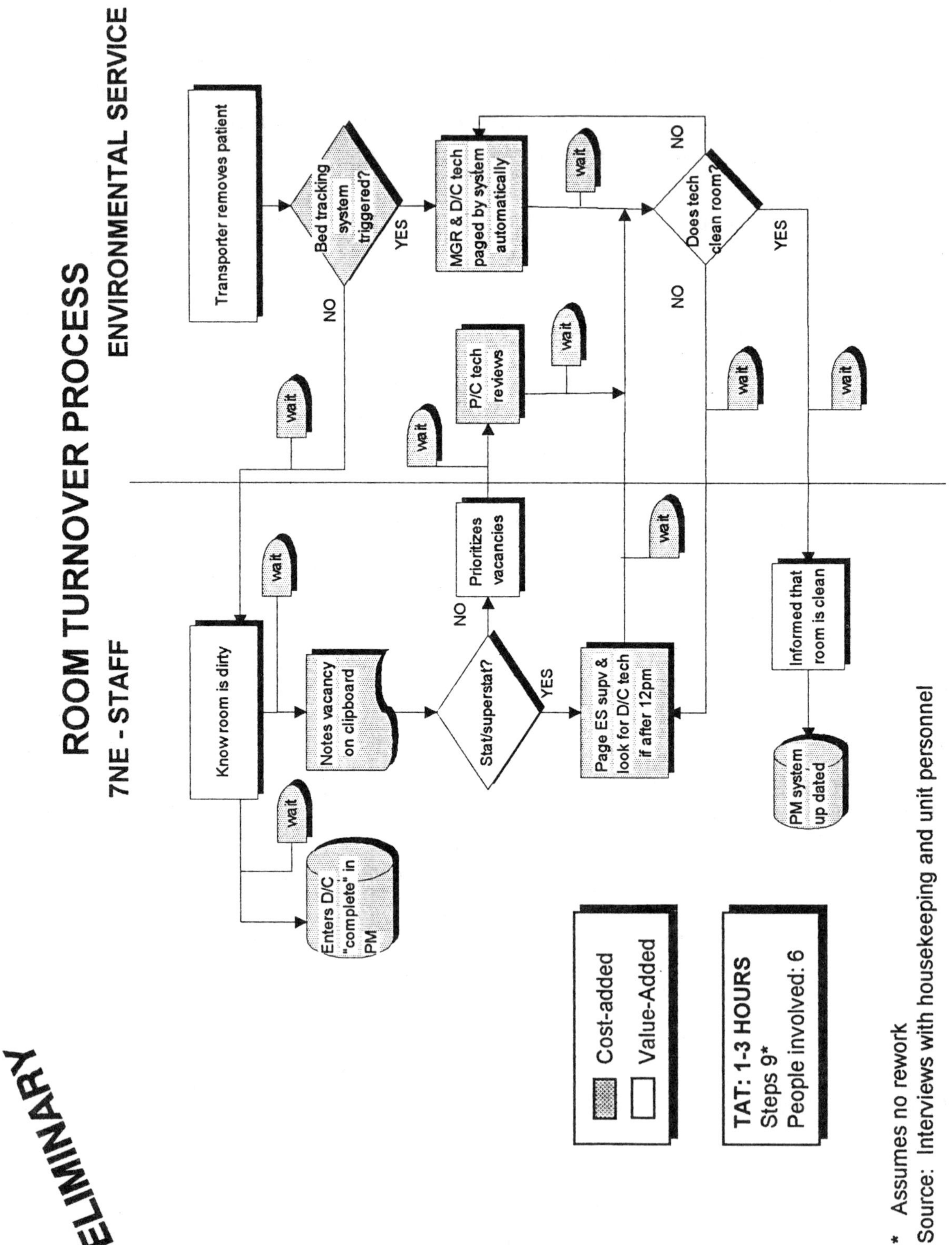

* Assumes no rework

Source: Interviews with housekeeping and unit personnel

Figure 3.4: Restructuring Ground Rules

- ❒ Cedars' mission and values will guide the process
- ❒ There are no hidden agendas
- ❒ There are no sacred cows; all ideas will be reviewed
- ❒ Communications will be open, fair and honest
- ❒ Interdepartmental cooperation is critical and expected
- ❒ Full employee and staff physician participation is important
- ❒ Staff will be involved in changes affecting their departments
- ❒ Employees' dignity, rights and contributions will be respected
- ❒ The hospital remains in charge; the project team facilitates

Patient Aggregation

The concept of managed demand, one of the PFC design principles described in Chapter 2, requires that units remain as close to "full" as possible and that patients be grouped according to like clinical needs. Each of the PFC task forces was required to address patient aggregation and produce a reaggregation plan. The steps in creating such a plan include examining existing patient populations on each unit, closing units if possible and/or necessary to increase the occupancy rates for all open units, and grouping patients with similar needs.

Figure 3.5 illustrates the analytic process for patient aggregation on the orthopedics unit. The chart on the left indicates that only 76% of orthopedic patients were cared for on the orthopedics unit prior to patient-focused care while the remaining 24% were dispersed throughout the hospital. At the same time, as shown by the chart on the right, not all of the patients on the orthopedic unit were orthopedic patients. Chapter 4 **(Figure 4.2)** shows the final patient population definition for the orthopedic unit resulting from these and other analyses. **Figure 3.6** details the overall surgical task force aggregation summary.

Figure 3.5: Patient Aggregation

While most orthopedic patients are concentrated on 7-NE, there is some potential to make the unit even more focused.

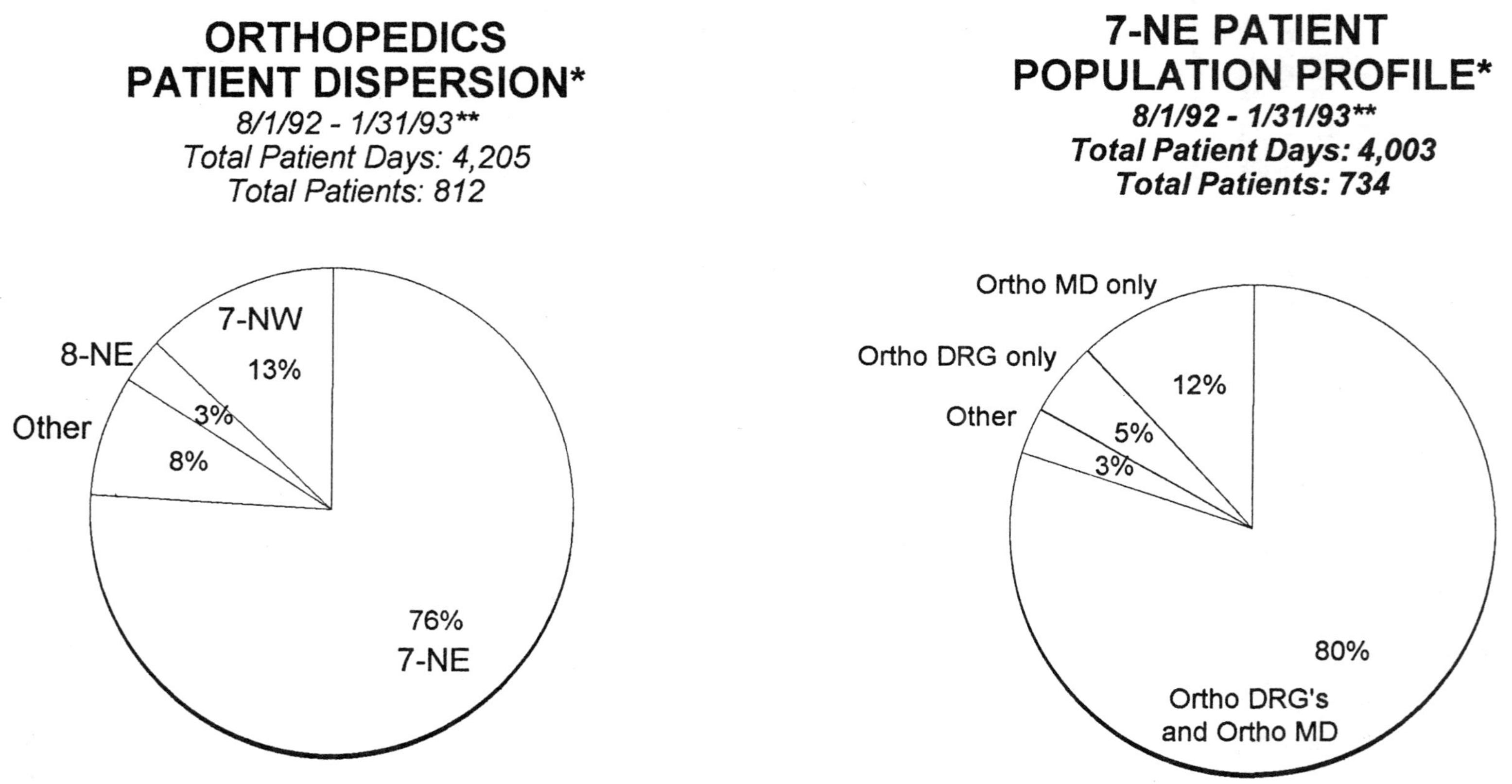

* Calculated based on Patient Days
** Excludes 10/5/92 - 10/29/92 when 7NW was closed
Source: CARDS Patient level Data
Note: An orthopedics patient is one who has contact with an ortho surgeon and has been assigned an ortho DRG

Figure 3.6: Surgical Task Force Aggregation Summary

	Historic			Projected		
Unit	Patient Type	YTD ADC	Percent Occupancy	Patient Types	Projected ADC	Percent Occupancy
6NW	CVT Surgery	21.7	67.7%	CVT Surgery Liver Patients	25.8	81%
6ICU	CVT Surgery	2.1	26.1%	CVT Liver Stepdown	2.5	31%
6NE	CVT Surgery Monitored beds for transplants	19.4	80.5%	Same	17.7	74%
7SW	General Surgery Liver patients	21.0	65.3%	General Surgery Flex	0	0
7SE	General Surgery Trauma	24.4	76.0%	Same	29.0	91%
7NW	Closed	---	---	Rehab	23.5	73%
7NE	Ortho Trauma	26.9	83.7%	Same	29.0	91%
8NW	Urology Eye Deluxe	13.6	56.5%	Urology Eye Deluxe General Surgery	17.6	73%
8NE	Neuro ENT Head/Neck Deluxe	18.7	77.8%	Same	19.6	82%
	Surgery Units Only Total	**145.7**	**73%**		**138.7**	**82%**

Care Model Development

As they began their work on care model development, task force co-chairs received assistance in planning agendas, leading the group, and setting the tone for the discussions. **Figure 3.7** provides an example of the types of questions the group members asked themselves and each other during the care model design process. While task force co-chairs led the brainstorming sessions and group discussions, project and APM staff provided support as needed. In their work, the task forces were instructed to follow the process detailed below, although the order in which some of the steps were undertaken could vary.

1. **Describe the current care model** on the unit using boxes/lines/circles to illustrate the way care is currently delivered and who is involved. Then use the same method to illustrate the desired future care model. **Figure 3.8** shows a typical diagram produced by the surgical task force during this design step. As with all of the housewide task forces, the surgical task force had the advantage of being able to build upon the orthopedics pilot care model design, and the generic job descriptions for clinical partners (CPs) and support partners (SPs) had already been developed. Chapter 4 details this development process as it took place for the pilot unit while Chapter 13 describes the education required for each job class.

2. **Identify all tasks performed** on each unit and which departments perform those tasks. Using the orthopedics task list (see Chapter 4), cross out all tasks not per formed on the unit and add tasks not already listed. Be sure to include tasks per formed by individuals from central clinical and support departments (e.g., transportation, phlebotomy, physical therapy, etc.). The representatives of those dep-departments on the task force can work with the group in developing this detailed information.

3. **Categorize tasks into classifications/staff types** (2+ years licensure, 1 year licensure, nonlicensed). In addition, determine the amount of education required to perform each of the tasks, i.e., lots of education (2+ years) or little education (1-2 weeks on the job education). Examples of the different types of caregivers with different levels of licensure and education might include RNs, LVNs, PTs, PT aides, RTs, care partners, etc. Involved in this step is research on licensure, certification, legal regulations, and technical skill required. Chapter 4 provides additional detailed examples.

4. **Identify high volume and low volume tasks** to use in Step 5 below to determine those tasks to redeploy to the unit, cross-prepare, or remain centralized. Sources include ancillary resource consumption and FTE data, census, and DRG information supplied by data anaysts. These data must be considered together since some ancillary department tasks may be high volume on the resource consumption reports, but they actually take little time as indicated by FTE data from ancillary departments. This step involves fully allocating ancillary and support services costs to the units. Project leaders and analysts can work with representatives of centralized departments to allocate their costs to individual units. The housekeeping, transportation, or other depart-

Figure 3.7: Questions To Assist Brainstorming

Overall—How would Patient-Focused Care "look" on your unit?

- Empowered Employees
  - •What services are needed by the patient that might be deployed to the unit?
  - •Where might cross-training be appropriate?
  - •What tasks could be performed by others?
- Managed Demand
  - •What workload fluctuates the most? Why?
  - •How could you predict workload?
  - •What work could be delayed or postponed?
- Redesigned Work
  - •What activities consume the majority of the day? Can they be automated? Streamlined? Eliminated?
  - •Where are there delays or bottlenecks in doing work?
  - •What activities might be redundant or "low value-added"?

Figure 3.8: Surgical Care Model

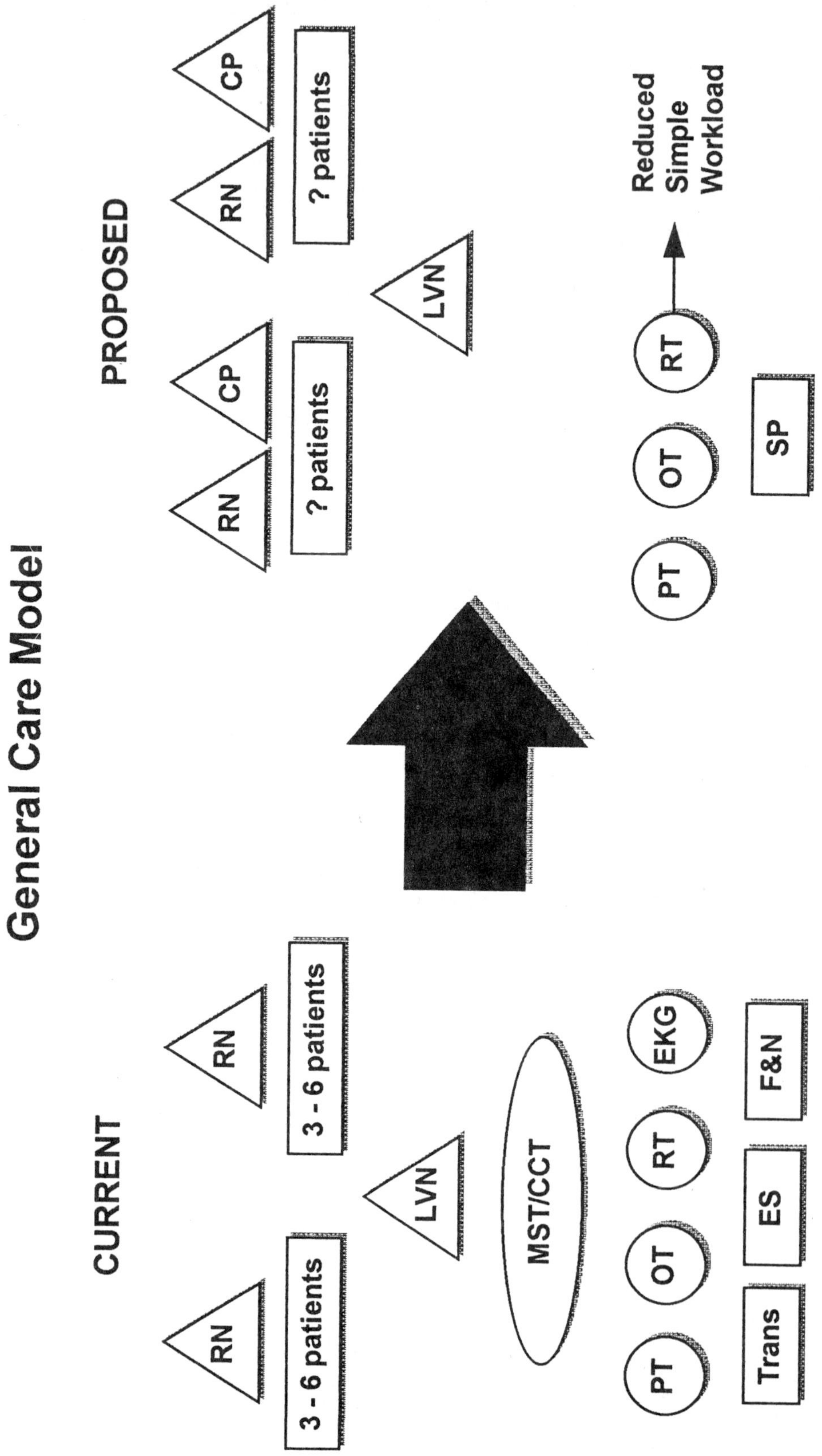

ments, for example, will need to designate the number of FTEs they currently require to serve each individual care unit, taking into account the differing needs of the units. If the tasks are subsequently redeployed to the care unit, then the FTEs are also transferred to the unit, a process that requires negotiations between the project management team and the involved central departments. The same process applies to clinical departments such as laboratory, physical therapy, respiratory therapy, etc. (See Chapter 7 for an example of the respiratory therapy FTE analyses for different types of units.) Departments may require analytical assistance in determining the appropriate unit allocations. PFC work redesign principles assume some reduction in FTEs when tasks are transferred to the unit because cross-preparation and decentralization can reduce or eliminate travel time, down time, and other inefficiencies. Detailed and careful analytical work is required in this phase of the project. Most institutions do not have information systems designed to provide the type of information required and care must be taking in using output from billing and other systems to determine the volume of tasks. Billing systems, for example, may attribute laboratory tests or other procedures to the patient's discharge unit, rather than to the patient's unit at the time the test was performed. Close collaboration between consultants and internal analysts who are familiar with the information systems is required to obtain valid and reliable data.

5. **Use the grid in Figure 3.9 to determine which tasks should be cross-prepared** to the care team, which tasks require a caregiver to be redeployed to each unit, and which tasks should remain in a central department. Volume is measured by the number of FTEs utilized per shift, while complexity is determined by licensure and/or the amount of education required to perform the task in question. Simple respiratory therapy procedures (see Chapter 7 for definitions of simple and complex procedures), for example, were assumed by cross-prepared unit staff on all units, while complex procedures continue to use dispatched central staff on units with low volume and respiratory therapists redeployed to the unit and cross-prepared to perform other tasks as needed where volume was high. Again, these task arrangements, with their matrix reporting relationships, require specific negotiations detailing task responsibilities. These negotiations involve the task force co-chairs, project management team, and department administrators. A cross-functional education needs list is then provided to the Education Task Force.

Figure 3.9: Redesign Framework

High Volume	REDEPLOY AND CROSS PREPARE	REDEPLOY AND/OR CROSS PREPARE
Low Volume	CROSS PREPARE CARE TEAM	USED DISPATCHED CENTRAL STAFF
	Low Complexity	*High Complexity*

6. **Determine the amount of time required to perform the tasks** in order to decide on the number of FTEs needed in the care team. Include the number of times the task is performed (derived from the information collected in Step 4 above) and the time of day. Central departments can help with information on how long it takes to perform specific tasks, i.e., cleaning a room, drawing blood, taking an EKG.

7. **Determine which classifications/staff types (skill mix)** are needed on the unit to perform the tasks based upon licensure and education requirements, volume of tasks, and the amount of time needed to perform each task. Make adjustments as needed. The pilot unit analyses established the staff classifications of RN, LVN II, clinical partner, and support partner. Later units were required to use these same classifications, although the specific tasks could vary by unit. The time of day tasks are performed is also essential. Be sure to estimate the number of admissions and discharges per day and the time of day (and day of the week), taking into account recent trends toward shortened lengths of stay. The amount of time required to perform each task throughout the day, combined with the skill mix determination will provide the information needed to outline a new staffing model.

8. **Determine the cost of the current model vs. the proposed model.** The first proposals will probably be too expensive and adjustments should be made until a model that meets both patient care needs and financial targets is reached. The product is a new patient care model with positions and job descriptions (clinical and support partners and revised responsibilities for RNs/LVNs and other team members deployed to the unit, e.g., physical therapists, respiratory therapists), number of FTEs, and costs.

As the task forces completed the analyses outlined above, the co-chairs reported their progress to the oversight and steering committees on a regular basis. Final patient aggregation recommendations and patient care models, including progress toward the design principles and financial targets, were approved by the steering committee. A formal sign-off process was also instituted in which the central clinical and support departments and patient care services agreed upon the tasks and FTEs to be transferred and assumed by each—PT and RT both experienced reductions in FTEs and some therapists entered into matrix reporting relationships; transportation—along with all FTEs—was moved to the units; materials management services remained centralized and received some additional FTEs to perform additional tasks.

Formal sign-offs on all task shifts is essential to ensure that important functions do not "fall through the cracks." The elevator operator for the patient elevator, for example, was a member of the transportation department, which was eliminated when the transportation function was moved to the units. Responsibility for the patient elevator, an important off-unit function, however, had to be allocated. The agreement with the laboratory addressed the reduction of approximately four laboratory FTEs because most nursing units were assuming responsibility (by licensed staff) for "stat" and "timed" blood draws. The laboratory asked for a "grace period" of two months before the FTEs were eliminated to assist the nursing units until the laboratory could document that the units were performing all of the designated blood draws. The impacts of these changes and agreements on the central clinical and support departments are described in their respective chapters later in this book.

Conclusion

The heart of the organizational change effort was the interactive planning process. This engaging and consequently comprehensive process required each stakeholder to forgo cynicism, power struggles, and professional ideologies to create a system where individuals from all disciplines and departments work together to improve patient care. Cedars-Sinai's overriding desire to create patient-focused models with interactive, multidisciplinary planning, and communication was facilitated by the structure of the project organization. Diverse task forces at the executive, operational, and staff levels formed the backbone of the project. The task forces collaborated to create a unified team committed to creating change beneficial to patients and the organization.

The project structure and task forces described above accomplished their purpose by reaggregating the patient populations at Cedars-Sinai and designing new models for each patient care unit. Housewide, the financial targets were also met. The next chapters provide detailed examples to clarify the processes further as leaders of model development teams describe the steps undertaken by their task forces and the final patient care models produced.

References

1 Ackoff RL. *Creating the Corporate Future.* New York: Wiley, 1981.

2 Ackoff RL, J Gharajedaghi, and EV Finnel. *A Guide to Controlling Your Corporation's Future.* New York: Wiley, 1984.

3 Lathrop JP. *Restructuring Health Care: The Patient Focused Paradigm.* San Francisco: Jossey-Bass, 1993.

Chapter 4

The Orthopedic Pilot Unit Care Model

Brigitte Failner, MN, RN, CON

This chapter describes the model development process for the orthopedic pilot unit. The experience described in this chapter was Cedars-Sinai's initial effort in the patient-focused care restructuring process. The discussions and analyses follow the general model building steps detailed in Chapter 3, and the outcome provided a framework for the development of care models for Cedars-Sinai patient care units housewide. The care model features, assumptions, and structure; task lists; and job descriptions produced by this design team were the starting point for each of the task forces that were to follow.

The Orthopedic Unit Before Patient-Focused Care

The orthopedic care unit was a thirty-two private bed unit with a preoperative and post-operative patient population comprised of musculoskeltal trauma and musculoskeltal surgery patients. The patient care delivery model on the unit prior to restructuring was a combination of primary nursing and team nursing with a ratio of 80% licensed to 20% nonlicensed staff. The patient communications center was covered by a nursing communication technician (NCT) seven days a week from 7:00 am to 11:00 pm. At the time of restructuring, the unit had a budgeted occupancy of twenty-four beds. All traditional non-nursing services were delivered by central departments. The physical therapy department provided both licensed and nonlicensed staff to carry out the physical therapy treatments and as many as six different therapists might be working on the unit at any one time. **Figure 4.1** illustrates the pre-PFC model. Within the circle are those caregivers actually based on the unit. They included the licensed RNs and LVNs and unlicensed medical-surgical technicians (MST), nursing communications technician (NCT, or unit secretary), and nursing services technicians (NST). All of the other patient services were provided by individuals from central departments serving the entire medical center.

Brigitte Failner, MN, RN, CON—Unit Manager, Orthopedics, Clinical Nurse Specialist, Neuroskeletal and Orthopedic Nursing, Department of Surgical Nursing, Cedars-Sinai Medical Center.

Figure 4.1: Pre-PFC Care Model

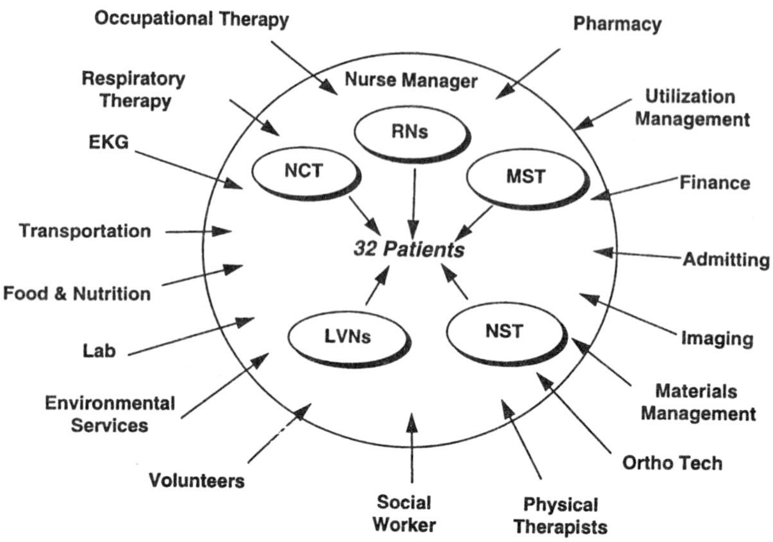

Figure 4.2: Patient Flow Task Force
The Patient Organization Subgroup identified the following patient populates to be placed on 7NE:

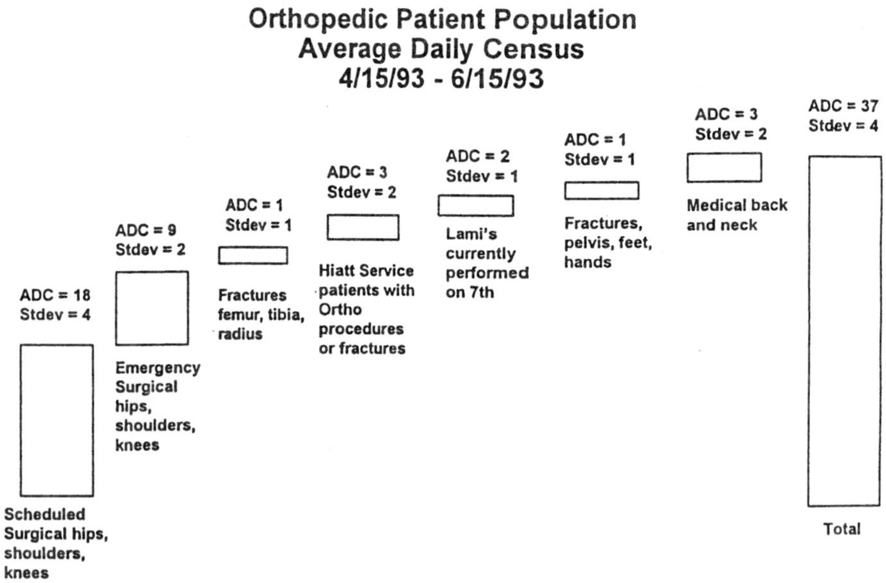

The above population will fill 32 beds 90% of the time and 31 beds 95% of the time.

Restructuring Phase I

Defining the Patient Focused Environment

Restructuring was based upon the three fundamental building blocks, or design principles, introduced in Chapter 2:

Managed Demand. Reorganizing into patient-centered units entails an important departure from conventional structures. Demand variations are minimized and workload becomes more predictable. During the design phase for the pilot unit, a patient organization design team was formed to look into patient placement practices and their implications. While it had been assumed that all orthopedic patients were coming to the orthopedic unit, analyses of computer billing records showed that orthopedic patients were actually dispersed throughout the hospital. Thus the team recommended concentrating all orthopedic surgical patients on the orthopedic unit (7NE), since the patients utilize similar services and resources. Cost analyses also indicated that it would be more cost-effective to maintain a 90% or higher occupancy rate on the unit. Since there were not enough orthopedic patients to accomplish this goal, the team identified other diagnoses and/or procedures that would utilize similar services and resources and recommended that those patient populations also be admitted to 7NE. **Figure 4.2** provides details on the patient groups designated for the orthopedic unit under the PFC reaggregation plan.

Redesigned Work. Redesigning the work involves determining how to best allocate resources to meet the new demand pattern. A second design team examined the integration of support services and identified the services utilized by patients on the orthopedic unit. They also brainstormed issues and problems with how these services were being provided. **Figure 4.3** provides an overview of the results of these brainstorming sessions, as well as identifying the additional data required to determine how to improve the delivery of service to orthopedic patients. The team then identified methods for improving the delivery of these services. Their preliminary recommendations are detailed in **Figure 4.4.** Many of these recommendations were explored as the project continued. Some of these recommendations were implemented for the pilot orthopedic unit and the housewide implementation as well (e.g., consolidating materials tasks into materials personnel as described in Chapter 12). Others were not found to be appropriate to orthopedics, but they were later implemented in other selected areas (e.g., cross preparing unit staff to perform EKGs and draw blood). Others were investigated further and found not to be cost-effective (e.g., satellite labs). These preliminary recommendations provide examples of the types of changes to consider when exploring ways of improving the delivery of care and service to patients.

Figure 4.3: Support Services Integration

The Support Services Integration Design Team identified the services utilized by patients on 7NE. They then brainstormed issues and problems with how these services are currently provided.

BRAINSTORMING RESULTS

TOPIC	EXAMPLES
• **Services utilized by Orthopedic patients**	• Housekeeping • Physical Therapy • Respiratory Therapy • Transport • Pharmacy • EKG • Others
• **Issues with how these services are provided**	• Too much documentation • Services are not coordinated • Too many people entering patients room • Too much time spent in transport • Service providers and caregivers need to listen to patients more actively • Inter departmental communication needs to be improved • Others
• **Data required to determine how to improve service delivery**	• Flow diagrams of key processes • Work sampling of select areas • FTE's by department required to support 7NE • Costs of providing services to 7NE • Skill levels of FTE's providing service to 7NE • Number of procedures performed on 7NE patients • Others

Figure 4.4: Support Services Design Team Preliminary Service Delivery Recommendations

SERVICE	PRELIMINARY RECOMMENDATIONS
EKG	• Cross train on unit staff to perform EKG's • Place EKG machine on unit
Transportation	• Reallocate transport resources to unit • Cross train transporter to transfer/transport patients • Designate additional tasks when activity is low
Physical Therapy	• Maintain PT staff in gym on 7NE • Explore potential for a satellite treatment area on 7NE
Materials Management	• Separate clean tasks and dirty tasks into only two distinct job descriptions • Consolidate all materials tasks into materials personnel
Nursing	• Remove materials tasks from NST role • Cross train staff to perform multiple on unit tasks
Pharmacy	• Evaluate the use of a Pyxis machine on unit • Pilot pyxis unit on 7th floor
Laboratory	• Explore cross training feasibility of on unit staff to draw blood • Explore feasibility of a satellite lab • Evaluate feasibility of upgrading pneumatic tube system • Examine other methods of specimen collection
Environmental Services	• Consider cross training care team member to perform environmental tasks
General	• Explore the possibility of developing a central scheduling system

Note: The design team determined that other departments examined should maintain their current method of delivering services to 7NE, these services include: Food & Nutritional Services, CT-Ultra Sound, MRI, Nuclear Cardiology, Clinical Nuclear Medicine, and Radiology 5th Floor.

Empowered Employees. To operate in an environment where decisionmaking and accountability are dispersed, people must feel valued, well-prepared, and empowered. Working toward this end was the care model design team. This team, as well as the two listed above, were made up of both management and staff of all departments interacting with 7NE in any way. The care model design team developed a set of desired features for the delivery of patient-focused care. These desired care model features are listed in **Table 4.1.**

Table 4.1: Desired Care Model Features

- Tasks performed where individual is capable *when* task is required (few hand-offs).
- Clear understanding and acceptance of unique responsibilities among care team members.
- Care team is "small" and can accomplish the "majority" of patient needs on the unit when possible (preadmission to post-discharge).
- Patient schedule well-coordinated.
- Excellent communication among team members and across teams
- Minimal travel, movement of patient and staff.

Identifying Tasks, Treatments, and Services

With the desired care model features established, the design team set out to identify all the tasks, treatments, and services needed or utilized by the 7NE patient population. These items were categorized by the type of caregiver currently performing the task and the type of skill needed to perform the task. This step led to the identification of three types of caregivers to be considered for the orthopedic care team: (1) licensed caregivers with two or more years of formal education, (2) licensed caregivers with one year of for-

Figure 4.5: Care Model Structure

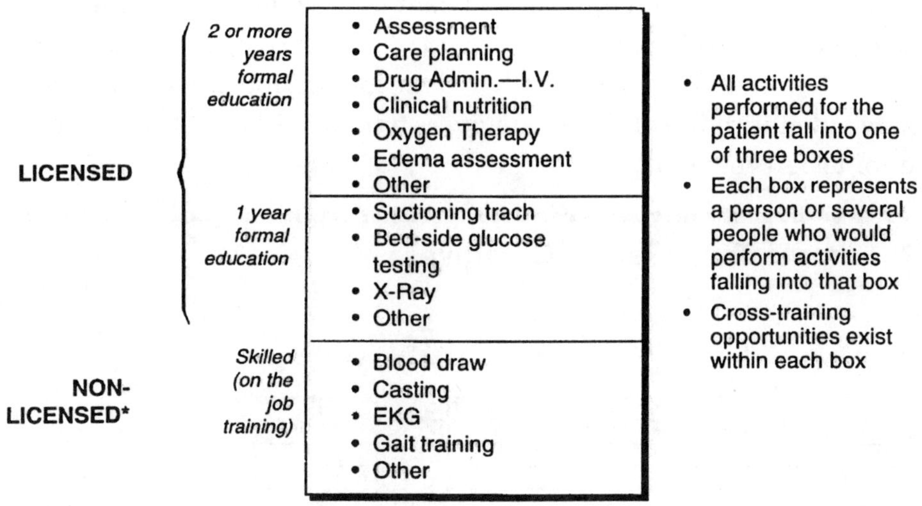

* Also includes some activities covered by certification

mal education, and (3) nonlicensed individuals. **Figure 4.5** gives examples of the tasks that could potentially be performed by each category of caregiver, although further exploration was still required to determine California regulations governing specific tasks (e.g., phlebotomy). The key assumptions that would drive the care model staffing structure are listed in **Table 4.2.**

Table 4.2: Key Assumptions

- All staff are responsible for assuring that all needs of the patient are met.
- Licensed staff (registered nurse, physical therapist, medical social worker) will be minimally cross-prepared.
- Some mix of licensed staff (LVNs and/or licensed respiratory care practitioners) will be utilized on the unit.
- Nonlicensed staff will be fully cross-prepared to perform clinical activities that will encompass current MST tasks, PT aide tasks, and simple respiratory therapy procedures.
- Nonlicensed staff will also be cross-prepared to perform many support activities presently performed by environmental services and transportation.

The next step involved examining the lists of tasks in greater detail to identify exactly which types of employees in the licensed categories would be able to perform the identified tasks. Involved in this step were all of the issues related to licensure, certification, technical skill, volume, and cost of education and equipment needed. **Table 4.3** shows sample portions of the task lists for licensed-1 year, licensed-2+ years, and unlicensed caregivers. Each column represents a specific type of caregiver (e.g., RN, LVN, PT, PT aide, RT, care partner, etc.), and the shaded boxes in the columns indicate those tasks that the specific caregiver is able (via licensure and/or education) to perform. The columns were initially identified by number rather than identifying the caregiver to allow for more objective identification of those caregivers who would be able to perform the greatest number of tasks on the unit.

Table 4.3: Sample Task List for Caregivers

LICENSED - 1 YEAR

TASK	STAFF TYPE 1	2	3
Oxygen Therapy	X	X	
drug admin-po,IM,SC,ear,/eye drops	X	X	
tube feedings	X	X	
check emergency cart	X	X	
check one touch	X	X	
catherization(bladder)	X	X	
vascular checks	X	X	
trach care	X	X	
narcotic count	X	X	
Neuro checks	X	X	
suctioning trach	X	X	
sputum induction	X	X	
bladder irrigation	X	X	
Glucose testing	X	X	
transfusions		X	
verbal orders		X	
placement/removal of drains/catheters		X	
skin testing		X	
IV start		X	
Verification of transcribed orders		X	
X-Ray			X

LICENSED - OTHER/ 2+ YEARS

TASK	STAFF TYPE 4	5	6	7	8	9	10
Oxygen Therapy	X						
assess for adaptive equipment /medical equipment		X	X	X		X	
assessment		X	X	X	X	X	X
bed mobility- assessment, evaluation		X	X				
care planning		X	X	X	X	X	X
clinical specialist consult		X	X	X			
debridement		X	X				
discharge planning*		X	X	X	X	X	X
drug admin-IV		X					
edema management- assess, evaluation		X	X				
Enterostomal consult		X					
follow up on lab		X			X		X
gait training- assessment, evaluation		X	X				
hyperalimentation		X			X		X
infection consult		X			X		
med/allergy history		X			X		

SKILLED - NON-LICENSED

TASK	STAFF TYPE 11	12	13	14	15	16	17	18
ADL assistance	X	X	X	X	X	X	X	
complaint handling	X	X	X	X	X	X	X	
spiritual care	X	X	X	X	X	X	X	
stock replacement	X	X	X	X	X	X	X	
interactions with family		X	X	X	X	X	X	
oxygen administration		X	X	X	X	X	X	
assist with procedures(MD)		X	X	X	X		X	
compression (JOBST)		X	X	X	X		X	
equipment delivery (to room)		X	X	X	X		X	
pain management modalities- application	X	X		X	X		X	
application & care of TEDS/SCDs		X		X	X		X	

Tasks were also classified according to the redesign framework (see **Chapter 3, Figure 3.9** for more information). This framework was used to weigh both the complexity (i.e., licensure and/or amount of education required to perform the task) and the volume (measured by the number of FTEs utilized per shift) in determining which caregivers should perform each task. According to this framework, for example, tasks falling in the upper left cell (i.e., high volume and low complexity) would be performed by all caregivers, including cross-prepared unit staff and staff redeployed from central departments. On the orthopedic unit, performing activities of daily living (ADLs) and ambulating patients might fall in this category. All caregivers could both learn the tasks and maintain their competence in performing them. It was particularly important to examine the volume of tasks to ensure that individuals would have enough opportunity to maintain competence in the cross-prepared tasks.

The design team spent many hours with the task lists and redesign framework to ensure that all licensed staff categories received equal consideration. Could a physical therapist handle the required tasks instead of a RN? Could a licensed respiratory therapist handle the tasks instead of a LVN? The group also considered the cost of appropriate cross preparation, as well as equipment costs and the costs of education required to ensure-maintenance of the competency/skill needed to perform tasks if the volume was low. The care model design team's work resulted in the recommendations for the unit team staff types detailed in **Table 4.4.**

Table 4.4: Care Model Staff

- Appropriate mix of care practitioners
  - –Licensed staff (RN, PT, RT, LVN, etc.)
- Clinical Partner
  - –Nonlicensed clinical staff
- Support Partner
  - –Nonlicensed support staff

Restructuring Phase II

Task Force Deliverables

Phase I of the restructuring process for the pilot unit set the stage for the more detailed work of Phase II by defining the patient-focused environment, identifying the tasks, treatments, and services used by the orthopedic patient, and designating the categories of caregivers to be included on the unit team. In Phase II, the patient care task force was charged with actually creating this new environment by using the fundamental restructuring principles and design team recommendations to rethink/redesign core processes.

The patient care task force was given the following objectives:

1. Develop the details of the care model based on the work of the Phase I care model design team. Deliverables were to include staffing, hours per patient day (HPPD)

ratios, job descriptions, and plans for cross preparation of the care team
2. Operationalize the recommendations of the service integration design team (see **Figures 4.3 and 4.4**).
3. Brainstorm and operationalize additional patient-focused care ideas not identified by design teams.

Defining the Care Model

The patient care task force used the task lists (**Table 4.3**) and the care model staff types (**Table 4.4**) to create a detailed list of potential team members and the tasks each was capable of performing, either currently or with appropriate cross preparation. The end product was the list of unit team tasks by staff type detailed in this chapter's appendix. This list was then presented to the orthopedic staff for their input. Based upon all of these steps, the patient care task force members finally defined a unit team consisting of RNs, LVNs (rather than respiratory therapists, because of the high volume of medications and low volume of respiratory treatments), clinical partners, support partners, and receptionists. In addition, the physical therapists and social worker would be permanently assigned to the unit by their central departments. Other staff would be deployed-from a central department as needed for specific treatments or tasks. **Figure 4.6** illustrates the resulting care model.

Figure 4.6: The Orthopedic Care Model

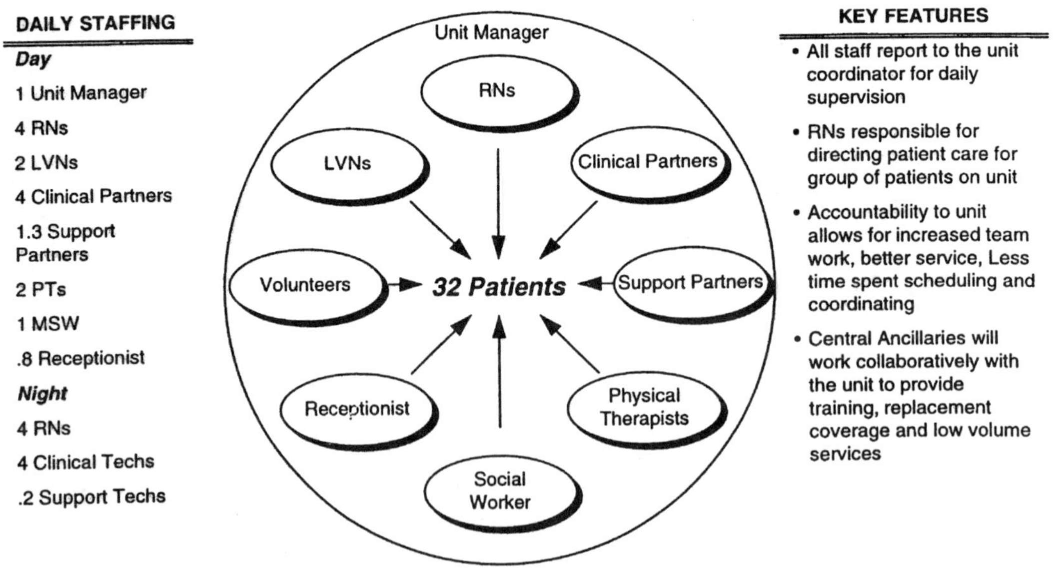

Note: A multidisciplinary, cross-prepared team of caregivers work on the units providing almost all care needs for a group of 32 patients.

Figure 4.7: FTE Changes

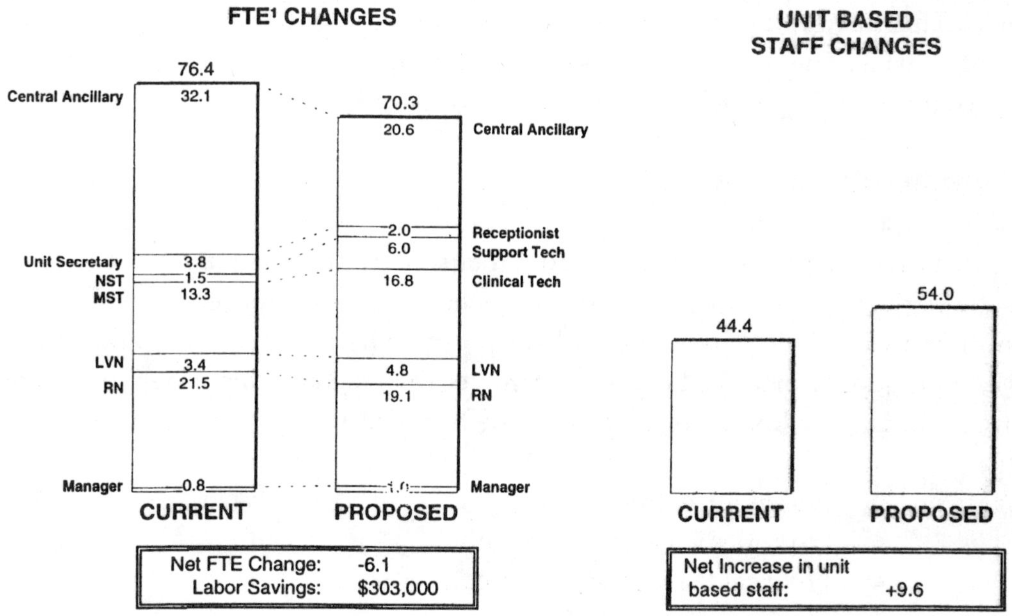

1 All FTE figures include 13.8% for VHS; all dollar figure include 20% for benefits.

Note: The PFC model structure reduces total staff required to support 7NE, allowing for an annual savings of $303,000. Unit based staff increases by over 9 FTEs; this will improve service provided to patients.

Once the care model team was defined, the group needed to determine the exact number of FTEs for each staff type needed on the unit team based upon patient aggregation design team recommendation of a 90% occupancy rate. Patient acuity, cross preparation of team members, and the average number of daily tasks per unit were used in determining FTE needs. **Figure 4.7** details the number of FTEs both on and off the unit before and after PFC. As shown in **Figure 4.7**, the number of FTEs on the unit increased with this model, since unit staff members were taking on tasks that had been done by central staff in the past. However, the total FTE usage by central departments for the unit decreased. The new HPPD were 5.79 for the morning shift and 3.72 for the evening shift, for a daily HPPD of 9.51.

Implementation

Once the FTEs were determined, job descriptions were written with the assistance of the ancillary departments and approval of the unit manager and clinical director and were posted for job applicants. The education task force developed the education program (see Chapter 13 for details), and all staff attended the initial team building and common cross preparation sections on environmental, food and nutrition, and PFC requirements. Each staff type also attended the appropriate classes for needed cross preparation. The current unit staff was divided into two groups to ensure that competent orthopedic staff remained on the unit at all times. Each group attended the class with a number of the newly hired staff.

Implementation of the new model occurred on October 5, 1993, the day after the second group finished class. To help all unit staff accept the change, a farewell party for the old system and a ribbon cutting ceremony on the day the new PFC model was implemented were held. This helped the staff realize that the old way of doing things was gone and would not be back. The new model was here. Although the unit could and would make changes to improve the model, 7NE would not go back.

The Orthopedic Care Model

Figure 4.8 shows the orthopedic care model focused around the patient. The team caring for the patient consists of physicians, registered nurses, licensed vocational nurses, physical therapists, clinical partners, and support partners. The model allows for cost-effective, high quality orthopedic patient care because the care team delivers all appropriate treatments, coordinated during all of the hours of the day. These include the following:

- Nursing treatments
- Orthopedic basic treatments
- Physical therapy simple treatments
- Respiratory simple treatment
- Environmental tasks

Figure 4.8: PFC Care Model

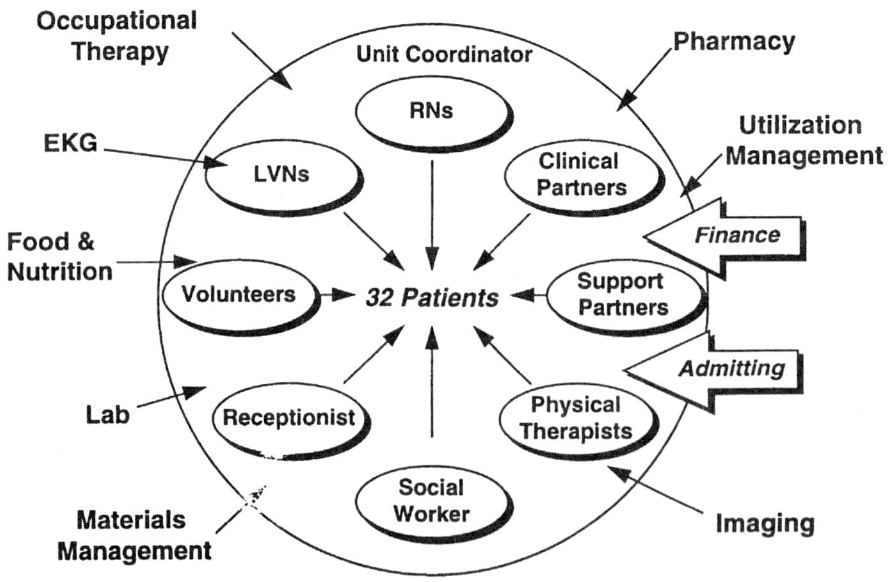

New Communication Patterns

The biggest change was in communication. In the past, shift report was given to a group, sitting in a conference room. With the new model, report takes place at the bedside, licensed staff to licensed staff and clinical partner to clinical partner. Thus, staff members remain near their patients and available for physician questions. The clinical partners go into patient rooms and get patients up for breakfast together. A team (RN, LVN, CP, and PT) report/conference is then held at 7:45 am for each side of the unit. At that time, PT tasks are assigned to clinical partners and PTs and RNs discuss appropriate treatment schedules for the patients in order to coordinate ADLs, treatments, and tests. The team meets again in the afternoon for any updates. RN and clinical partner teams meet periodically to review patient issues and orders.

Enablers

The modular desks, personal computers, and space for patient charts installed outside each quad, or four patient rooms (see Chapters 11 and 12 for details), created an environmental change allowing RNs to enter orders in a computer located close to patient rooms. This change brought the care team closer to the patient, allowing caregivers to answer call lights in a more timely manner. All parts of a patient's chart were also located in one place near the bedside.

Staffing Mix

The team staffing mix detailed above allows for the appropriate level of caregiver (whether licensed or unlicensed) for each task. For increased teamwork, if one member of the care team is busy in one room, another member is able to respond to the rest of the patients in the team assignment. Most important, since physical therapy tasks are no longer performed only by physical therapists between 9:00 am to 4:00 pm, this new model allows physical therapy activities to be scheduled on a twenty-four hour a day basis. PT treatments or tasks are now performed by cross-prepared caregivers and spaced out during the whole day, as well as being incorporated into activities at night (e.g., gait training while helping a patient get up to go to the bathroom or exercises while doing evening care).

Figure 4.9: Care Model Function Distribution

FUNCTIONAL AREA	ON UNIT STAFF	OFF UNIT STAFF
Basic Nursing	All	None
Physical Therapy	All	None
Environmental Services	Daily Tasks	Project Cleaning
Occupational Therapy	Simple Procedures	Complex Procedures
Respiratory Therapy	Simple Procedures	Complex Procedures
EKG	All	None
Food & Nutrition	Simple Tasks	Complex Tasks
Transportation	All	None
Pharmacy	None	All
Utilization Management	None	All
Social Work	All	None
Finance	None	All
Admitting	None	All
Imaging	None	All
Lab	None	All
Ortho Tech Tasks	Simple Procedures	Complex Procedures

Shading indicates a change from current practice

Conclusion

The patient care model developed for orthopedics provided a starting point for the housewide model development process detailed in Chapter 3. The housewide task forces adopted the desired care model features, key assumptions, and general staffing principles in beginning to plan their own care models. The care model function distribution summary in **Figure 4.9** also provided a starting point for other task forces, although the resulting models varied according to unit needs. Chapter 5 provides an example of how the critical care units used these pilot unit principles and task analyses to develop PFC models for critical care.

Appendix: Unit Team Tasks by Staff Type

RN		Non Licensed (clinical tech)	Non Licensed (support tech)
assessment		check emergency cart	transport pt./specimens
care planning		♦ ADL assistance	♦ pass juices
IV-drug admin.		♦ vital signs	♦ pass H2O
central line specimen collection		♦ bedpans	♦ prepare Clear liquid trays
central line hyperalimentation		neuro-vascular checks-basic	♦ pass snacks
○ verbal orders		dermal ulcer care	clean pt. room/bathroom
○ order transcribe		application of pressure relief devices	discharge room clean
○ order entry		application & care of TEDS/SCDs	application & care of ortho fram
○ order/schedule- tests/studies		foley care	replenishing of paper & soap
follow up on lab/assess/plan action		removal of catheter	trash & sharps removal
pain management assessment		tube/drain emptying	vacuum or dust/wet mopping pt.
pre-admit Ed		♦ feeding pt.	logging of shampooing needs
teaching/ed. pt./SO		♦ application & care of restraints	cleaning nurses station
		non invasive specimen collection	delivery of equipment to room
		transfers, bed to chair	belongings/valuables, security
		♦walking pt.	clean staff restroom
		♦application of hot/cold therapy	♦ report running
		#application and care of CPM	♦ filing
		#application of slings/immobilizers/braces	♦ clearing trays from room
		#ROM	
		#transfer training	
		#progressive exercise & mobility	
		#equipment training /equip adjusting	
		#gait training	
		#bed mobility training	
		#application of skin traction	
		#assist with casting/splints	
		#EKG	
		ostomy care	
		tap H2O enema	
		#pulse Ox	
		#care of residual limbs	
		post-mortom care	
		assist with procedures	

Legend

○ Tasks under own license
♦ All team members
\# New task for job class

Appendix: Unit Team Tasks by Staff Type (cont.)

LVN	1 year licensed (respiratory tech)	1 year licensed (PT Assist)
drug admin. po/IM/SC/ear/eye/pr	narcotic count with RN	narcotic count with RN
IV start/D/C/hang IV	tube feeding- refilling	tube feeding- refilling
transfusion	central line care	central line care
narcotic count	neuro-vascular checks -basic	neuro-vascular checks -basic
check one touch	dressings	dressings
glucose testing	wound care	wound care
° verbal orders	chest tube care	chest tube care
° order transcribe	trach care	trach care
° order entry	suction oral/nasal/trach	suction oral/nasal/trach
catherization(bladder)	sputum induction	sputum induction
dressings	#Oxygen Therapy	#Oxygen Therapy
wound care	#hand held nebulizer/MDI	#aerosol therapy-intermit/continue
invasive specimen collection (urine)	#aerosol therapy-intermit/continue	#chest percussions/vibration
#Oxygen Therapy	#chest percussions/vibration	#postural drainage
incentive spirometry	#postural drainage	incentive spirometry
central line care	incentive spirometry	° verbal orders
chest tube care	° verbal orders	° order transcribe
trach care	° order transcribe	° order entry
suction oral/nasal/trach	° order entry	
tube feeding -assess, check for residual		
sputum induction		
#hand held nebulizer/MDI		
#aerosol therapy-intermit/continue		
#chest percussions/vibration		
#postural drainage		
quiaic testing		
peripheral hyperalimentation		
bladder irrigation		
skin testing		

Appendix: Unit Team Tasks by Staff Type (cont.)

Physical Therapist	MSW	Receptionist	
assessment,evaluation, performance &/or delegation of: -bed mobility -gait training -transferring -therapeutic exercise/manual therapy care of prosthetics&orthotics (education) electrical stimulation-assess,evaluation,application edema management recommendations for adaptive devices pre-admit Ed teaching/ed.pt./SO ° order entry	discharge planning referrals / continuity of care psycho social interventions assessment for -information & resource referrals -placement in community	directing traffic information communicator ♦ answering telephone ♦ respnding to intercom ♦ phone calls to obtain: -old charts -transcriptions -items from central issue -name plates & facesheet -security for valubles pickup/delivery -copies of X-Rays from file room ♦ phone calls to: -order ambulance -order repairs -have belongings picked up -have belongings delivered ♦ phone call to obtain consults ♦ call Admit Supervisor for direct admit ♦ Patient chart activity	

Chapter 5

Patient Care Models for Critical Care

Maria Fe M. Mangila, RN, MSN, CCRN
M. Michael Shabot, MD
Bernice Coleman, RN, MN, CCRN
Joey Zimmerman, RN, BSN
Sue Kelman, RN, BSN, CCRN
Berdie Justice, RN, BSN
Karen Morris, RN, MPA, CNA
Lawrence Maldonado, MD

This chapter describes the development of specific patient-focus care (PFC) models for the Cedars-Sinai Medical Center adult critical care areas, including planning, model design, and implementation processes and outcome measures. Included are critical care models for medical and respiratory intensive care, cardiac surgical intensive care, general surgical intensive care, and cardiac intensive care units.

Planning the Change Process

The role of the staff nurse is crucial to the successful implementation of change in the intensive care unit (ICU) setting, a fact that was recognized from the outset at Cedars-Sinai. Since there were no models available from other institutions for patient-focused

MARIA FE M. MANGILA, RN, MSN, CCRN—Clinical Nurse Specialist, Department of Surgical Nursing, Cedars-Sinai Medical Center.

M. MICHAEL SHABOT, MD—Associate Director, Department of Surgery, Cedars-Sinai Medical Center.

BERNICE COLEMAN, RN, MN, CCRN—Clinical Nurse Specialist, Cardiac-Thoracic-Liver Service Line, Cedars-Sinai Medical Center.

JOEY ZIMMERMAN, RN, BSN—Assistant Director, Cardiac-Thoracic-Liver Service Line, Cedars-Sinai Medical Center.

SUE KELMAN, RN, BSN, CCRN—Unit Manager, 7 & 8 Surgical Intensive Care Units, Cedars-Sinai Medical Center.

BERDIE JUSTICE, RN, BSN—Unit Manager, Cardiac Intensive Care Unit, Cedars-Sinai Medical Center.

KAREN MORRIS, RN, MPA, CNA—Unit Manager, Medical and Respiratory Intensive Care Unit, Cedars-Sinai Medical Center.

LAWRENCE MALDONADO, MD—Director, Medical Intensive Care Unit,General Internal Medicine, Cedars-Sinai Medical Center.

care in the ICU setting, the process of "rethinking" the intensive care paradigm was a particular challenge. ICU nurses are, by nature, typically vigilant and goal directed. This vigilance is reflected in the excellent patient outcomes common to this practice setting. However, the ICU setting also has a tight connection with tradition and, to some degree, regimentation, attributes that can make envisioning "what could be" from "what is" more difficult. Thus careful thought was given to creating a change process that would include staff nurses and enable them to deliberately challenge current practice and bring about the paradigm shift required to provide quality care in a cost-effective manner.

To that end, a change process was planned that would allow staff nurses to participate, while the role of key visionary was assigned to the unit manager on each intensive care unit. The unit manager was to assist staff nurses in planning and implementing the new PFC models. The critical care task force, which met weekly, provided general direction in developing a generic model for all critical care units. (See Chapter 3 for a discussion of project organization.) This multidisciplinary group, which included representatives from pulmonary medicine, laboratory, pharmacy, food and nutrition, materials management, environmental services, medical directors of the various ICUs, nursing administration, and nurse managers of the ICUs, provided coordination and allowed collaboration and the sharing of experience among staff from the different ICUs. Each unit manager was encouraged to invite staff nurses to attend meetings as appropriate. Attending these meetings gave the individual staff nurses exposure to the overall process and an opportunity to become familiar with each of the steps in the development of the care model.

Developing the Care Model

Pre-PFC Critical Care Model

The first step in any model development process is to review the way care is currently being delivered. At Cedars-Sinai, critical care technicians (unlicensed personnel) and licensed vocational nurse IIs (LVN IIs) were already used in the intensive care units. (Chapter 13 details the educational program in place for critical care technicians prior to PFC implementation.) The multidisciplinary critical care task force began the change process by devoting several meetings to "sharing." That is, staff from each of the critical care units, as well as other departments such as respiratory therapy, were given time to present details of their patient populations and current practice to the group. A picture of the existing generic care model emerged, but even more importantly, the process gave staff from the individual units the opportunity to point out the ways in which their practice and concerns differed from those of other units. This recognition of care unit similarities and differences was a key element in the change process. **Figure 5.1** provides an example of the existing (pre-PFC) generic critical care model including the on-unit and off-unit staff.

Figure 5.1: Generic Critical Care Model (Pre-PFC)

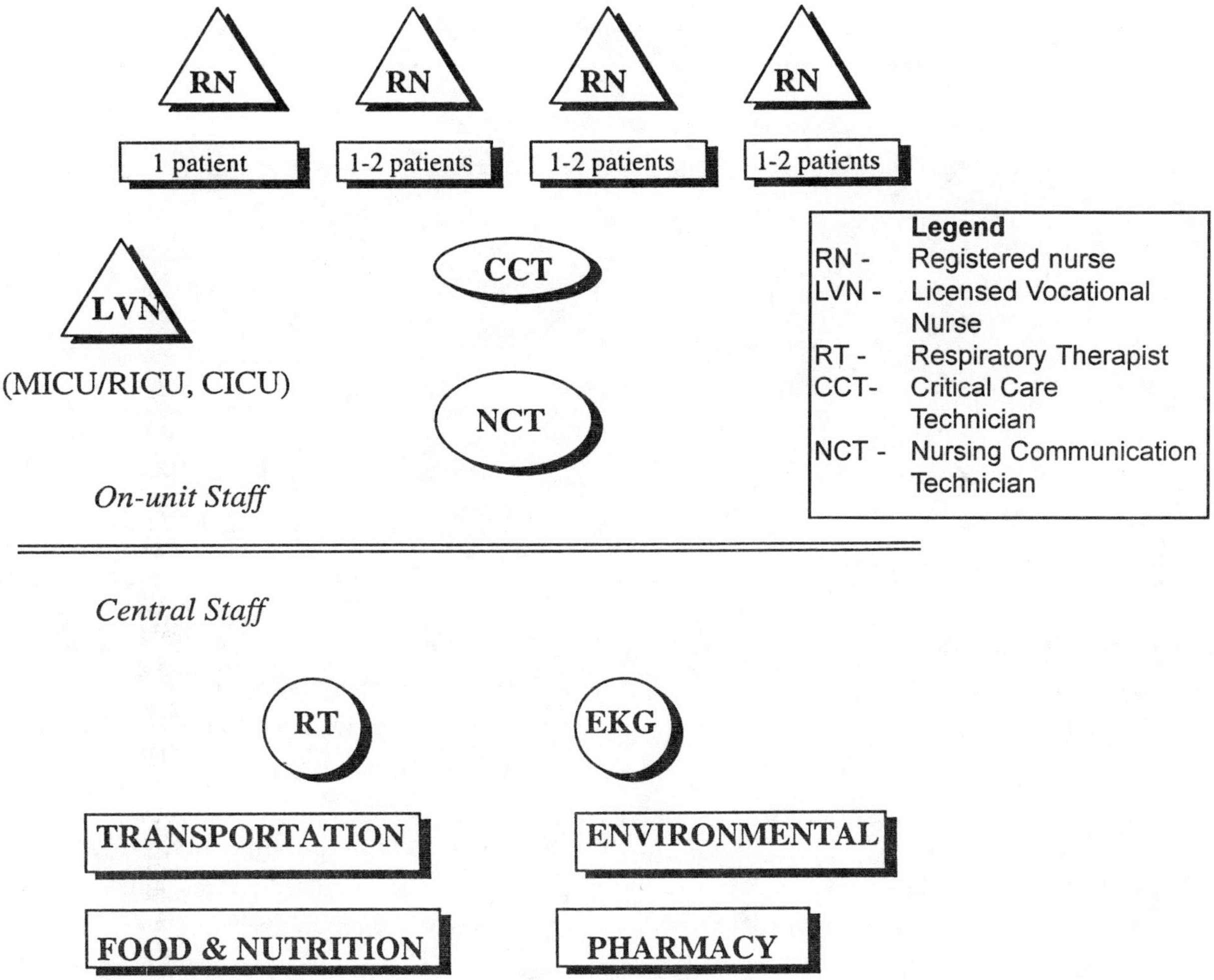

Applying the PFC Design Principles

Following the review of the existing care model and recognition of individual variation, the next steps were devoted to developing proposals to change the critical care delivery system integrating the PFC design principles. Numerous multidisciplinary meetings followed to address the three main design principles—managed demand, work redesign, and employee empowerment. The overall results of these meetings are presented in **Table 5.1**. While the design principles themselves were common throughout the PFC project, the proposed changes differed by area. In critical care, for example, potential reaggregation of patients was limited by the physical plant, but halves of units could be closed to accomodate the fluctuating census. Redesigning the work required a number of steps, beginning with the construction of task lists as described in the following section. The proposals for empowering employees were consistent throughout the PFC project housewide.

Table 5.1: Patient-Focused Care Design Principles

DESIGN PRINCIPLES		PROPOSALS
MANAGED DEMAND		
1. Patients grouped by clinical similarity to enable customized care and predictable scheduling.	•	Service lines are aggregated in present models. Physical plant limitations prevent reaggregation. Reassessment will be done after clinical pathways are instituted.
2. Units designed to be "full" with less work load fluctuation.	•	Continue to close halves of units as census fluctuates.
3. Clinical pathways to ensure quality, cost-effective care.	•	Clinical Pathways are being developed.
REDESIGNED WORK		
1. Cross-prepared teams, redesigned jobs, proper skill deployment.	•	Cross-prepare non licensed unit-based staff to perform many clinical and support activities. Increase LVNs and non licensed staff.
2. Capital resources and ancillary, administrative, and support services on the unit where clinically and economically feasible.	•	Move all or part of functions of EKG, RT, Environmental Services, and Transportation to unit staff.
3. Processes simplified.	•	Streamline documentation, charts, supplies, and computers moved closer to patient.
EMPOWERED EMPLOYEES		
1. Authority, responsibility, and accountability for patient care resource allocation appropriately aligned, minimal responsibility and hand-offs.	•	All staff are responsible for assuring that all needs of the patient are met.
2. Fewer workers interacting with any one patient.	•	All staff working on the unit will report to the unit coordinator for daily supervision.
3. Overall service improved.	•	Each RN is responsible for managing all of the care needs of a group of patients in the unit.

Constructing Task Lists

The PFC design principles required a model with cross-prepared teams of caregivers working in redesigned jobs with proper skill deployment. Furthermore, the task forces were to use and adapt the roles already delineated during the pilot unit design process (e.g., RN, LVN II, clinical and support partners, respiratory therapists, etc.) as appropriate to their areas. The actual tasks performed by each role could vary according to unit needs, as long as they were appropriate to the skill level, and education and licensure requirements. Thus, LVN IIs and respiratory therapists, as well as unlicensed personnel, would be incorporated into the individual unit care models as appropriate.

In order to determine the optimal skill mix, the task force set out to identify all of the individual tasks required to deliver patient care in each of the ICUs and to determine, for each task, the level of education and professional licensure requirment in the state of California. (See Chapters 3 and 4 for additional details on the design process.) To eliminate rework, the units began with the task lists developed for the orthopedic pilot unit and adapted and added to them for critical care.

To capture the valuable perspective of the staff nurse in implementing PFC work redesign, each nurse manger selected key nurses from the unit to participate in reviewing the typical tasks carried out by RNs and determining which functions might be carried out by a non-licensed person. In addition to the orthopedic task list mentioned earlier, the staff nurses also listed all the tasks or functions they performed in their practice. (Please refer to the Nursing Sample Task List located in this chapter's appendix for further information.) For each task, the second column shows the type of licensure required (i.e., 1L=1 year license, 2L=2 year license, RN, Pharmacist, etc.), followed by columns delineating who had been performing the task and who might perform the task in the new model. Defining the task list is an important and time-consuming step that must be thoroughly exhausted before moving to the next step in the design process. Although all of the ICUs are governed by the same policies and procedures, recognition of unit culture is key in beginning to change practice. Nurses from all units came together to work on the task list, providing a forum in which to discover how other nurses viewed the practice of nursing. By providing an opportunity for nurses to share with their counterparts in other units, they actually became the challengers of each others' practice. This strategy was key later in the design and implementation process.

Once all the typical nursing practices were listed, each staff nurse and unit manger was given a copy and advised to meet with their individual staffs to review them. The representatives who had worked together as a group to develop the initial lists acted as the champions of the process with their peers. Each unit further defined the list and held lengthy discussions on which tasks they felt could be accomplished by someone other than a registered nurse. The importance of this process cannot be underestimated as it provided the essence of change and staff nurse "buy- in." Once each unit was satisfied with their own list, the groups met together to construct one generic list built upon a foundation that included state regulations, projected cost savings, and nurses' perceptions. Maintaining high quality, cost-effective care was the driving force for the model development.

Applying the Redesign Framework

Once the task lists were completed, the group turned to the redesign framework, which consisted of two variables—volume of services or tasks provided on each unit and (2) the level of complexity for each task. For each task a redesign grid was utilized (see **Figure 5.2**) to determine whether deployed central staff or cross-prepared unit staff would be used. The four categories in the grid included (1) redeploy and cross prepare, (2) redeploy and/or cross prepare, (3) cross prepare care team, and (4) use dispatched central staff.

Figure 5.2: Redesign Framework

High Volume	(1) REDEPLOY AND CROSS PREPARE	(2) REDEPLOY AND/OR CROSS PREPARE
Low Volume	(3) CROSS PREPARE CARE TEAM	(4) USED DISPATCHED CENTRAL STAFF
	Low Complexity	*High Complexity*

Using this grid, any tasks falling into the upper left cell (i.e., high volume as measured by the number of FTEs utilized per shift.) and low complexity (i.e., no licensure and mimimal education required) would be performed by cross-prepared unit staff as well as other staff redeployed to the unit. Activities of daily living (ADLs) would fall in this category. Because of their low complexity and high volume, all caregivers could both learn the tasks and maintain their competency in performing them. Tasks falling into the lower right cell (low volume and high complexity), however, would require the use of centrally dispatched staff since the complexity and/or licensure requirements would make cross preparation difficult and, because of the low volume, unit staff would be unable to maintain competency. Complex respiratory treatments would fall into this category. This grid was used to develop the task assignments for the individual care unit models. **Tables 5.2** and **5.3** show the generic unit-based caregiver roles as well as the services to be decentralized and brought to the unit as designated by the critical care task force. The following sections describe each of the unit care models, along with the rationale for each model and the implementation strategies employed and lessons learned.

Table 5.2: Unit-Based Care Giver Roles

POSITION	PRINCIPAL ACCOUNTABILITY EXAMPLES	
RN	• Assessments • Care Planning • Evaluation • Supervision • Patient Education • Discharge Planning • Order Entry • Medication Administration	• Assists with: – Simple Respiratory Therapy – Phlebotomy – EKG
LVN II	• Med Administration: PO, IM, SC, Eye/Ear Drops, IV • IV Starts • Trach Suctioning/Care • Central Line Care • Transfusions • Order Entry	• Simple Respiratory Therapy • Bladder Irrigation/Catheterization • Dressing/Wound Care • Chest Tube Care • Neuro/Vasc Checks • Invasive Specimen Collection • Phlebotomy (STAT and Timed) • EKG • Glucose Testing
RT	• Complex Respiratory • Inhalation Meds • Trach Suctioning/Care • Pulmonary Assessments • Pulse Oximetry	• Phlebotomy/Line Draws • EKG • Vital Signs
Clinical Partner	• Basic Patient Care Tasks • EKG • Activities of Daily Living (ADL) • Vital Signs • Order Entry/Clerical (SICUs)	• Transportation • Assist MDs with Procedures
Support Partner	• Transportation • Daily Environmental Service • Activities of Daily Living (ADL)	• Equipment/Supplies
Nursing Communication Technician	• Organize Charts (all units except 8SICU) • Orders • Supplies	

Table 5.3: On-Unit Decentralization Recommendation Summary

DEPARTMENT	ACTIVITIES	UNITS AFFECTED	WHO PERFORMS (PREDOMINANT ROLE)
Respiratory Therapy	• Simple: MDI, Pulse Oximetry, SMI, Free flow O_2 delivery • Complex and Expanded Simple	• All • 8SICU, 7SICU, MICU/RICU	• LVN, RN • Deployed RT
Transportation	• To all areas except Radiology, Nuclear Med, MRI, Pathology	• All	• Support Partner
Environmental Services	• Daily cleaning of Patient Care Units, Conf. Rooms and Nursing Station	• All	• Support Partner
Pathology and Lab	• Phlebotomy – Stat and timed • Phlebotomy – Routine • Line draws	• All • SICU, MICU/RICU, CSICU • All	• RN, LVN, RT
EKG	• EKGs	• All	• Clinical Partner, RN, LVN, RT, Rad Techs

Critical Care Models

Medical and Respiratory Intensive Care Units

Planning for PFC. The Medical and Respiratory Intensive Care Units (MICU/RICU) previously utilized an all RN staff for patient care. Respiratory therapists (RTs) provided treatments centrally as did other departments (e.g., EKG, housekeeping, transportation). The patient-focused care goal was to restructure operations so that patient care could be delivered in a less costly manner without jeopardizing quality. An additonal goal was to reduce the number of individuals to come in contact with patients and family members during the hospital stay.

In order to achieve these goals, it was necessary for MICU/RICU staff to examine the patient's entire length of stay in the unit from admission to the unit to transfer, or discharge. These analyses including examining what tasks were being performed by the all RN staff and what could be delegated or assigned to other licensed or non licensed personnel. Task force members had to ask the following quesitons:

- Who is doing what?
- Why is it being done?
- Is it appropriate?
- Is there a better way of doing it?

The group began by evaluating the allocation of all resources and attempting to determine whether tasks were being performed by specific individuals because of licensure, and if they could be delegated to other licensed personnel and/or assigned to unlicensed staff. Ultimately, the question was "Is this change going to benefit the patient by reducing cost, shortening stays, and improving outcomes?"

In evaluating these parameters, it became apparent that there could be no uniform care model for all ICUs. Different units required different models based not only on the needs of patients and families, but also on the practices of the physicians and the flexibility of the nursing staff. The patients in the MICU may and usually do have multisystem medical problems, while the RICU patients are generally intubated patients with complicated respiratory disease problems and include long term ventilator patients. The needs of both populations differ from patients in the surgical ICUs. In addition, physicians and nursing staff in the different ICUs have different practice patterns and preferences concerning the ways in which the work might be redesigned.

Structure and Process Changes. The PFC model for MICU/RICU includes four levels of nursing personnel—RN's, LVN's, clinical partners, and support partners—as well as an expanded role for the respiratory therapists. The licensed and unlicensed staff are supported by a unit manager (RN), nursing communication technician (unit secretary), and materials management storekeeper (supply order entry). The PFC Model for the MICU/RICU was based on the following assumptions: the nursing staff would do routine and STAT phlebotomies; RNs, LVNs, and CPs would do all EKGs; and RT would assist in doing phlebotomies, drawing blood for labs from invasive lines, ABGs, suctioning, EKGs, and would be available to participate with "assistive" patient care (i.e., turning patients and moving them up in bed, helping with water and juice, etc.) Having the respiratory therapist assigned to the unit would minimize calls to respiratory therapy services for ventilator or respiratory changes and treatments would be done in an expeditious manner because the therapists would remain in the unit. These changes would also decrease the need for two nursing communication technicians (NCTs) on the day and evening shift and completely remove the NCT from the night shift. Calls to support areas would no longer take place since unit staff would be providing transportation and environmental services functions and doing phlebotomy and EKGs. In addition, most of the blood drawn for the laboratory would be transported through the pneumatic tube system.

Implementation. Considerable thought and discussion went into the development and implementation of the model for the MICU/RICU so the staff could be prepared, ask questions, and voice concerns. Care was taken to be sure that patient care was not being jeopardized by changing the skill mix. A job description for each category of personnel utilized in the unit was posted for all staff to review. Also, as a senior project, nursing students assigned to the unit made posters listing duties that could be assigned to the various categories of personnel. These lists contained examples of delegated or assigned tasks, but were not all inclusive. The posters allowed the staff to understand which duties could be performed by both licensed and unlicensed staff. The staff could then become familiar with the new roles, reference the lists easily, and ask appropriate questions concerning the changing environment before implementation of the model took place.

In preparation for implementation it was necessary to hire LVNs, CPs, and SPs—4.8 FTEs for each category. In addition to hiring new personnel, it was also necessary to change the NCTs' shifts from days, evenings, and nights to one NCT from 7:00 am-3:30 pm, one from 12:00-8:30 pm, and one from 3:00-11:30 pm. This schedule would provide adequate coverage during peak admission, transfer, and physician ordering times. The nursing staff and the clinical partners would all be educated to do order entry in case the NCT was deluged with orders.

In order to develop the "team" concept, current RN staff in the MICU/RICU interviewed the personnel that they would work with the closest, the LVNs and the CPs. The unit manager interviewed the support partners, and the respiratory therapists were assigned by their department, with individual RTs' preferences and suggestions from the nursing staff being taken into consideration in making the assignments.

All new personnel were required to go through PFC education in addition to hospital and unit orientation. Orientation for CPs and SPs lasted approximately four weeks, but it was individualized to meet the needs of each employee. The LVNs were all new graduates without critical care experience and were given a six-month orientation, both practical and didactic. All current personnel were required to complete the three-day PFC educational workshop. All personnel were required to pass competencies for the various new tasks they would need to perform or that they would supervise others in doing. (See Chapter 13 for further details.)

Lessons Learned. The transition for the MICU/RICU from an almost all RN staff to a PFC model with varying skill levels proceeded smoothly because of the preparation that occurred before implementation. As with any change, some staff members were resistant and looking for any excuse for the project to fail. In reviewing the experience, the project leaders felt they would have benefited from having had a firmer guarantee from respiratory therapy services that they would fulfill their commitment in assisting the nursing staff. Also, when the materials management staff took over the responsibility for ordering unit supplies (see Chapter 12 for details), the unit should have made sure that the storeroom technician and his/her replacement person were familiar with all of the supplies, their location, and the par levels needed to maintain a smooth, consistent operation.

Cardiac Surgical Intensive Care Unit (CSICU)

Planning for PFC. Preparation for change in the CSICU began with educating staff on the need for change. Over the previous year, the census in the unit had fallen from close to 100% occupancy to about 65% occupancy. According to the physician staff, the change was due to a decrease in the referral base related to new health care contracting procedures and the increase in managed care in Southern California. In this new environment, the Cedars-Sinai cost per case was too high to be competitive. Wanting to be competitive in the marketplace and to secure their jobs, the staff was motivated to look for ways to reduce costs, utilize present staff more effectively, and to look for new ways to accomplish the work.

Several CSICU staff members were involved in hospital committees prior to planning the PFC care model. One committee was considering eliminating whole departments such as inpatient cardiology and shifting the workload to the unit level. Other staff were involved in patient reaggregation committees that were looking at grouping patients by clinical similiarities or by service lines, thus making each unit a center of care for a well-defined case type with common therapeutic goals and a staff properly trained to care for those specific patients. Other staff were involved in committees that were looking for ways to decrease costs by measures, such as standardizing housewide supplies, equipment, and medications, and changing staffing ratios and workloads, in the CSICU for the coronary artery bypass graft (CABG) patient population.

Having staff involved in housewide committees made the process easier when it came time to develop the new patient-focused care model in the CSICU. The staff were aware of the need for change and had some idea of the housewide goals. They were excited that they were being asked to participate and also excited that their ideas were being heard. Staff leaders were chosen to participate in the unit design committee, but any staff member interested in participating was allowed to join the discussions. Even the most resistive staff were encouraged to voice their concerns. Since the meetings were held in the unit conference room, they were easily accessible and anyone on duty that day was welcome to join the discussion.

One of the first steps taken by staff in the development of the model was to describe the normal course of the CABG patient and to examine the needs of that patient while in the intensive care unit. The discussions took into account the new changes that were being discussed in other committees, such as the fact that patients would be admitted to the hospital the morning of surgery rather than the night before, with patient education done primarily by the cardiac liaison nurse several days before admission, and patients would receive a pre-operative videotape to review at home. The patients would continue to come directly from the operating room to the unit, but the expectation that the patient would be extubated during the post-operative night was changed to being extubated within the first six hours following surgery. Other cost-effective changes included transferring patients out of the unit the following morning between the hours of 10:00-11:00 am instead of the more customary afternoon transfer, thus reducing the patient stay in the unit to slightly less than twenty-four hours.

The staff quickly realized that the patients would be in the intensive care unit less time and that every minute that the patient was in the unit was critical. They realized that, in order to accomplish their goals, all of the staff would have to work together as a team with each player knowing his/her job and what was expected. They planned to start their morning shift with all patients doubled up (i.e., two patients assigned to each nurse) and then to add nurses at 11:00 am to accomodate the admissions, keeping in mind the number of transfers out of the unit as well, in order to have enough nurses to admit new cases from the operating room.

Structure and Process Changes. Keeping all of the above in mind, the staff set out to develop their model. Since patients would be arriving between the hours of 10:00-12:00 am, the staff decided to create a new twelve-hour shift from 11:00 am-11:30 pm. Depending on the number of surgical cases scheduled, the staff would decide the number of staff needed to come in at 11:00 am the following day. The goal was to admit, recover, and extubate the patient within six hours of surgery, thus enabling the patients to be safely doubled up during the night shift. Since the night shift had to continue to stabilize the patients, bathe them, and mobilize them so that they would be ready for transfer early in the morning, a decision was made to add a second clinical partner to the night shift in order to accomplish this goal.

Similiar to the other intensive care units, PFC staffing for the CSICU would be composed of RNs, clinical partners, support partners, and respiratory therapists. Utilizing LVNs was considered, but was voted down by the staff because they felt that they did not have sufficient information at that time regarding the functions of the LVN and were concerned about role confusion. Like the other ICUs, the staff also decided that all members of the team should be cross-prepared and multiskilled.

The ICU RN staff was to be trained in respiratory therapy, phlebotomy, EKG, and cardiac rehabilitation. The clinical partners were to attend classes in cardiac rehabilitation, housekeeping, transportation, and so forth (see Chapter 13 for details). Since the unit had been using clinical partners (called critical care technicians prior to PFC) for some time, the staff was familiar with their skill level and abilities. The clinical partners would continue to do the room setups, assist with basic patient care needs, vital signs, admission, and transfers to the step down area. The addition of the support partner to the unit was also a new concept in name only. The staff had always had a good rapport and working relationship with their nursing service technician (NST) and housekeeping personnel. The NST had been involved with simple patient care responsibilities, transfer of patients to the step down area, room cleaning, and equipment checks. The creation of the new support partner role simply combined these tasks into one role.

The idea of respiratory therapists being redeployed to the unit was also accepted wholeheartly by the staff. The concept of having the RT unit-based and cross-prepared to do other patient care tasks appealed to the staff. Prior to PFC, the staff had to call the RT when they needed him/her and many times patient care was delayed while the RT traveled from another unit after completing a task there. With this change in philosophy, the RT would be working toward the same goals and helping the unit staff meet patients' needs in a timely manner.

Based on the task list, the unit committeee also decided that the NCT (unit secretary) would only be needed twelve hours a day as compared to the previous model of twenty-four hour coverage. NCT's primary responsibilities would be to transcribe orders, answer the telephone, and direct traffic. She/he would work from 8:00 am -8:00 pm each day and the clinical partners would assist with these tasks when the NCT was not on duty.

Implementation and Lessons Learned. The CSICU model was implemented in August 1994, with only a few changes made in the original design following implementation. The second clinical partner on the night shift was eliminated, since the staff was able to accomplish their goals through better teamwork and felt that the addition of a second person was unnecessary.

Staff education was the same as that detailed for MICU/RICU. It was originally planned to have CSICU staff attend the same respiratory therapy class as the staff from the cardiac surgery floors, but the length of that class prompted a decision to reduce the class to one day and have all the ICU nurses attend the same class. In retrospect, it would have been better for the CSICU nurses to have attended the longer respiratory therapy class, since they float through the service line, but have not been educated to perform the respiratory treatments done by the staff on the floors. Plans are in place to cross prepare them for these tasks in the near future.

Surgical Intensive Care Units (7SICU and 8SICU)

Planning for PFC. Prior to PFC, the surgical intensive care unit RN nursing staff provided all direct patient care. Both units (7SICU and 8SICU) implemented their PFC models simultaneously in September 1994. Preparation began the previous March, however, and included the existing staff in those units along with the medical staff. Forums to discuss the process included staff meetings, multidisciplinary PFC critical care task force meetings, and joint practice committee meetings. Initially these meetings were educational and included agenda items such as the definition of PFC and the critical care targets for dollar savings after implementation.

Structure and Process Changes. The biggest decision the SICUs made concerned the addition of other licensed personnel. The biggest staffing adjustment was the decrease in the number of patients staffed one to one (i.e., one RN for one patient). Since the PFC charge included making appropriate changes to the skill mix, the staff began the design process by weighing the pros and cons of adding respiratory therapists (RTs) to the unit staff vs. adding LVNs. It was difficult initially for the staff to be objective about the role of the LVN. If LVNs were to become part of the model, fewer RNs would be needed, creating a real feeling of job insecurity for the current staff. Once those feelings were overcome, however, the staff was able to examine the functions that could be performed by RTs and LVNs for the unit's patient population.

The majority of patients in the SICUs are ventilated. The population has a high incidence of sepsis and staff are frequently managing acute respiratory distress syndrome (ARDS). Thus, the expertise of a respiratory therapist in the staffing model would be invaluable. The average salary of the respiratory therapist was comparable to the LVN. Therefore, a decision was made to include RTs in the model based on the number of ventilator days, the complexity of the patients, the potential tasks they would be cross-prepared to perform, and the large number of respiratory treatments required by the patient population. Some of the tasks RTs were cross-prepared to perform included drawing off of lines, changing simple sterile dressings, assisting with ADLs, sending off blood work, and doing EKGs. They are responsible for all respiratory management of the patients inclusive of treatments and chest physiotherapy and are truly an asset to the staffing, making the transition to staffing the patients one RN per two patients easier.

Three years prior to the PFC implementation the SICUs began using clinical partners, formally called critical care technicians, so the staff had already faced some of the challenges of adding assistive personnel. Clinical partners (CPs) assist the RN with ADLs, are trained to set up transducers for line insertions, and can function as a unit secretary. This role was carried over into the new staffing model, and there is usually one CP per unit per shift. The CPs were also cross-prepared to do EKGs, and the unit has significantly cut back on unit secretaries since the CPs are cross-prepared for this function. The need for a unit secretary was determined based upon the peak hours of the operating room schedule Mondays through Fridays.

The final job classification added was the role of the support partner, essentially a housekeeper/transporter assigned to the unit. This individual was also cross-prepared to assist with ADLs and simple secretarial functions. There is one SP scheduled in each unit 7:00 am-7:00 pm. **Figure 5.3** shows a sample staffing model for the surgical intensive care units.

Figure 5.3: Sample Staffing Model for the SICUs

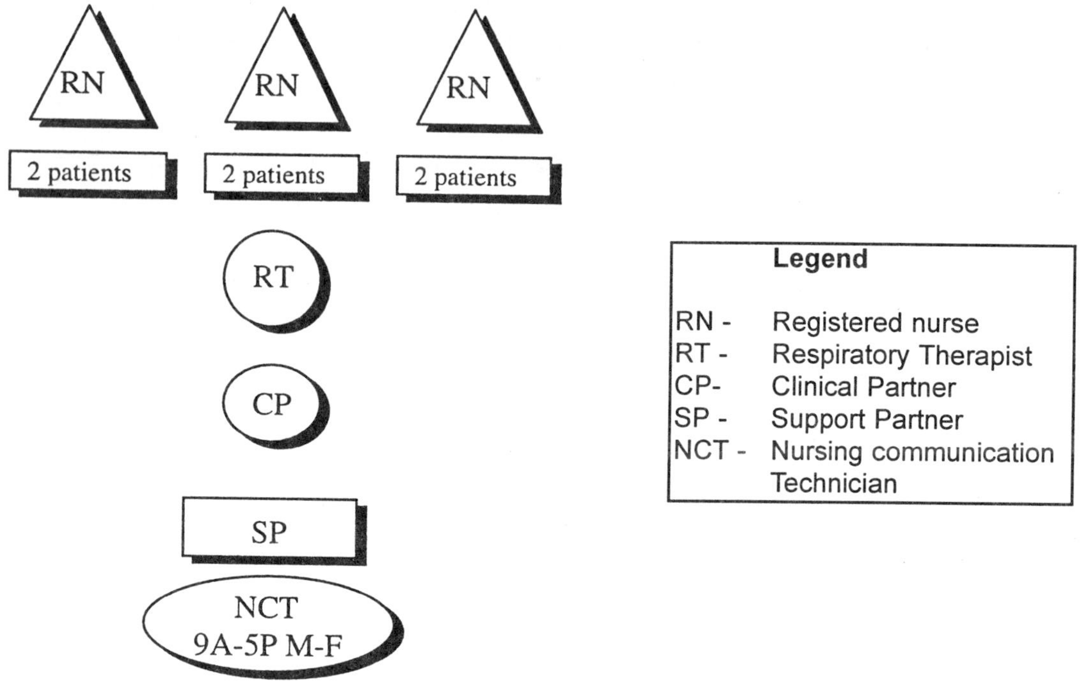

Implementation and Lessons Learned. The staff was very involved in the interview process for the new roles—a key factor in the success of the project. The more involved the staff, the easier the assimilation process. Many of the new clinical partners were former unit secretaries. One difficulty encountered was that the employees who moved into the new positions found that the staff did not allow them time to make the transition into their new roles, resulting in an overwhelming feeling of frustration for all.

The senior staff who were educated in the era of team nursing had an easier time delegating the tasks formally done by RNs to the other members of the staff. Nurses educated in primary nursing had a more difficult time developing trust in the new roles, and, therefore, did not assign work as readily. At six months post-implementation the staff was continuing to work through some issues. For example, several RNs might ask one of the support personnel for help at the same time. The support person may not yet have enough confidence or experience to prioritize the demands. The RNs are working to be sensitive to this point and try to coordinate the workload. The nurse manager meets with the staff as a whole and also meets with the support personnel separately to give them another forum to discuss their concerns. The strongest recommendations for success, however, include ensuring that (1) the staff is involved from the very beginning and (2) the education is completed for all personnel before implementation. Ideally the new roles themselves will be implemented gradually before the actual implementation of the entire PFC model.

Cardiac Intensive Care Unit (CICU)

Planning for PFC. Due to specific requirements mandated by the California Department of Health, the care delivery model in the cardiac care unit differs significantly from those in medical-surgical nursing units. At all times the nurse patient ratio must be 1:2 or fewer. According to these standards and those of the American Heart Association, licensed vocational nurses (LVNs) may constitute up to 50% of the licensed nursing staff. The CICU began using LVNs as part of the care model in 1992. At that time, 10% of the total staff were LVNs, increasing to 25% in 1993.

Structural and Process Changes and Lessons Learned. Patient-focused care's impact on the unit primarily involved the cross preparation of nursing staff to assume the respiratory and EKG functions. This change decreased delays and enabled patients to receive faster treatment. The incorporation of the support partner role for transportation and room cleaning decreased room turn around time and delays in transfers. It has, however, taken a long period of time to learn to use the skills of the clinical partner properly, and the challenge of motivating registered nurses to direct, assign, and supervise the clinical partner remains. Patient care has not changed, however, and continues to be excellent. Staffing has been adjusted to meet demand and the cross prepared team performs patient care functions in an efficient and effective manner. The final CICU model is depicted in **Figure 5.4.**

Education and Cross Preparation of Critical Care Staff

Chapter 13 describes the Cedars-Sinai education program developed for PFC housewide in detail. The following sections present the education and cross preparation specific to the critical care units.

Licensed Staff

All critical care registered nurses and LVN IIs completed the PFC critical care education program (see Chapter 13). In addition, all licensed staff were educated to perform twelve-lead EKG, phlebotomy, and, in some areas, respiratory functions such as hand held nebulizers (HHN), metered dose inhaler (MDI), and other simple respiratory tasks. The decision to add respiratory functions to the core PFC critical care program was made on a unit by unit basis according to the volume of respiratory services in each unit. For instance, the CSICUs patient population required HHN and simple respiratory services; therefore, all CSICU RNs were educated to perform these functions. Ventilator management and other complex respiratory functions remain the responsibility of the respiratory therapists assigned to each ICU.

Figure 5.4: CICU Care Model for Census of 10

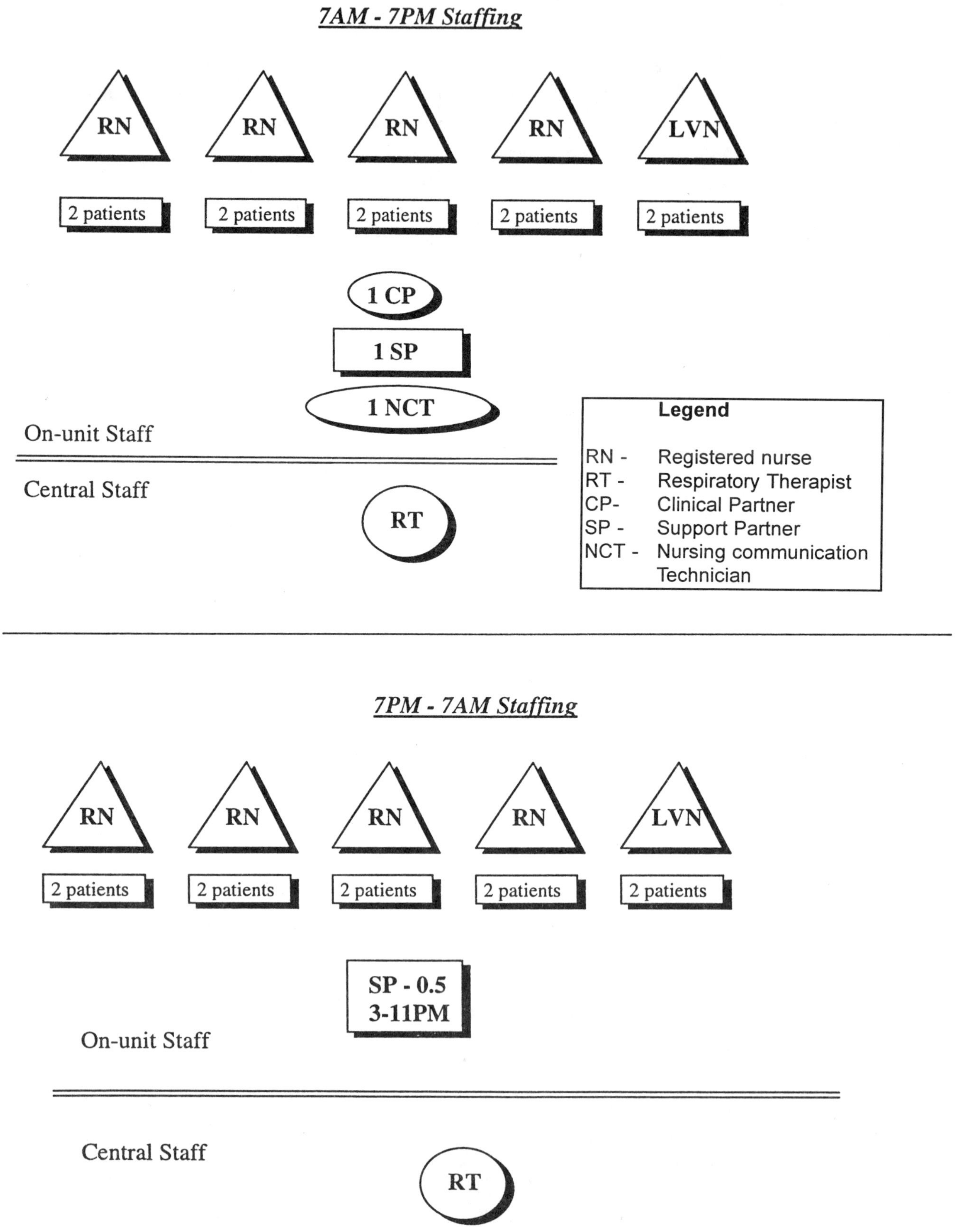

Respiratory therapists also attended the PFC critical care class and, in addition, received education in blood drawing from A-lines and phlebotomy. The respiratory therapists also received education in assisting patients with activities of daily living. These functions were added to their role to operationalize the "minimal hand-off" principle of PFC.

Unlicensed Staff

All clinical partners and support partners were required to attend the critical care PFC course for unlicensed staff. The course included education in environmental and transportation functions and simple functions such as assisting patients with activities of daily living. In addition, clinical partners received education on twelve-lead EKG, quality control for bedside testing, procurement of supplies, and hemodynamic setup. Preceptors and supertrainers were available to assist with actual clinical training, which lasted from three to six weeks, according to the individual's previous clinical experience. All unlicensed personnel were required to complete a basic life support course. **Table 5.4** summarizes the education and cross preparation for each member of the unit team. Competency checklists were developed and used to ensure staff competency with new skills. The supertrainer staff development strategy was also utilized to develop new skill competencies and cross preparation.

Table 5.4: Critical Care Education and Cross Preparation

Education and Cross Preparation	RN	LVN	RT	CP	SP	US
Patient-Focused Care Class	X	X	X	X	X	X
Environmental Function				X	X	
Transportation Function	X*	X*		X	X	
Phlebotomy Training	X		X			
Blood Drawing from A-line	X*		X			
Assist Patient with Activities of Daily Living	X*	X	X	X	X	
12-Lead EKG	X	X	X	X		
Simple clerical functions	X*			X	X	X*
Equipment and supplies for Patient Use				X	X	

* previous training

Outcomes

Report Cards

The evaluation of the PFC initiative was designed to be multidisciplinary with measurement along service lines. A sample of the "report card" initially developed for critical care is shown in **Table 5.5**. The complete PFC evaluation plan and findings are detailed in Chapters 15 and 16.

Table 5.5: Sample QA Report Card: Outcome Measures

Key Indicators/Measurements	Targets	Comments
I. Staff Competency	100%	
A. Orientation Checklist analysis	100%	
B. Preceptor/Self-evaluation of Performance	100%	
C. Skills Assessment of Cross-prepared Staff	100%	
II. Clinical Outcomes		
A. Length of Stay per Diagnostic Guidelines		According to Service Line
B. Patient Care Quality Indicators per ICU		To be determined by each unit
1. Readmission to ICU	TBD	
2. Dermal Ulcer Rate	TBD	
3. Unattended Falls Rate	TBD	
4. Surgical Site Infection Rate	TBD	
5. Medications Errors	TBD	
6. Code Blue	TBD	
7. Patient Education	TBD	Per Patient Satisfaction Survey
8. Post-op Pneumonia	TBD	
9. Delays in Transfers	TBD	
III. Service Outcomes		
A. Responsiveness		
B. Teamwork/Coordination		
C. Environment/Amenities		
D. Information/Communication		
IV. Customer Satisfaction		
A. MD Satisfaction	TBD	
B. Patient/Family Satisfaction	TBD	
C. Employee Satisfaction	TBD	
V. Financial Impact		
A. Average Daily Census	TBD	
B. Total Operating Cost per Case	TBD	

TBD – To Be Decided

Patient/Family Satisfaction

As described in Chapter 16, Cedars-Sinai measures patient/family satisfaction using national surveys which allow comparison with other hospitals nationwide. However, these surveys do not specifically reflect patient/family concerns when patients are in the ICUs. In particular, concern about nursing availability and meeting the needs of families using the new PFC models prompted the development of a Critical Care Family Needs Survey. The eleven-item survey exploring how well critical care personnel met the needs of patients' families was first administered one month prior to PFC implementation and again six months after implementation. The results are presented in **Figure 5.5.** The goal was to maintain and/or increase family satisfaction with services provided. Although, the findings varied among ICUs, the overall findings indicated a statistically significant increase in family satisfaction with nursing availability to the family (t [85.9] = -2.09, $p<0.05$). The results of the survey also indicated areas for improvement (e.g., MD availability, explanation of ICU environment, and providing information on how to reach the ICU).

Figure 5.5: Cardiothoracic and Surgical Intensive Care Unit: Patient/Family Satisfaction

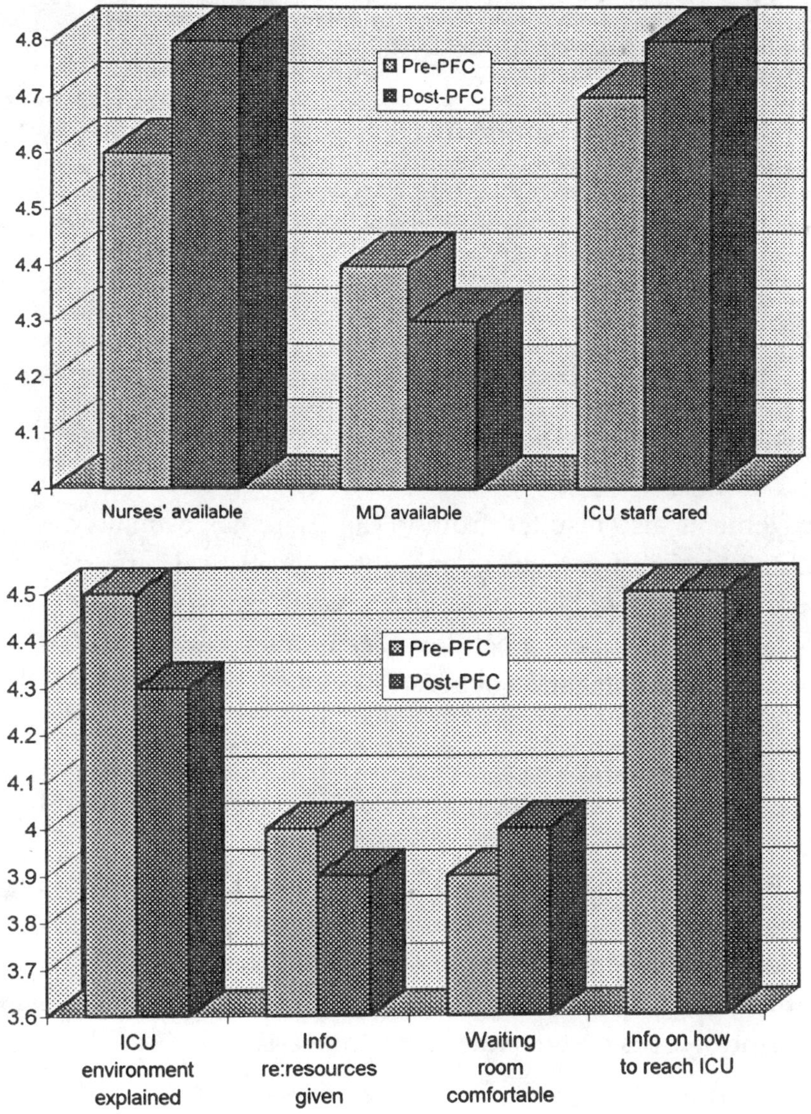

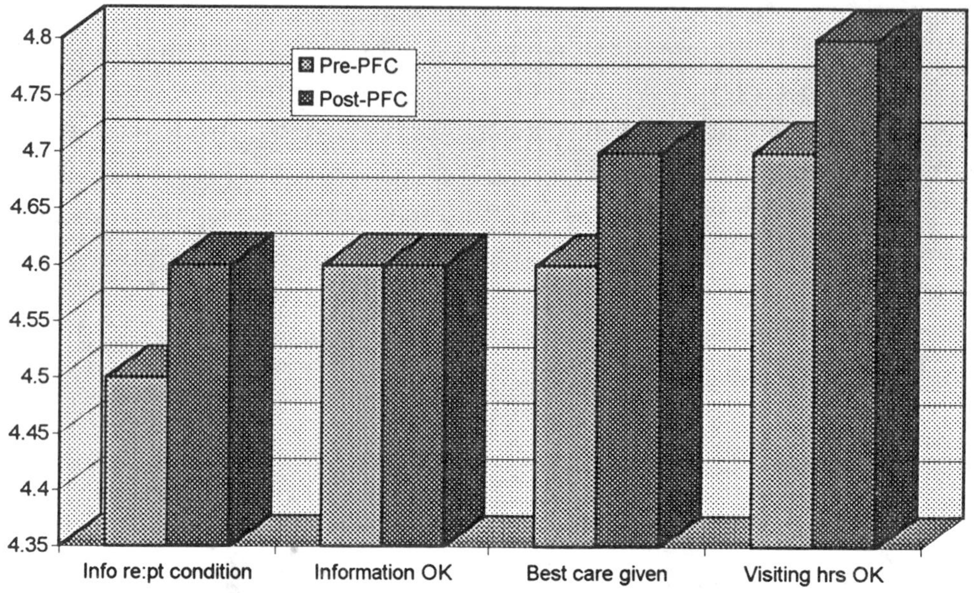

Process Improvements

Process improvements also resulted from PFC. There has been an overall reduction in delays related to transfer of patients in and out of the critical care areas due to the presence of personnel who have been cross-prepared to transportation and housekeeping functions. Because all ICU personnel have been cross-prepared to assist patients with ADLs, there is improved delegation of tasks as evidenced by increased RN availability to patient's families.

Summary

In conclusion, work redesign in the critical care areas had been challenging to implement, but the ultimate outcome has been a rewarding and positive experience for patients, their families and Cedars-Sinai staff. With cross-prepared staff, the ICUs have increased efficiency and are better able to manage processes and ensure that the patient's needs remain as the central focus of the patient care process.

Appendix

TASKS	REQ LIC?	CURRENTLY PERFORMED BY:	PROPOSED TO BE PERFORMED BY:	NOTES:
Belongings/valuables security		RN; LVN; CCT	NL	
Bladder irrigation-without meds	1L	RN; LVN	NL	
Blood draws - peripherial		RN,Techs	RN/LVN/Med Tech/Phle	
Burn care - simple		RN	RN	Unit Specific
Catheterization(bladder)		Non-licensed	NL	
Check emergency cart (locked)	1L	RN; LVN,MST	NL	
Check one touch	1L	RN; LVN,MST	NL	
Chest tube care	1L	RN;LVN	NL	
Chest tube set up			NL	
D/C Peripheral lines		RN	NL/LVN	
Data entry on pt flow sheets			NL/LVN/RN	
Dressings - simple wound		RN, LVN	NL	
Ear Irrigation		RN	RN/LVN	
Enemas - non-medicated		RN; LVN	LVN	
Enter orders	PHARM	PHARMACIST/TE	NL	
Equipment acquisition		RN; LVN; CCT	NL	
Equipment delivery (to room)		RN; LVN; CCT	NL	
Equipment- adjustment/fit		RN; LVN; PT AIDE	NL	
Eye Irrigation - non-medicated		RN	NL/LVN	
Feeding Patients		RN; LVN; CCT	NL	
Foley care	1L	RN; LVN; CCT	NL	
Glucose testing	1L	RN; LVN	NL/LVN/RN	
Incentive Spirometry	1L	RT	NL/LVN/RN	
Med/allergy	1L	RN	NL	
Moving beds		RN,Techs	NL	
PT order entry		PT	NL	
Patient education - Tasks		RN	NL	
Patient transport		RN/Techs,LVNII	NL	
Placement of IV w/ saline flush		RN, LNV II	NL	unit-specific
Placement/removal of foley			NL/LVN	
Post-mortem care		RN; LVN; CCT	NL	
Procedures - assist MD (lumbar, pelvic-simple, suturing, I&D)		RN	NL/LVN	unit specific
Pulse oximetry - application	1L	RT,RN	NL/LVN/RN/RT	
Quiaic testing	1L	RN; LVN	NL	
ROM		RN; LVN; CCT	RN; LVN; CCT	
Set up room		RN,CCT	NL	

Appendix

TASKS	REQ LIC?	CURRENTLY PERFORMED BY:	PROPOSED TO BE PERFORMED BY:	NOTES:
Simple ostomy care		RN; LVN; CCT	RN; LVN; CCT	
Skin Prep		Techs	NL	
Speciality bed operations		RN,CCT,LVNII	RN,CCT,LVNII	
Specimen collection non-invasive & straight cath		RN; LVN; CCT	RN; LVN; CCT	
Splinting - application		RN	NL	
Sputum induction - non complicated	1L	RN; LVN	RT	
Suctioning mouth/nasal	1L	RN; LVN	RN; LVN	
Suctioning trach	1L	RN; LVN	RN; LVN	
Teaching crutch walking		RN,ORTHO TECH	NL	
Trach care - old	1L	RN; LVN	RN; LVN	
Traction non-invasive		RN; ORTHO TECH	RN; ORTHO TECH.	
Transcribing orders	L	RN,PCC,LVNII	RN,PCC,LVNII	
Transfer training- training		RN; LVN,PT AIDE	RN; LVN,PT AIDE	
Transfers, bed to chair		RN; LVN; CCT	RN; LVN; CCT	
Tube drain/care		RN; LVN; CCT	RN; LVN; CCT	Unit specific
Tube feedings	1L	RN; LVN	RN; LVN	
Vital signs		RN; LVN; MST	RN; LVN; MST	
Walking		RN; LVN; MST	RN; LVN; MST	
Weighing patients	NL	RN,LVNII,CCT	RN,LVNII,CCT	
Wound care - simple		Non-licensed	NL	
Arterial puncture	RT	RT/RN	RN	
Artificial Liver		RN	RN	
Assessment	RN	RN	RN	
Attend code blues	PHARM	PHARMACIST/RN	RN	
CAVH or CVVH		RN	RN	
CPR		RN	RN	LVN II/NL
Calculate IV drip rates	PHARM	PHARMACIST,RN	RN	or Pharmacist
Cardiac Hemodynamic Monitoring/Cardiac outputs		RN	RN	
Care patients on vent - awareness,setting alarm,Abg's		RN/RT	RN	or RT
Care planning	RN	RN	RN	
Central line care	1L	RN	RN	
Close loop monitoring		RN	RN	
Complaint handling		RN; LVN; MST	RN	(all)
Complex ostomy care		RN; LVN; CCT	RN	ET nurse
Critical Thinking			RN	
D/C Central Line		RN	RN	

Appendix

TASKS	REQ LIC?	CURRENTLY PERFORMED BY:	PROPOSED TO BE PERFORMED BY:	NOTES:
D/C Planning	2L	RN; MSW	RN	
E-Wall placements		RN	RN	
ET tube care	2L	RN/RT	RN	or RT
Extubation		RN	RN	
Follow up on lab/assess	RN	RN	RN	
Gait training - assessment, evaluation	PT	PT; RN	RN	Unit specific
Hyperalimentation	1L	RN	RN	
IApb Monitoring		RN	RN	
ICP Monitoring		RN	RN	
Local Monitoring (PARU)		RN	RN	
Lumbar drainage & pressure monitoring		RN	RN	
Mass trouser monitoring		RN	RN	
Monitoring vaso active drugs		RN	RN	
Narcotic count/adding meds to stock	1L	RN	RN	
Neuro checks/monitoring		RN	RN	
Patient Medication Education		Pharm/RN	RN	
Patient education - Concepts		RN	RN	
Pre-admission education	RN	RN	RN	
Prepare IVs at unit level		PHARMACIST/TECH,	RN	
Psychosocial			RN	
Referrals/cont of care	2L	RN/SW/PT/OT	RN	
SPUN HCT (7/8 CSICU)		RN	RN	
Skin testing	1L	RN	RN	
Splinting - monitoring		RN	RN	
Systemic temperature control		RN	RN	
Teaching/education-patient/SO	RN	RN	RN	
Triage		RN	RN	
Verbal orders	L	RN	RN	
Sexual Assult data collection		RN	RN	
Child, elder abuse		RN	RN	
Domestic violence reporting		RN	RN	

Appendix

TASKS	REQ LIC?	CURRENTLY PERFORMED BY:	PROPOSED TO BE PERFORMED BY:	NOTES:
Interactions with family		RN; LVN; CCT	All	
Aerosol Therapy	1L	RT	LVN II	
Bladder irrigation-with meds	1L	RN; LVN	LVN II	
Check IV pump rate settings	PHARM	PHARMACIST,RN	???RN/Pharm	
Chest Physiology	1L	RT	LVN II/RT	
Chest percussion vibration	1L	RT	LVN II/RT	
Dermal ulcer care		RN; LVN; PT AIDE	LVN II/RN	
Dressings - complex wound	1L	RN; LVN	LVN II	
Drug admin-IV & piggy backs	RN	RN	RN	
Drug admin-po,IM,SC,ear,/eye drops	1L	RN; LVN	LVN II	
Equipment- training		RN; LVN; PT AIDE	LVN II	PT; OT; Ortho
Gait training- training		RN; LVN; PT AIDE	LVN II	PT; PT aide; OT
Gastric lavage		RN	LVN II	
Hand held nebulizers	1L	RT,RN	LVN II	
IV pump settings		RN,LVNII	RN	
IV start w/ solution	1L	RN; LVN	LVN II	
MDI Instructions	1L	RT	LVN II	
NG tube placement		RN	LVN II	
Narcotic count		RN; LVNII	LVN II	
Neuro-vascular checks	1L	RN;LVN	LVN II	
Oxygen therapy	1L	RT	LVN II	
Pain management modalities- assess, evaluation	RN	RN	RN	
Placement/removal of drains/catheters	1L	RN; LVN	LVN II	
Postural drainage	1L	RT	LVN II	
Specimen collection - invasive	1L	RN;LVN	LVN II	
Trach care - new	1L	RN; LVN	LVN II	
Transfusions - perpherial	1L	RN	LVN II	
Verify orders in computer	PHARM	PHARMACIST,RN	LVN II	
Wound care - complex	1L	RN; LVN	RN	
ADL assistance		RN; LVN; CCT	NL	
Application & care of TEDS/SCDs		RN; LVN; CCT	NL	
Application & care of restraints		RN; LVN; CCT	NL	???
Application of hot or cold therapy		RN; LVN; CCT	NL	
Application of pressure relief devices		RN; LVN; PT AIDE	NL	Licensed to monitor
Application of traction; Buck's,pelvic,cervical,skeletal		RN; ORTHO TECH	NL/Ortho	Licensed to monitor
Bed mobility- training		RN; LVN; CCT	NL	PT; PT AIDE

Chapter 6

Work Redesign and Performance Improvement Strategies in the Operating Room

Randy Cook, RN, CNOR, MBA
J. Louis Cohen, MD
Gerry Popolow, RN, MSN

The current demand for reform in health care provides those who work in operating room services, as well as in other aspects of health care, with the opportunity to redefine the processes of providing care. Health care reform in the operating room (OR) translates into the need for behavioral and process changes involving everyone who directly or indirectly affects patient care. Future generations of health care providers will function using the processes and systems currently being developed.

This chapter describes the operating room performance improvement strategies undertaken at Cedars-Sinai Medical Center and the ways in which the institution combined the work of multiple groups to avoid duplication of effort and bring about measurable improvements in operating room services. The operating rooms at Cedars-Sinai perform approximately 20,000 procedures annually, routinely utilizing 25 operating suites in 4 locations. The institution provides for a broad range of specialties including, but not limited to, heart, lung, kidney and liver transplantation, open heart, orthopedics, neurology, pediatric, GYN, general, urology, plastic, thoracic, vascular, ophthalmology, and trauma surgery. The operating rooms are staffed seven days a week, twenty-four hours a day. The performance improvement strategies described in the following sections encompass the work of both the OR quality action team (QAT) and the OR nurse operations committee (NOC) and also employ the patient-focused care (PFC) concepts of work redesign to achieve measurable improvements in the OR care delivery process at Cedars-Sinai.

OR Quality Action Team

Defining the Customer

Health care is a service industry, and perioperative services is a very specialized component of that industry serving multiple customers. Nursing team members provide service to each other. The perioperative department provides services to other departments

RANDY COOK, RN, CNOR, MBA—Director, Nursing Operating Room Services, Cedars-Sinai Medical Center.
LOUIS COHEN, MD—Medical Director, Operating Room Services, Cedars-Sinai Medical Center.
GERRY POPOLOW, RN, MSN— Vice President, Patient Care Services, Cedars-Sinai Medical Center.

and likewise is a recipient of their services. In some sense, everyone who comes into contact with perioperative services, including the patient, surgeon, other departments, OR team members, etc., provides and receives services. The primary external customer is the patient, and the primary internal customer is the surgeon. Furthermore, while the patient is the most important and easily defined customer, internally the majority of the work the team performs directly relates to the surgeons' needs. Thus performance improvement at Cedars-Sinai began with a decision to focus the reform efforts on defining and meeting the needs of the surgeon.

Determining Customer Expectations

Phase I of the OR performance improvement process began with a retreat involving all key players, including physicians, administrators, nursing, and ancillary department representatives. The retreat focused primarily on surgeon perceptions of issues in the OR. The brainstorming discussions were both emotional and constructive. The outcome of the retreat was the identification of seventy-five performance, service, efficiency, and cost issues, and the creation of a multidisciplinary quality action team (QAT) to follow through on the issues. In evaluating the seventy-five issues identified during the retreat, the QAT grouped them into key points to simplify the process. By grouping similar issues, five primary surgeon-customer expectations were developed. These included the following:

- Start on time/quick turnovers between cases
- Well prepared patient
- Access to the OR schedule
    - Scheduling guidelines
    - Triaging of add-on cases
- Well trained and service-oriented staff
- Equipment and supply issues

The QAT decided that improving "start time/turnover time" issues would provide the greatest impact on service and made it the first priority. Since first case starts and turnover time are very similar in their issues, they were addressed together.

OR Nurse Operations Committee

Simultaneous to the QAT, the OR Nurse Operations Committee (NOC) was looking at the issues and preparing for the QAT recommendations. The OR NOC consists primarily of the OR management team. Three individuals were members of both the QAT and OR NOC and it was through the OR NOC that the nursing staff was kept abreast of issues as they developed. (**Table 6.1** details the QAT charter and the membership of both teams). NOC also developed and implemented an OR Newsletter through which challenges and issues are shared with the OR team directly.

Table 6.1: TEAM CHARTER

TO: QUALITY COUNCIL
INITIATOR: Randy Cook, CNOR, MBA
DATE: AUGUST 2, 1994

Problem Statement:
Benchmarking Study (April 1993) indicates that for ***CSMC*** the average turnover time in the Operating Room on "to follow" cases was 42.6 minutes with a range from 35 minutes to 118 minutes.

Champion: G. POPOLOW, RN, MSN
Process: Operating Room Turnover
Project: Reduction of Turn over Time

Expectations: This project should:	What To Measure / Frequency
Improve performance of the process	Patient Turnaround Time - Reduce To 25 Minutes / Monthly
Reduce costs/generate revenues	Variance To Budget / Monthly
Improve physician satisfaction	Physician Satisfation Survey 4.5 (scale 1-5) / Quarterly/Annually
Improve staff satisfaction	Team Satisfaction / Monthly/Annually

---

Coordination With Other Teams: Operating Room Advisory Committee, OB/GYN Advisory Committee, Surgical Advisory Committee, Management Team, Admitting Q.A.T.

Membership:

Surgical Quality Action Team

Leaders: Lou Cohen, MD and Gerry Popolow, RN
Anthony Alter, MD
Jean Beavers, OR
Arnold Cinman, MD
Myles Cohen, MD
Randy Cook, RN
Pat Eastman
Emma Harper, RN
Randy Harris, MD
Jonathan Hiatt, MD
Gary Hoffman, MD
Barbara Johnson, RN
Steve Keleman
Larry Platt, MD
Tomm Webb, MD

O.R. Nursing Operations Committee

Leader: Randy Cook
Tita Agorrilla
Jean Beavers
Charito Bernal
Emma Canicula
Agnes Dizon
Michelle Goode
Robin Hudson
Doug Johnson
Barbara Johnson
Ning Tan-Joyce
David Keymel
Lina Lapid
Esther Yu-Lim
Beth Lytton
Jeanne Markey
Jeri Mays
Melanie Miller
Faith Millman
Denise Morrissey
Sandra Olsen
Barbara Paige
Michael Siller
Algy Stanton
Tommie Thompson
Kathy Velasquez
Tony White

Projected Schedule:
Start: Data analysis and recommendations 11/93 — **Completion:** 3/94
Start: Implementation of recommendations 7/94 — **Completion:** Ongoing

Reporting Cycle to Quality Control: Semiannually

Developing a Vision Statement

OR NOC's first order of business was to develop the context and parameters within which change could be implemented. The group needed a vision statement. With a defined goal, the group could refer to it periodically to track its course. NOC developed the following vision statement:

> *"Position ourselves for the rapidly developing managed care environment by providing service of excellent value."*
>
> *"Value = Providing quality services that exceed our customers' expectations in a cost competitive manner."*

The vision statement's key was the definition of value. As decisions regarding changes in service were made, each decision was compared to the definition of value to see if it was congruent. Thus each decision is formulated in a manner that keeps the group on track and provides value to the defined customers.

Coordinating Team Efforts

As the QAT and NOC teams began their work on first case starts and turnover time, it soon became evident that the issues involved were closely related. An unprepared patient affects the ability to start on time, lack of equipment and supplies can affect turnover time, etc. Since quality action teams are intended to focus on a single identifiable issue and the resulting measurable outcome, the QAT needed to concentrate on specific turnover time issues. The OR NOC, on the other hand, needed to take a broader approach. Both teams, however, utilized similar methods, including those listed in **Table 6.2**.

Table 6.2: Methods Used by Performance Improvement Teams

- Brainstorming
- Literature searches
- Validating definitions
- Benchmarking
- Evaluation tools
  - —flow charting
  - —fishbone diagrams (see **Figure 6.4**)
- Identifying opportunities
- Developing recommendations
- Identifying anticipated outcomes
- Developing feedback tools

Defining Opportunity

As both teams began evaluating the input from the retreat, a picture of the current situation in the OR was developed. A snapshot of the operating room revealed the following characteristics:

- Varying demand— the volume of procedures fluctuates from day today.
- Separate autonomous units—each operating room site (four) functioned independently.
- Heavy and redundant patient preparation and nursing documentation.
- Support staff—not integrated into the care team, fragmented duties.
- Culture of lateness—A trust issue. Each group (nursing, anesthesia, surgeon) did not trust that the other would be on time, so no one was.
- Disjointed pre-op patient preparation—admitting, patient accounting, the pre-op testing program, discharge planning, ancillary testing, etc. were all in separate areas of the hospital functioning independently of one another.
- Long term employees - resulted in the following:
  - Well skilled and knowledgeable team.
  - Need for frequent, consistent communication in various formats (newsletters, team meetings, presentations, etc.).
- Disjointed management of supplies and equipment.
- Broad and intricate OR administration.
- Extended decisionmaking process for triaging add-on and emergency procedures.
- Multiple phone calls required of customers to arrange an OR procedure.
- Cumbersome decisionmaking process for multidisciplinary issues.

Taken in aggregate, these issues resulted in the following:

- **High cost**
  - Rich RN skill mix.
  - Staffing which did not match demand.
  - Excess overtime.
  - Excess support staff.
  - Redundant and overstocked supplies.
- **Poor service**
  - Late starts.
  - Extended turnover times.
  - Add-on procedures inappropriately triaged.
- **Frustrated staff**
- **Dissatisfied customers**

Each of these issues provided opportunities for improvement. In order to set priorities, however, it was apparent that NOC first needed to identify the operating room services core business (i.e., the basic components of operating room services) as well as the critical factors required for success in the identified core business.

Critical Success Factors

NOC's vision statement provided the direction and context within which to function. Key surgeon customer expectations and the current situation had also been defined. The next agenda item was to determine what OR services does and how to measure success. It was time for the team to take a step back and define the key issues that make the operating room a success. After much discussion, the success factors broke out into four categories:

- Service
- Quality
- Team and Customer Satisfaction
- Financial Parameters

Service issues related to processes and customer expectations. Quality issues were those that affect patient outcomes. Team and customer satisfaction were the issues that contribute to team building, service ethic, the ability to match service to expectations, work environment, etc. Financial parameters were budget related issues involving wage and non-wage costs as well as revenues.

The team felt that each factor was equally important. If one of the categories was not successful, the operating room service was failing. By determining these success factors, the team had established a direction in which to go, including definitions of customers' expectations, the current situation, and the core business. Each of these items was referred to as the group progressed into developing and implementing improvement strategies.

Improvement Strategies

Improvements in the operating room can only be achieved through multidisciplinary activity. Each discipline has a role to play and expectations to achieve. There are, however, components that must be addressed by individual disciplines. Each discipline had a specific role to play in developing and implementing the following identified change strategies:

- New Nursing operating structure
  - Implement a philosophy of acting as one unit.
  - Centralize triaging of urgent and add-on procedures.
  - Streamline decisionmaking committees and process.
  - Flatten the OR organizational structure.
  - Create direct accountability of managers for specific issues.

- Revised staffing design
  - Redesign of work shifts to match patient demand.
  - Increase the number of available schedule hours utilizing fewer full time equivalents (FTEs).
- New "on time" start policy
  - Communication of expectations.
  - Enforcement.
- Restructuring of support staff roles
  - Broaden the role of support staff for greater flexibility.
  - Redesign of support staff shifts for better coverage.
  - FTE reduction.
- Restructure of documentation
  - Consolidation of forms required for pre-op patient preparation (reduced from 11 to 3).
  - Computerization of intra-operative documentation.
  - Elimination of redundancy between pre-op, intra-op and post-op nursing documentation.
- RN/OR technician skill mix change
  - Was 82% RN/18% OR tech, currently 70%/30% with a goal of 60%/40%.
- RN/LVN Post Anesthesia Care Unit (PACU) skill mix change
  - Creation of LVN role in PACU.
  - Goal of 80% RN/20% LVN.
- Simplified necessary reports
  - Streamlined required reports to only the most pertinent.
  - Looked at each report to determine if the report had value.
- Materials Management (MM) teams

Three approaches were taken to address materials issues in the OR:

- OR/MM liaison team: Example issues:
  * Addressing issues of process and control.
  * Supply flow/just-in-time/stockless inventory.
  * Automated and accurate preference cards.
  * Security and theft prevention.
  * Forecasting tools.
  * Par level supplies.
  * Stock/Non-stock designation.
  * Case cart protocols.
  * Rush shipping.
  * Instrument tray processing.
  * Automated requisitioning process.
  * Redefining of cost centers and subaccounts.
- Sacred cow program (a grass roots nursing process): Example issues:
  * Utilization of drapes.
  * Selecting appropriate gowns.

        * Shoe cover usage.
        * Opening of supplies.
    - Resource Management initiatives: Example issues:
        * Clinical pathway implementation.
        * Standardization issues.
        * Supply bid process.
        * Identifying and implementing a "new" product decision tree.
        * Implement a return on investment decision tool.
- Set productivity measures
    - Advance review of OR schedule intensity tied to staffing hours and skill mix.
- Creation of admission and testing center
    - Aggregate all departments/functions that need to deal with the patient prior to the day of surgery into one centralized unit (e.g., nursing, discharge planning, admitting, patient accounting, ancillary testing services, utilization review, etc.)
    - Create centralized accountability for pre-op patient preparation.
- One stop shopping for Central OR Scheduling and related needs
    - One phone call achieves:
        * Booking of OR procedure.
        * Bed reservation.
        * Admission and Testing Center appointment.
        * Pre-op order collection.
    - Recommendation of ancillary department central scheduling (radiology, lab, etc.)
- Restructured patient flow process
    - Eliminate all but the most essential steps required of patient and family on the day of surgery (parking, admitting center, pre-op, OR).
- Creation of surgeon specific block scheduling
    - Assists in the alignment of labor and supply resources.
    - Create ownership of nursing and anesthesia teams to efficient functioning.
- Accountable decisionmakers
    - Creation of an accountable empowered team, consisting of nurse director, chief of anesthesia, and surgeon medical directors to guide implementation, enforce policy and expectations, and act as a resource.
- Create performance improvement monitoring systems
    - Develop and implement report card that reflects the four key success factors with the issues to be measured grouped under each appropriate category (see **Table 6.3**).

Table 6.3: Cedars-Sinai Medical Center, Patient Care Services Performance Improvement - 1995 Operating Room Services

Indicators	Target/goal	Base line	Quarter Jan-March	Quarter Apr-June	Quarter Jul-Sept	Quarter Oct-Dec
Clinical Outcome Staff Competencies - OR/PACU	100%	100% Annual				
6, 7, and 8 Patient Preadmission Preparation and Education	80% of patients	8/93 - 64%				
Patient Preparation at Pre-op	98%	10/94 - 78.5%				
PACU L.O.S. - All floors (After discharge ready)	1 hour	10/94 - .5 hr				
Patient Preparation and Education	100%	TBD				
Customer Satisfaction Team Satisfaction (range 1-5)	4.5	8/94 - 3.52				
Physician Satisfaction (range 1-5)	4.5	8/94 ORS 2.91 PACU 4.52 OR 4.17				
Service Outcomes First Case Starts (5 min var. OK)	90% on time	8/93 - 21%				
Overall Delays	80% on time	10/93 - 68%				
Turnover Time (average patient out to patient in)	20 minutes	10/93 - 42 mins				
Turnover Time (average patient in to incision)						

Note: Turnover time goal changed from 25 minutes to 20 minutes 10/94.

Cedars-Sinai Medical Center, Patient Care Services Performance Improvement - 1994 Operating Room Services

Financial Impact	(Budget)	(FYE 3/31/94)	YTD-6/94	YTD-9/94	YTD 12/94	Comparison to target	Comparison to base line
Non-labor Expense/Unit (3, 6, 7, 8, SDOSC, Liver)							
Salary Unit (3, 6, 7, 8, SDOSC, Liver)							
Total Expenses/Unit (Ellis Eye							
Total Expenses/Unit (8SE)							

Appropriate teams and subteams were identified to address each of these improvement strategies. Each team and subteam followed similar processes. The start time/turnover time project undertaken by the QAT and described in the following section provides an example of the process used by each group.

Start Time/Turnover Time

Defining Turnover Time and Opportunities for Improvement

The OR QAT's first activity was to brainstorm start/turnover time issues. Everyone, the group discovered, had a different definition of start time (i.e., what the time on the OR schedule means) and a different perception of what was expected of them (i.e., who should be where at what time). A literature search uncovered recent data regarding turnover time.[1,2] Using this data and other sources the team agreed upon the definitions illustrated in **Figure 6.1.** In measuring total turnover time and its components, the group determined that, according to the benchmark data, the greatest opportunity for improvement was in the "patient out to patient in" timeframe (see **Figures 6.2** and **6.3**).

The group then used flow charting to clarify and identify key points of control and activity. The flow charting exercise was essential to determining which steps or activities could be combined, eliminated, or improved. Other management tools such as a fishbone cause and effect (see **Figure 6.4**) were utilized to clarify and help analyze the issues.

Figure 6.1: Quality and Service - Turnover Time

Operating room "turnover time" is defined several different ways. A nationwide benchmarking survey collected data on total "turnover time" and its two major components.

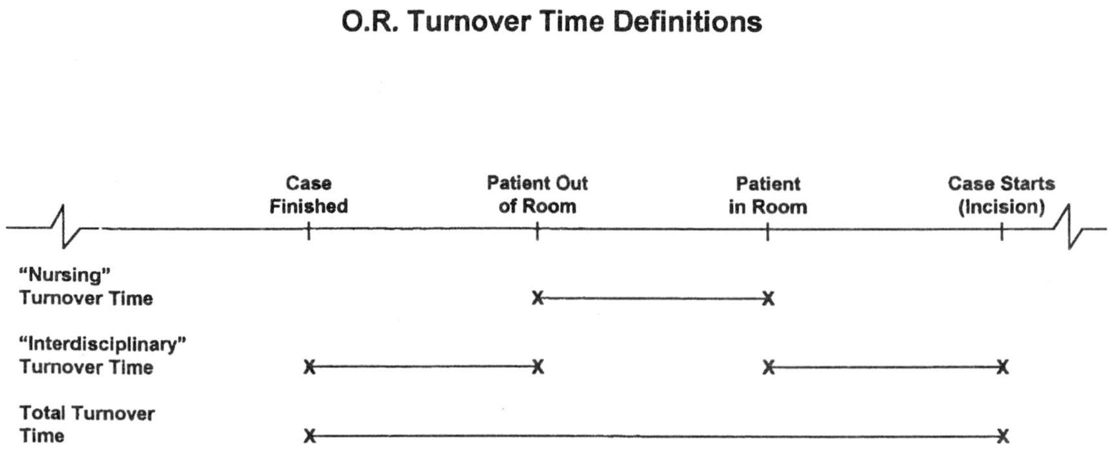

Figure 6.2: National Survey Information Used To Set Targets

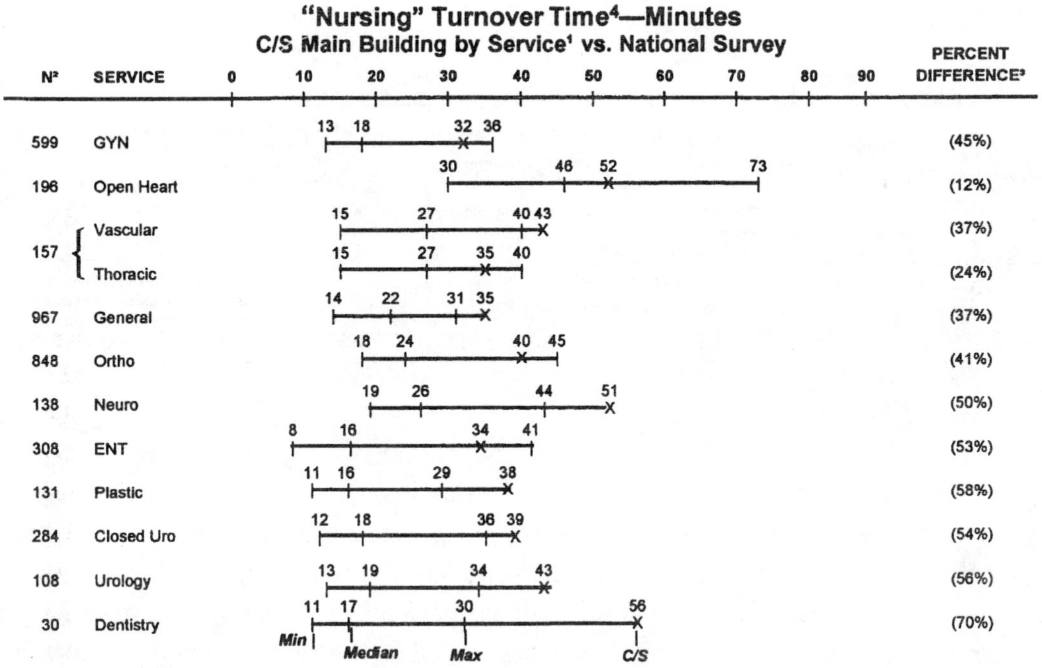

1 Avg. of C/S April 1993 & Nov. 1993 performance.
2 sample study volume.
3 (Median-C/S) (C/S)
4 Nursing turnover time defined as "patient out of room" to "patient into room."

Figure 6.3: O.R. Turnover Time

Overall comparisons of turnover time indicate that the greatest opportunity for Cedars is improve "nursing" turnover time.

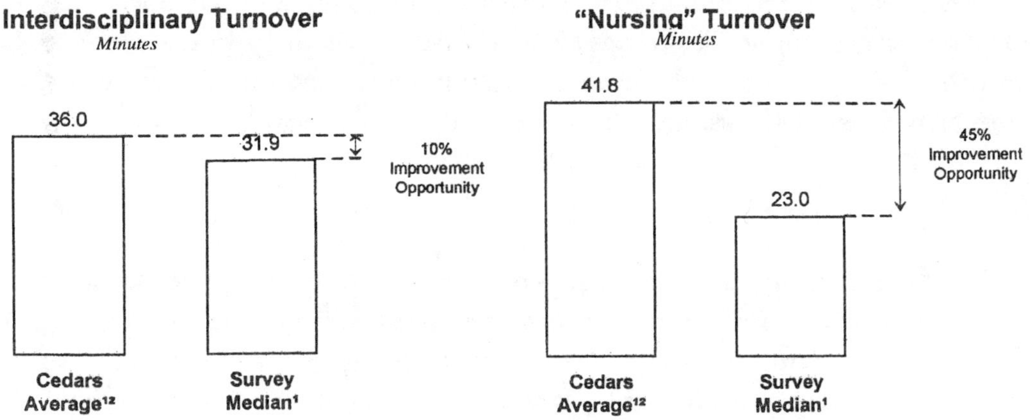

1 Simple average of turnover time by specialty.
2 Includes actual data from April and November of 1993.
Source: OR Manager; October, November 1993 and January 1994 issues; Cedars Sinai OR management reports.

Table 6.4: Cause and Effect Diagram
Conclusion: Multiple factors exist which result in extended time between procedures

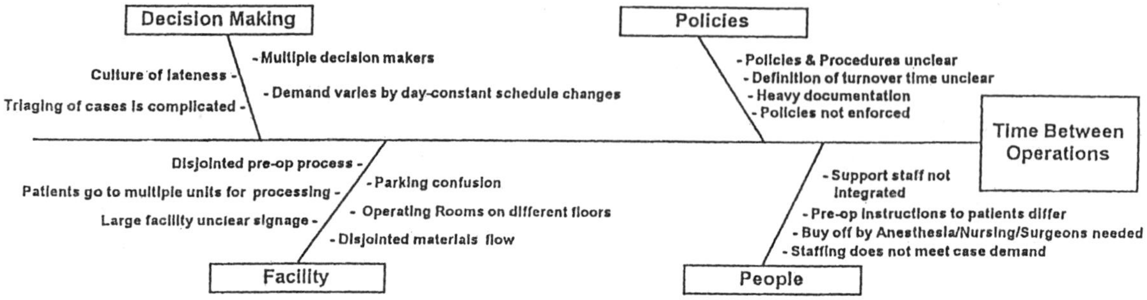

Recommendations

The QAT then made its recommendations regarding turnover time. It is interesting to note that, because issues in the operating room are extremely compacted and intertwined, the QAT recommendations went well beyond team expectations. A procedure will not start on time unless the patient, surgeon, anesthesiologist, nurses, ancillary departments, supplies, equipment, and data are all in the proper place and at the appropriate time. The QAT recommendations related to each of these issues.

The QAT agreed that the patient should enter the room at 0715 for a 0730 procedure. The nurses and anesthesiologist should be present at that time, with the surgeon arriving by 0730. It was decided that 0730 was not to be construed as cut-time, since the group felt that the procedure should begin when the patient is placed on the OR table and prep and positioning begins. The exact definitions are unimportant, however, *as long as everyone has the same understanding and knows what is expected.*

One of the primary issues in determining these expectations involved the fact that procedures have different prep and positioning timeframes. A major orthopedic or neurology procedure may require an extended timeframe once the patient enters the room, while a minor general or GYN procedure may have a very short timeframe. Because the team was setting expectations for people to remember, the group wanted to keep them as simple and clear as possible.

Implementation

The new definitions and expectations were shared with surgeon, anesthesia, and nursing staff at unit meetings and sent to each surgeon by direct mail. The new expectations were also shared at each unit meeting and manager meeting. Most importantly, accountability and authority was established by key decisionmakers to achieve the goal. Through changes in behavior and enforcing expectations, patient-out to patient-in turnover time was reduced from an average of forty-two minutes to below the original goal of twenty-five minutes (**Figure 6.5**) and first case starts from 17% on time to 54% (**Figure 6.6, Series**

1). When given a buffer of ten minutes, 82% of first cases are on time **(Figure 6.6, Series 2)**. The task force is now reviewing "interdisciplinary" turnover time with an emphasis on "patient-in to cut-time" as the primary focus. This was identified as the timeframe with the second greatest opportunity for improvement. The goal is to compact the timeframe from when the patient enters the room until the surgeon begins his/her portion of the procedure by doing more in pre-op and/or Post Anesthesia Care Unit (PACU).

Figure 6.5

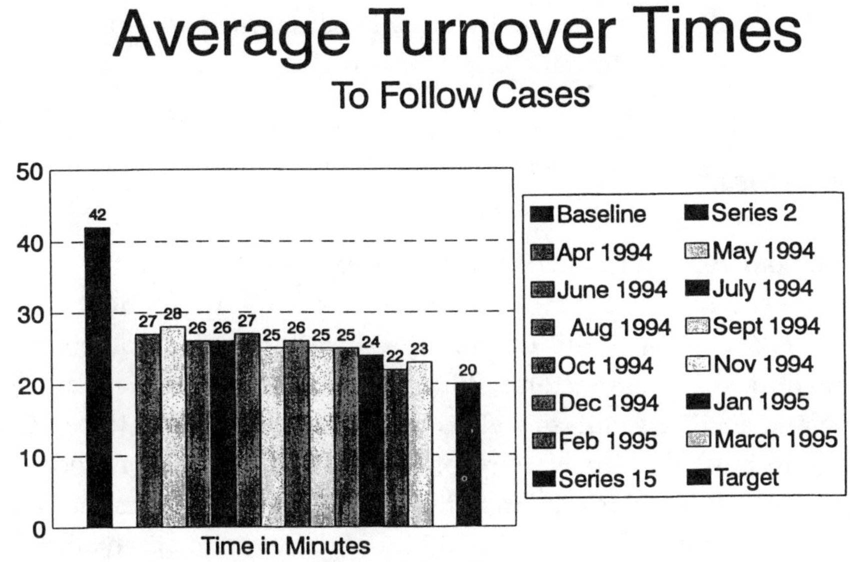

IOP Target = 20 Minutes
Baseline = 42 Minutes (October 1993)

Figure 6.6

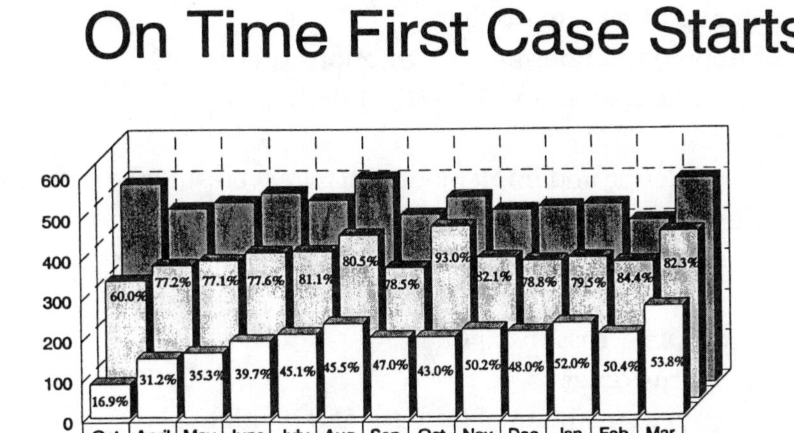

	Oct	April	May	June	July	Aug	Sep	Oct	Nov	Dec	Jan	Feb	Mar
Series 1	84	146	159	188	205	231	197	197	216	210	230	204	271
Series 2	298	336	347	367	369	409	329	430	353	345	352	341	415
Series 3	496	435	450	473	455	508	419	462	430	438	443	404	504

Series 1 = Actual On Time Starts 7:20/8:50 AM
Series 2 = Actual On Time Starts 7:30/9:00 AM
Series 3 = Total First Cases

Report Card

Each issue addressed by performance improvement teams must be measured to determine its success and/or to identify the need to re-address the issue if not successful. Cedars-Sinai's OR report card was adapted from a measurement tool outlined by Khadem and Lorber (**Table 6.3**). [3] The team had already identified the critical success factor categories of service, quality, team and customer satisfaction, and financial parameters. Each recommendation for change was placed in one of these four categories and each issue was measured for current status, benchmarked to determine goals, and is measured periodically to determine improvement.

Lessons Learned

Successful implementation of change is based upon maintaining the appropriate direction (vision statement), exceeding customers' expectations (patient and surgeon key expectations), following a multidisciplinary education and involvement process, and achieving the critical success factors. Buried in these issues is the management of people. Nursing and ancillary staff, as well as the medical staff, need to be willing to change their behavior to meet the expectations of their roles. The passion and enthusiasm displayed by key decisionmakers and implementation teams provides the single most motivating force in the change process. The ability of the team to act in a positive manner is directly affected by the manner in which the leadership (both formal and informal) presents and implements change recommendations.

Additional key points learned as a result of the change process include the following:

1. Fit services to meet customers' needs, instead of making customers fit the services.
2. The continued success of the OR must be based on partnering with medical staff and other departments.
3. Agreement upon definitions and assumptions is critical.
4. If it doesn't maintain or add value - don't do it!

It is also essential to define and implement a change *process* that encompasses the key elements listed below to enable the team to buy into the recommendations and understand their own processes at a more detailed level. Team leaders must ensure that the change process:

- Involves people across disciplines
- Involves the customer
- Relies on data to maintain objectivity and validate perceptions
- Improves efficiency by using multiple teams
- Communicates as frequently as possible, in as many formats as possible. Keep communication constant. No surprises.

  - Newsletters
  - Unit meeting
  - Medical staff meetings
  - One on one with informal leaders
  - Manager meeting
  - Posters and bullet points
- Simplifies work before staff is reduced
- Motivates team members and staff through education, communication, and involve ment
- Breaks large issues into their component parts and solves each part
- Lets people know the consequences of not being able to change
- Includes representatives on the teams who have a strong link to the groups they represent so they do not need to continually check the progress of the team against the needs of their group
- Includes agreement on accountability and empowerment for key issues
- Celebrates success and gives credit to the design and implementation teams

As operating room services moves forward to address the future in health care, systems will be redesigned and adjusted on an ever more frequent basis. There will be continued pressure to be more efficient with fewer resources and the possibility exists that the operating rooms of the future may be looked upon not as revenue generators, but as extremely expensive resources. The change management strategies described in this chapter, however, can help institutions respond to the needs of the future in a cost efficient manner while remaining responsive the needs of defined customers.

References

1. Schanilec JL. "Nursing Turnover Times Examined by Specialty." *OR Manager* 9(11) 1993:14.

2. Schanilec JL, LD Reynolds. "Turnover Time Data Show Times Vary Most in the Hospital Setting." *OR Manager* 10(1) 1994:10-12.

3. Khadem R, R Lorber. *One Page Management.* New York: Quill William Morrow, 1986.

Chapter 7

Patient-Focused Care Model for Respiratory Therapy Services

Zab Mohsenifar, MD
Mahmoud Samie, RCP, BMET
Brian Richards, RRT, BA
Spencer K. Koerner, MD, FCCP

Patient-focused care is based on the concept that the patient is the central focus and care should be provided by only a small number of workers who have been trained in a variety of health care disciplines.[1,2,3] This concept is not new and was the norm at the turn of the century. At that time, there were few specialists, no respiratory therapists, and very few dieticians. The various aspects of health care were delivered by a team consisting of a nurse and physician.

As technology progressed and the medical field became more sophisticated, it became difficult for one person to deliver all aspects of care. Thus, medicine became diversified, giving rise to different specialties and a variety of health care disciplines. Today, however, because of the need to reduce soaring medical costs, competition mandates that health care facilities reduce the cost of delivering care, while improving or maintaining the quality of care and patient satisfaction. To achieve this tri-fold goal, the patient-focused care design principles incorporate cross-prepared teams and redesigned jobs.[4] Fewer workers interact with the patient, creating a more personal hospital experience for the patient. In addition, clinical guidelines and pathways ensure quality and cost-efficient care.

Zab Mohsenifar, MD—Director, Respiratory Therapy for Cedars-Sinai Medical Center; Professor of Medicine, University of California-Los Angeles, School of Medicine.

Mahmoud Samie, RCP, BMET—Technical Director, Respiratory Therapy, Cedars-Sinai Medical Center.

Brian Richards, RRT, BA—Education Coordinator, Respiratory Therapy, Cedars-Sinai Medical Center.

Spencer K. Koerner, MD, FCCP—Director, Pulmonary Medicine, Cedars-Sinai Medical Center; Professor of Medicine, University of California-Los Angeles, School of Medicine.

Respiratory Therapy Before Patient-Focused Care

Historically, the Cedars-Sinai Medical Center Respiratory Therapy Department has provided a variety of therapeutic procedures and diagnostic services. The staffing needs fluctuated continuously according to the patient work load, acuity, and complexity of procedures required. Prior to the implementation of patient-focused care, the respiratory therapy department consisted of therapists and technicians. Per diem utilization complimented the full-time staff when necessary.

The technicians' duties included simple respiratory therapy procedures such as: pulse oximetry monitoring, hand held nebulizer therapy, metered dose inhaler instruction, chest physiotherapy, incentive spirometry, heated aerosol treatments, and free-flow oxygen therapy. Therapists, on the other hand, performed all of these simple duties plus more complex procedures associated with the management of adult and pediatric ventilator systems and related adjuncts.

Respiratory therapy orders were received by phone and entered into a computer that generated a treatment card for each patient. This sequence of events is demonstrated in **Figure 7.1**. The respiratory therapy manager was responsible for work assignments and staffing housewide, which included staffing for seven adult intensive care units (ICUs), a pediatric intensive care unit, a neonatal intensive care unit, and approximately ten general patient care floors.

Respiratory therapists and technicians were dispatched centrally from the pulmonary division, where they clocked "in and out" and picked up their assignments on preprinted patient treatment cards. These cards were returned at the end of the shift and became the billing document.

Methods

In order to implement patient-focused care, the task force examined the level of complexity for each procedure performed, studied the volume of procedures in each area, and identified the number of full time employees (FTEs) required to administer these procedures. The tasks were ultimately divided up into two categories—simple and complex.[5] Simple Procedures (**Table 7.1**), or simple tasks, were those that could be taught over a period of a few days to licensed health care workers with previous experience in bedside health care delivery (i.e., RNs and LVNs). Complex Procedures (**Table 7.2**) were identified as those tasks involving multiple component equipment and/or requiring extensive training periods for therapists already versed in respiratory physiology.

Figure 7.1: Respiratory Therapy Order Flow Chart

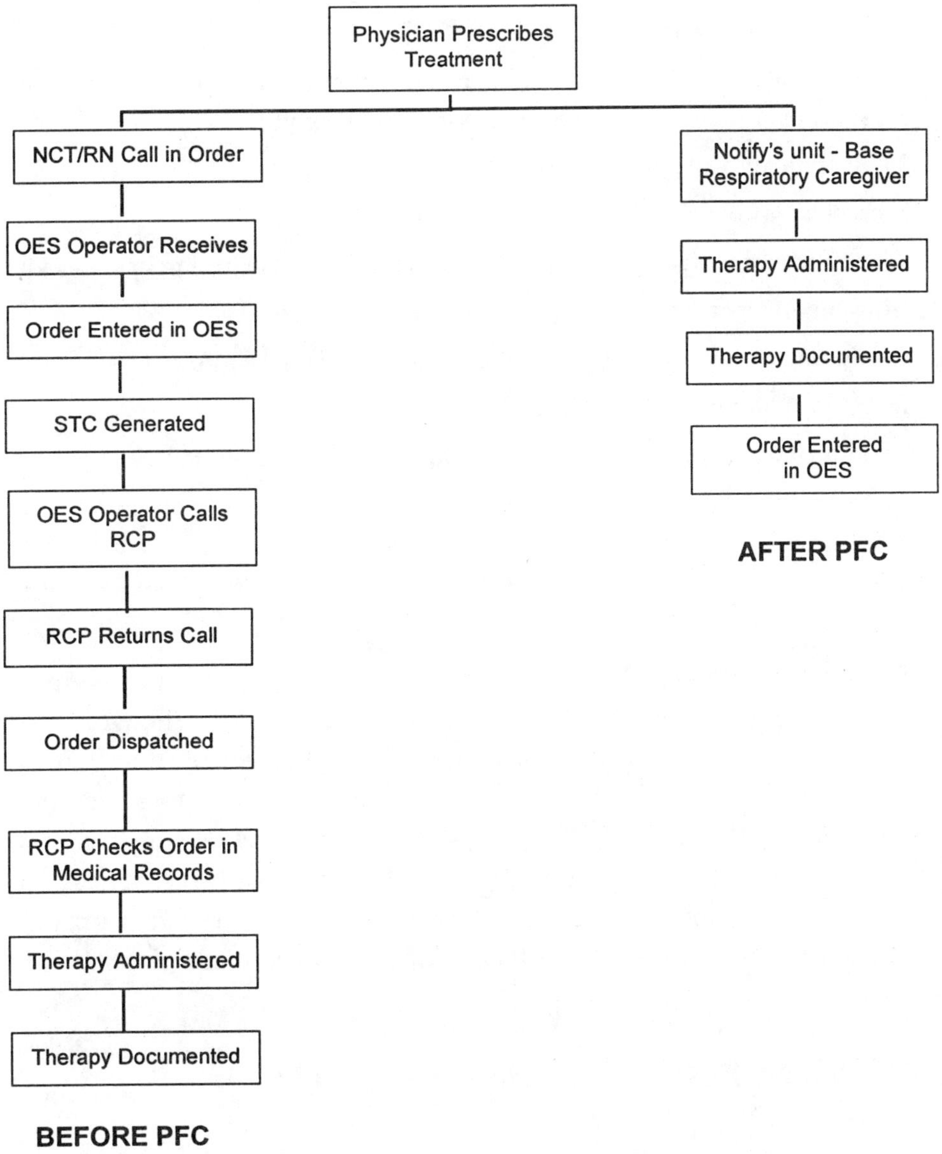

Legend:

OES=Order Entry System
STC=Shift Treatment Card
RCP=Respiratory Care Practitioner
NCT=Nursing Communications Technicians

Table 7.1: Simple Respiratory Therapy Procedures

- Set-up Oxygen Ventimasks.
- Set-up Heated or Cool Aerosol Generators (intermittent or continuous use; via aerosol mask, trache collar, trache tee, face tent, isolette, oxyhood).
- Medicinal Aerosol Administration - HHN, MDI, HHN to MDI conversion.
- Incentive Spirometry (first round instruction).
- Chest Physiotherapy (postural drainage with manual clapping or GK-3 vibrator).
- Coughing Instruction/Pursed Lip Breathing Exercise.
- Suctioning (nasal tracheal, orotracheal, via artificial airway).
- Insert oropharyngeal/nasopharyngeal airways.
- Sputum Induction, Routine (via x's Heated Aerosol Generator 20 to 30 minutes).
- Pulse Oximetry (continuous use with computer link or intermittent use without computer link).

The workloads for both simple and complex respiratory procedures were then analyzed by the patient care unit. **Figure 7.2** demonstrates an example of the workload in an intensive care unit with a high volume of complex procedures, predominantly mechanical ventilators. **Figure 7.3** demonstrates an example of workload on a medical floor with a high volume of complex and simple procedures. **Figure 7.4** demonstrates workload distribution on a floor with a varying volume of simple procedures. These analyses of the volume and level of complexity for respiratory therapy procedures provided the information needed to design the patient-focused care interventions described in the following sections.

Patient-Focused Respiratory Therapy Model

TRACK I

After reviewing the work complexity and distribution, the task force determined that complex procedures requiring more training and a higher level of skill (e.g., ventilator management) would continue to be done by therapists. Therefore, all ICUs with a high volume of mechanical ventilators (**Figure 7.2**) and the pulmonary floor with high volume of complex procedures (**Figure 7.3**) would be staffed by therapists. Since the work in these areas fluctuated (**Figures 7.2** and **7.3**), therapists in these areas would be cross-prepared to provide more comprehensive care by performing such tasks as veni-puncture, electrocardiogram (EKG), trache care, vital signs assessment, and patient procedures related the activities of daily living (ADL). The therapists stationed in the various ICUs and on the pulmonary floor would have a dual accountability—to the unit manager and to the respiratory therapy manager. During periods of low workload, they would be responsible for providing most respiratory care and, as time permitted, would carry out

Table 7.2: Complex Respiratory Therapy Procedures

- Bedside Spirometry
- Set-up Blender Driven, High Flow Non-rebreathing O_2 systems.
- Set-up USN's for PCP sput induction with 3% hypertonic saline.
- Respirgarde II Pentamidine Nebulizer Set-up/Administration.
- IPPB Set-up/Administration.
- CPR (including use of bag-valve resuscitators, airway suctioning, and intubation adjuncts).
- Arterial Puncture.
- End-Tidal CO_2 monitoring via portable unit.
- Set-up/use Metabolic Cart (AKA non-invasive calorimetry).
- Routine Ventilator Patient Assessment (RR, HR, BSds, Sputum, Sensorial Status, ETT placement/stability, cuff press assessment, Inline suctioning, Pulse Ox saturation, ABG evaluation, Q/A ratio and static compliance calculation/evaluation.
- Ventilator Management; continuous ICU ventilator systems include 7200a and 7200ae, Bear II, Bear Jet, Sechrist and Bunnell High Frequency Jet, Infant Star Vent/high frequency option, Bio med MVP-10, Siemens Servo 900C, Bird VIP, Newport Breeze, Infrasonics High Frequency Oscillator.
- Differential Lung Ventilation (separate ventilator system for each of one patient's lungs).
- Continuous Mask CPAP via Down's CPAP Generator.
- Continuous Nasal CPAP (Nasal Pillows or Nasal Mask) via Respironics BiPAP generator, home care ventilators (e.g., PLV $_{100}$, PLV $_{102}$, Bear 33, PB 2800, 2801; mechanically less complex than ICU ventilators but monitoring is clinician rather computer generated).
- Adjunctive Airway Management including Intubation Assist; Placement Assessment;
- Tube Stabilization; Cuff Vol/Pres Measurement; Applic of Passey Muir Speaking Valve.
- Ventilator Patient Transport.
- Mist Tent set-up/servicing.
- Intubation Assist with ETT suturing (NICU).
- Delivery Room Resuscitation (excluding intubation) during high risk pregnancies.
- Continuous Albuterol Administration via HEART Nebulizer (as unique to PICU).
- Exosurf/Survanta Installation via ETT side Port (as unique to NICU).
- Ribavirin Administration via SPAG II nebulizer and exhaust filtered infant vent (as unique to PICU).
- Inhalational Drug Administration via flow dependent bag or infant vent and in-line "flow-thru" micronebulizer.
- Heel Stick Blood Gas Sampling (predominantly NICU function).
- Blood Gas Analysis (including use of tonometer and cooximeter and related quality control tasks).
- 60/40 Heliox Therapy (H-Cyl, precision regulator, via hood, tent, infant vent (unique to PICU/NICU).

additional tasks in which they were cross prepared, either on unit or in adjacent care areas. As the work load increased, the ranks of unit designated therapists would be supplemented with more therapists dispatched from a central department personnel flex pool. Unit designated therapists would also periodically rotate to other areas in order to maintain proficiency in respiratory skills not commonly performed in their usual assigned stations.

TRACK II

Simple, less time consuming duties (**Table 7.1**), that were in the past performed by technicians would now be delegated to cross-trained RNs and LVNs particularly in areas with low volumes of these activities. With proper training, RNs and LVNs would perform these respiratory treatments on the patient-focused care medical and surgical

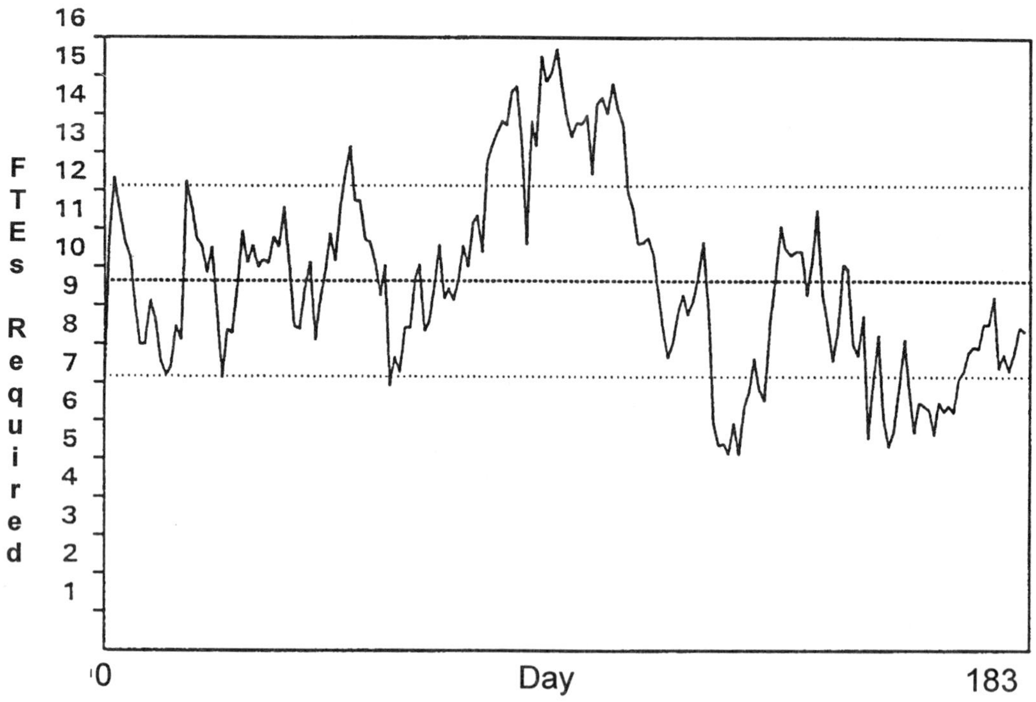

Figure 7.2: Workload example in a Intensive Care Unit with a high volume of complex procedures, predominently mechanical ventilators.

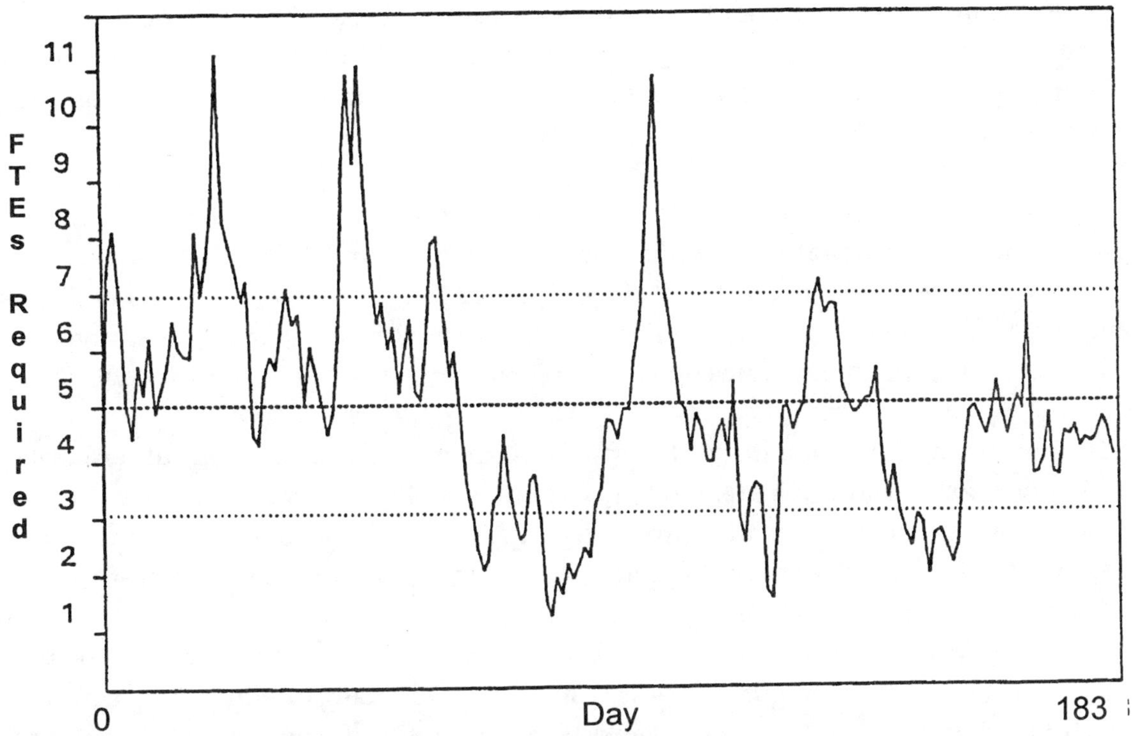

Figure 7.3: Workload example on a medical pulmonary floor with a high volume of complex and simple procedures.

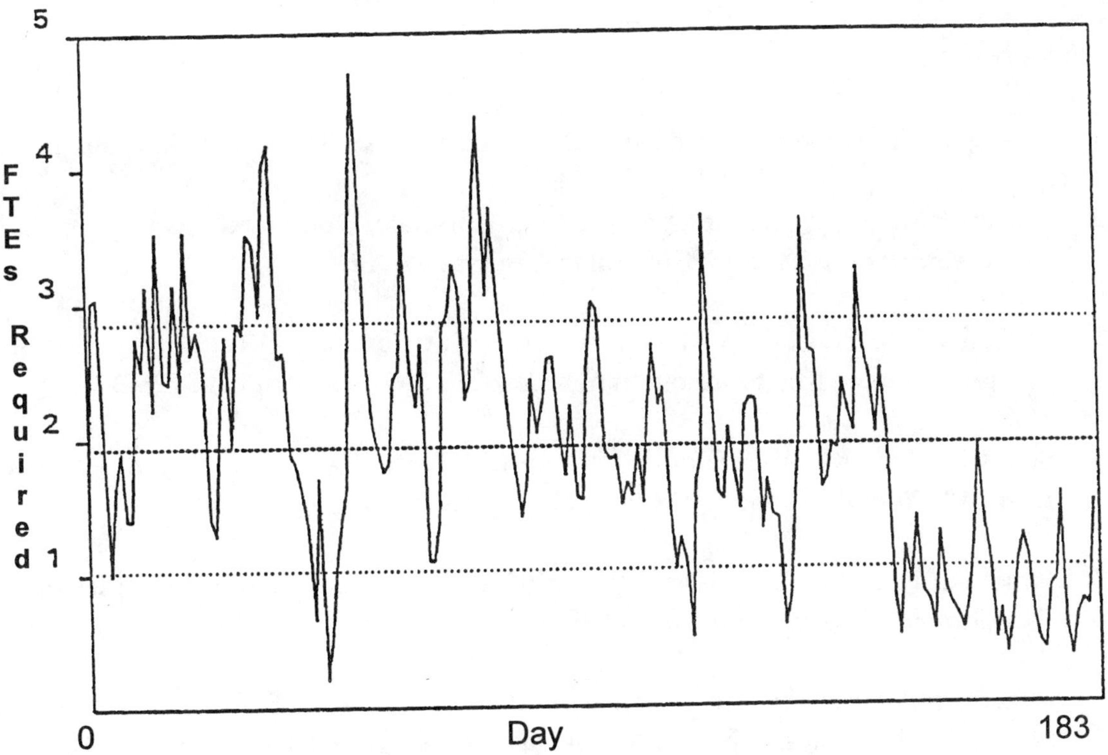

Figure 7.4: Workload example on a floor with a varying volume of simple procedures.

floors. Complex procedures on those floors would continue to be done by therapists dispatched from the central department flex pool. A significant amount of time would have been required to cross prepare RNs and LVNs to carry out these infrequent and complex procedures.

The cross-preparation of RNs and LVNs consisted of two-day, didactic education sessions taught by respiratory therapist clinical instructors and followed by hands-on skills labs. Thereafter, each RN and LVN was assigned to a therapist for further skills assessment for a one-day period or until deemed proficient in all "simple" respiratory treatments. This process continues on an annual basis to ensure skill proficiency.

In conclusion, the Respiratory Therapy Department remains the central authority and caregiver for respiratory care, while maintaining a close working relationship with the patient-focused care areas and providing support and education on an ongoing basis. With the simple tasks being delegated to RNs and LVNs on the patient-focused care floors, the department was able to reduce its staff by eleven FTEs (technicians and therapists). Further reductions in the number of FTEs in direct patient care may be realized as clinical pathways and guidelines are established, reducing or eliminating certain treatment modalities.[6] One of the key elements in the success of any patient-focused care program is the teamwork between nursing and respiratory therapy management.[7] By having an open line of communication, it is possible to minimize the anxiety on the part of both nursing and respiratory therapy staff when facing changes in their professional lives and in the delivery of patient care.

References

1. Lathrop P. "The Patient-Focused Hospital." *Healthcare Forum Journal* 1991; July/August: 17-23

2. Hammer M. "Reengineering work: Don't Automate, Obliterate." *Harvard Business Review* 1990;68 July/August 104-112.

3. Eubanks P, M Hagland, M Graywon, F Sadbatino . "Restructuring Care: Patient Focus in Key to Innovation. " *Hospitals* 1991; 65 (August 5):26-33.

4. Starrs C. "The Multi-Skilled Movement: A New Wave for Clinical Laboratory science." *Clinical Laboratory Science* 1989; 2 (July/August): 204-210.

5. Hmelo C, K. Axton. "Job Satisfaction and Task Complexity Among Respiratory Care Practitioners." *Respiratory Care* 1989; 34: 1129-1134.

6. American Association for Respiratory Care, Clinical Practice Guidelines Steering Committee. The AARC clinical practice guidelines. *Respiratory Care* 1991; 36: 1398-1426.

7. Snyder GM. "Patient focused hospital: An Opportunity for Respiratory Care Practitioners." *Respiratory Care* 1992; 37: 448-454.

Chapter 8

Patient-Focused Care Model for Physical Medicine And Rehabilitation Services

Terry Martin, PT
Mel Cohen, PhD
Zahra Ghasemi, MS, PT

With the current changes in health care, numerous facilities have engaged in restructuring of the entire delivery system. Many have called this new delivery system patient-focused care (PFC), but the meaning of the term may vary. This chapter outlines what PFC means from a Physical Medicine and Rehabilitation (PM&R) perspective at Cedars-Sinai Medical Center. The chapter reviews: 1) the rehabilitation department structure and operations before patient-focused care, 2) the departmental response to evolving changes in health care before patient-focused care, 3) participation in the design and implementation of patient-focused care within the institution, 4) the departmental structure and operations after patient-focused care, 5) strengths and weaknesses of the new structure, and 6) issues for consideration when embarking on the process.

Physical Medicine and Rehabilitation Before PFC

The Department of Physical Medicine and Rehabilitation (PM&R) at Cedars-Sinai Medical Center includes the disciplines of physical therapy, occupational therapy, speech-language pathology, therapeutic recreation, rehabilitation psychology, biofeedback, and physiatry. Therapy is provided in four major service areas—acute inpatient, sub-acute inpatient (skilled nursing care), inpatient rehabilitation, and outpatient. Although the patient-focused care design has been implemented in all areas except outpatient, this chapter will focus primarily on the largest and most costly level of care, the acute inpatient area.

TERRY MARTIN, PT—Manager, Physical Medicine and Rehabilitation Services in Acute Care, Cedars-Sinai Medical Center.

MEL COHEN, PHD—Finance Manager, Physical Medicine and Rehabilitation, Cedars-Sinai Medical Center.

ZAHRA GHASEMI, MS, PT—Senior Therapist, Acute Physical Therapy, Cedars-Sinai Medical Center.

Structure

The acute medical center, with 1,200 licensed pre-earthquake beds located in eight-story towers, provides medical and surgical care to patients within a broad range of programs such as orthopedic surgery, trauma, neurosurgery, pediatrics, general medicine, cardiology, and organ transplantation. Many of the patients are seriously ill and have multi-system involvement. Medical and other professional staff with specialized clinical knowledge and skills are needed to care for these patients. To properly deliver care, the staff must also be well-oriented and trained to the institution's policies, procedures, and personnel.

Prior to the implementation of PFC, the PM&R department was structured in much the same way that therapies were organized in other large facilities. Each discipline (referred to as "divisions" at Cedars-Sinai) had a division manager who reported to the administrative director. Each division manager had supervisors in each of the four service areas—acute, sub-acute, rehabilitation, and outpatient. Thus, the acute inpatient area

Figure 8.1: Physical Medicine and Rehabilitation Before PFC Implementation

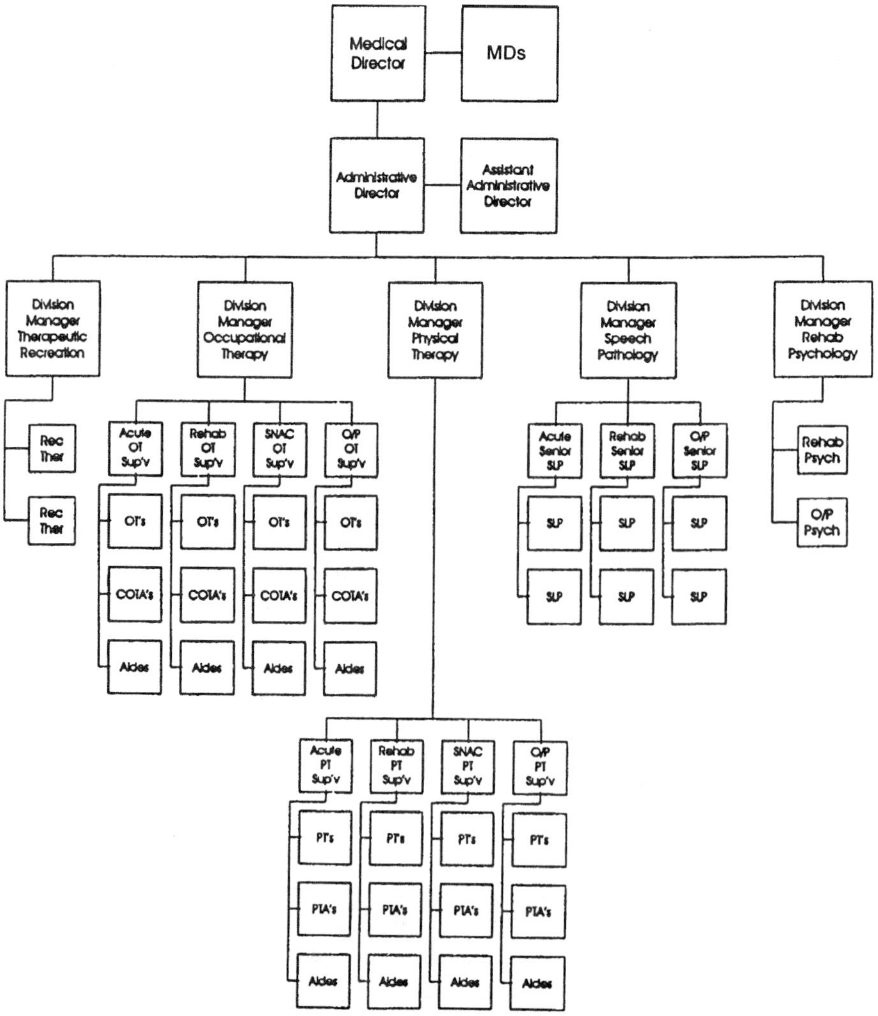

had a physical therapy supervisor, an occupational therapy supervisor, and a senior speech pathologist (see **Figure 8.1**).

Each supervisor was responsible for all operational issues, including staffing, training, equipment, and quality assurance within their respective areas. Communication and collaboration occurred across areas and divisions to ensure consistency and smooth opertions within the PM&R department. Accountability and reporting, however, were to one's own division manager, who was a professional with the same clinical background as the supervisor. Supervisors only managed staff in their own discipline.

Processes — Operations and Productivity

Therapy services in acute inpatient were provided from a central department. Historically, full coverage was provided to the inpatients on weekdays. This meant that all new and previously ordered therapy was performed and no treatments were missed. On weekends, Saturday and Sunday, staffing was reduced. Typically, five or six therapists were scheduled to work these days, and patients were prioritized based on their medical acuity, responsiveness to treatment, and likelihood of their discharge. Some patients were not seen by the therapies on the weekends, and treatment was resumed on the weekdays.

The central department had responsibility for providing adequate therapy coverage for the medical center, including backups and fill-ins when unscheduled staff absences occurred. The responsibility of the central department also included all issues relating to the quality of therapy services, staff recruitment and training, and acquisition and maintenance of therapy equipment. Staff reported to the area supervisor or charge therapist at the beginning of the day, obtained their assigned list of patients, and went to the nursing unit or units where their patients were located. Since the distance to the therapy gym made travel time to bring patients to the department prohibitive, the majority of treatment was provided in the patient rooms or on the units. Efforts were made to group each therapist's patients in the same geographic area of the medical center. This was dependent, however, upon a fluctuating patient census. One therapist, for example, may have had patients on three or more different floors as each of those floors had only a few patients requiring therapy. On such days, therapist efficiency decreased due to the added travel and elevator waiting time. Most therapists now choose to use the stairs instead of waiting for elevators.

Other factors contributing to nonproductive time included the following: patients not being available for therapy because they were receiving other services, patients taken off the unit for diagnostic or surgical procedures, patients transferred to other units, or patients discharged from the medical center. A project to create a central scheduling system involving all hospital departments proved difficult and was abandoned after many months of data gathering, group discussion, and investigation into the automated systems available in the industry at that time.

Productivity standards for the department were established in the early 1980s. Data collection, work sampling, logs, and other information was used to determine reasonable and appropriate expectations for all staff. At that time, it was generally agreed that most therapists should perform 4.5 to 5.0 billable hours of patient contact for every eight hours worked. "Constant" hours were built in the schedule to allow for continuing education, staff meetings, documentation, and other indirect time such as unavailability of the patient when the therapist was ready to provide treatment. The staff to supervisor ratio at that time was about eight to one, allowing time for intensive individual coaching and instruction, as well as new program development and sophisticated quality monitoring.

In an effort to streamline paperwork and free valuable therapist time for more direct patient contact, revisions in patient care documentation had been in process since 1988. Initial evaluation forms and daily treatment notes began to take on a pre-printed checklist format to avoid repetitive, time-consuming handwriting. These changes would also assist in moving to a fully automated medical record at some point in the future. A computerized order entry and charge system was implemented in 1990. It helped significantly in the relay of new orders and information, and in reducing delays in the start of therapy services for individual patients.

In addition, the department began an aggressive planning and development program to increase the numbers of patients who could be seen in a group setting. Group treatment was provided successfully in cardiac rehabilitation, with orthopedic surgical patients, with general deconditioned patients, and with liver transplant patients. Also successful were the outpatient back class and the chair dancing program in sub-acute. Preoperative training and education for total joint replacement patients began in 1992. This program was seen as an effective means of preparing patients for hospitalization, perhaps leading to a shorter, less costly hospital stay.

The department periodically assessed and revised its productivity standards, often with the help of an objective outside consultant, and always with community practice standards in mind. Periodic adjustments were made in response to the growth of managed care and increasing discounts commanded by payers. As a result, the standards were increased to 5.25 - 5.75 billable hours for each eight hours worked.

Skill Mix

On a typical weekday in the acute inpatient area, there were approximately sixteen to eighteen physical therapy staff working, seven to eight occupational therapy staff, and two to three speech pathologists. The typical staffing pattern consisted of licensed therapists, each with a bachelor's or master's degree, plus four non-licensed physical therapy aides, two licensed physical therapy assistants, and two certified occupational therapy assistants (COTAs). The department had recognized the need to reduce costs and improve efficiency. This skill mix represented the result of converting licensed staff positions to aides and assistants (through attrition) over the six-year period prior to implementation of PFC. Before that time, the use of aides and assistants was minimal.

Traditionally, PM&R aides were assigned routine tasks including patient transportation, hydrotherapy preparation and cleanup, pain management modalities, and assisting therapists as needed in their treatment sessions. Identification of additional tasks to be delegated to the physical therapy aides was the first step once the decision was made to increase their role in patient care. The possibility of training aides to carry out activities which they had previously not performed (e.g., some types of exercise and the supervision of high level ambulation) was considered. This move seemed logical and appropriate since family members were already being trained to do these tasks with patients once they went home. With much staff discussion, compromise, and anxiety, the group finally agreed on the direction to take with the aides. This step was taken many years prior to the implementation of PFC.

Physical Therapy Aide Education Program

In 1988, an extensive education program was designed to provide physical therapy aides with both didactic material and time to practice new skills. Didactic sessions were generally scheduled in blocks of one to two hours, for a total of twelve hours. Printed materials were distributed for independent study, and tests were given after each module. Hands-on lab sessions totaling seven to ten hours were arranged to follow each module (except terminology training) with a licensed therapist observing, directing, and coaching.

PM&R aides were taught basic terminology, body mechanics, posture, safety awareness, basic active exercise programs, bed mobility, transfer training, and methods for appropriately supervising the ambulation of patients using a variety of assistive devices. In addition, they received information regarding typical patient problems such as orthopedic surgical procedures and movement precautions for these patients, various disease processes, and commonly used diagnostic procedures and medications. They were given clearly defined limits, and at no time were they to vary from the activities as specifically identified and delegated by the therapist.

Newly trained aides were closely supervised and coached for approximately six weeks. All patient contact was observed by a licensed therapist during the first few weeks following training, documentation was audited, and routine discussion was held regarding their specific patient care activities. Comfort levels gradually increased as the aides became more skilled and confident and as the therapists learned to trust and let go. After all, the aides were essentially performing activities that the patients and their caregivers were to do themselves (i.e., the home programs and the routine practice of exercise and gait already taught by the therapist).

Therapists then needed to learn to become better delegators and to find ways to coordinate patient care activities with the aides to allow for appropriate supervision. The aides were functioning so well that new tasks were identified. Aides were trained to assist with group exercise sessions involving multiple patients and to perform some routine activities in cardiac rehabilitation. Again, training and supervision were intense until safety and competence could be demonstrated.

Not every aide was selected for training in these areas. They first needed to perform basic tasks safely and effectively. Individuals with a high degree of personal motivation, a strong desire to learn, and a commitment to excellence in their work were selected. These qualities, as well as previous patient care experience, were the attributes expected in newly hired aides. The department also specifically recruited individuals enrolled, or intending to enroll, in professional physical therapy training programs at local universities. This ensured that the department would hire dedicated individuals, for their career focus was rehabilitation.

With the success of the aide training, an ongoing program was instituted in 1989. The department was more able to rotate staff between the areas, and a structure was established for training new staff in the specialty services such as cardiac rehabilitation. The department was also able to meet the growing demand for therapy at a more reasonable cost to the medical center.

Patient-Focused Care Design and Implementation

Designing the Pilot Unit

Implementing PFC at Cedars-Sinai represented the prospect of changing, both philosophically and practically, the way that patient care was delivered. This enormous project would require total commitment at all levels of the organization, beginning with the executive management group, and including all levels of staff in each of the departments. When the initiative was announced and the orthopedic unit was identified as the first unit to be restructured, it was apparent that PM&R would play a key role, since physical therapy was a vital part of the orthopedic patient's medical or postoperative recovery. The medical center needed to emphasize cost savings and to improve efficiency while achieving its clinical and service goals. Cedars-Sinai's caregivers worked hard to ensure that the proposed new efficiencies did not negatively impact effectiveness. Task forces and, later, small work groups were formed, and the project's basic design principles were established.

Primary goals for the restructuring were to improve patient/customer satisfaction, maintain or improve clinical outcomes, eliminate unnecessary and repetitious work, improve overall operating efficiency, and reduce the cost of delivering patient care services. Time frames for planning and implementation were established and cost reduction targets were identified for each department and nursing unit. Preliminary meetings began in April 1993. The training for the pilot unit (orthopedics) took place in August and September 1993, and full implementation on that first unit occurred in October 1993. All other units were phased in over the next twelve months. By October 1994, the entire medical center was operating in the new patient-focused care structure. Cedars-Sinai was clearly on a "fast track"!!

The PFC planning process was a difficult period, with many hours spent collecting, organizing, analyzing, and discussing data. Work groups examined everything in the most minute detail. How many staff per job type (PT, Assistant, Aide) delivered how many units of service on each nursing unit? How many treatments were missed on each unit, each day of the week, for the last year? How did service change on the weekends? How did missed treatments affect patient outcome and length of stay? What were the salary costs for each job type? What specific activities were performed by aides, assistants, and therapists? How were decisions made regarding which activities were assigned to aides? Which activities were covered by licensure in this state? Which activities could and could not be performed by other non licensed staff with training? How much time each day did a therapist spend in direct patient care, in documenting, scheduling, transporting (self or equipment), and coordinating with others? There was no automated system in place that would allow for easy retrieval of most of this information. There were too many questions and too few answers.

Task force members were asked to participate in creative group problem solving as they developed the pilot patient-focused care model. Many of the initial group participants were not involved in direct patient care (i.e., administrators, managers, and outside consultants) and had no knowledge of a nursing unit's daily operations. PM&R had to provide an accurate presentation of patient rehabilitation needs. Therapists had also been accustomed to a delivery model and hospital length of stay that allowed the discharge of patients when they were walking, talking, and often functionally independent. Task force members, and therapists alike, needed to "think outside of the box." It was necessary to look at discharging patients at a safe level and for therapists to accept that major functional gains would happen with other therapists in other care settings.

Two of the basic PFC design principles were: 1) to reduce the number of different hospital staff who needed to directly interact with the patient and 2) to provide as much of the patient's required care as possible on the unit rather than moving the patient to various departments throughout the hospital. To meet these challenges, it was agreed that some staff would be cross prepared to perform tasks that were neither part of their traditionally assigned duties nor contained in their psychological contracts. It was also important to adopt the philosophy that patient care and customer service tasks would not be passed to others by a staff member who was present, educated, and available to perform the task at the time. These two principles proved to be the most challenging for the therapies in design, principle, and follow-up.

In agreeing with the PFC principles, therapists saw them as having the potential to help achieve greater patient, customer, physician, and staff satisfaction; improved clinical outcomes; increased efficiency; and reduced non-productive time. The principles also helped to create the framework for improved communication and collaboration among caregivers. Guidance would be needed in dealing with problems that related to each employee's psychological contract. Individual staff acceptance of new work hours and schedules, as well as the expectation that they perform tasks not included in their jobs at the time of hire, were problems that were easier to discuss in committees than to address in the work arena.

After extensive discussion and analysis of the data, it was determined that some of the patient care tasks currently performed by physical therapy aides would be performed by caregivers directly on the unit. As part of the core education program, RNs and LVNs, as well as the cross-prepared care partners, were to receive a module on physical and occupational therapy tasks specific to the needs of the orthopedic patient population. Since the majority of the orthopedic patients required therapy and since physical therapy aides currently performed some of the tasks, it seemed reasonable to train nursing personnel (in particular care partners whose skill level and hourly pay most closely matched those of the aides) for some of these routine, high level activities.

Processes of Care

Therapy Guidelines. Before embarking on any education, some clear guidelines needed to be established and agreed upon regarding the patients' therapy programs while they were hospitalized on the orthopedic unit. These guidelines included the following:

1) The licensed therapist would be responsible for performing an initial evaluation, establishing functional goals, setting up the treatment plan, and determining the most appropriate equipment to be used for each patient.
2) The licensed therapist would identify which portions of the patient's treatment program could be delegated to the care team and would discuss the treatment program with the individual care partners on a daily basis.
3) The licensed therapist would see each patient at least once a day and, depending on the complexity of the patient's medical and functional status, delegate the second treatment for some patients to the care partner. Not every patient would have activities delegated to the care partner. These individual decisions needed to remain within the realm of the therapist's professional judgment.
4) The care partner would be responsible for carrying out the tasks/activities as del egated to them by the therapist and for documenting what was performed. Verbal exchange of information regarding patient response and status was also expected.
5) The licensed therapist would be responsible for monitoring the patient's progress and for modifying individual programs as needed. They would remain a key contributor to the discharge planning process.

Delegation and Supervision. Discussion and planning evolved naturally into the areas of supervision and the reporting structure. Therapists were expected to delegate patient care tasks to staff for whom they had no direct supervisory relationship and be accountable to the manager on the orthopedic unit. This model was new to everyone. It demanded that each individual re-think the way the work would be performed and the way they related to those with whom they worked most closely. This model would also require greater communication between managers from PT, OT, and nursing. A matrix structure was agreed upon in which the therapists who were permanently assigned to the orthopedic unit would report both to the unit manager and to the manager in physical or occupational therapy. Therapy managers would retain responsibility for quality, performance reviews, education and training, and counseling as needed with the therapy staff. The unit manager would be responsible for daily unit operations, assuring that patient care happened appropriately and that necessary communication occurred with the therapy staff. The nurse/unit manager would have input on therapists' performance reviews. Therapists would have input on the reviews of unit personnel as they related to their performance of therapy tasks.

Tasks to be delegated to the unit personnel were much the same as those delegated to physical therapy aides. They included the following: proper patient positioning, bed mobility, transfer activities from bed to chair, high level supervised ambulation with various assistive devices, some basic range of motion (ROM) and conditioning exercises, and the use of adaptive equipment in patient grooming, dressing, and bathing. Information was provided concerning weight bearing precautions, positioning and movement precautions for various orthopedic surgeries, and the rehabilitation philosophy of encouraging patients to learn to care for themselves rather than "doing it for them." This approach would obviously take longer, but it would have greater long term benefit to the patient than the custodial approach that is quicker in the short term but creates perpetual dependency.

PFC Education Program. Developing, planning, coordinating, and executing the PFC education program proved to be a challenging, costly, and time-consuming project. The physical and occupational therapy aide training program already in place in the department could not be plugged "as is" into the proposed patient-focused care education. The program was far more comprehensive than what was necessary for the care partners on the unit. Therapy activities comprised only a few of the items on a list of duties these new caregivers were expected to perform. Time had to be allotted for education in the other tasks as well. Senior therapy staff, charged with creating the education materials, had endless questions about what to include as they considered the actual tasks care partners would be performing in the new model. Finding answers to these questions was difficult, since committee members had varying interpretations of what had been agreed upon by the design group. The size of each class, as well as the dates and times allotted for the therapy modules, was also changed frequently to accommodate all care partners.

The final education program consisted of ten eight-hour work days to competently cross prepare the new care partners. (See Chapter 13 for a detailed description of the education program.) Initial class sizes were twenty to thirty people. For all staff on the orthopedic unit to complete the education, a time frame of six to eight weeks was projected. This included staff from all shifts, some per diem staff, and the physical and occupational therapy staff regularly assigned to the unit. PT and OT modules, including didactic material, lab sessions, and competency check outs, were completed in two and one-half days—a total of sixteen hours. Actual practicums with patients and observed by a PT or an OT were difficult to schedule with all care partners. Additional training and coaching had to take place on the unit once caregivers actually began to perform the new tasks. In addition, some of the patient care partners were not only new to patient-focused care and the orthopedic unit, but they were also new to the medical center and had varying levels of patient care experience. Combining these new recruits in classes with experienced staff posed an additional challenge to educators.

Although the complexity of the process and need for flexibility were acknowledged, it was also difficult to properly cover the patient care areas and provide adequate therapy to patients during the education program. The department faced some hard decisions regarding the provision of education and the provision of direct patient care with limited resources. Efforts to enhance coverage with registry and per diem personnel revealed that temporary staff simply were not available. Regular therapy staff offered overtime hours to help with the project. Some staff came in during a series of evening sessions to provide coaching and supervised practice time with the evening nursing staff.

Physical Medicine and Rehabilitation After PFC: Outcomes of Redesign

The new model developed for patient care on the orthopedic unit was finally implemented in October 1993. Model design and education had been completed, but putting the plans into practice would also prove to be an ongoing and challenging process. All caregivers would be expected to shift their attitudes and perceptions about their work, their coworkers, and about how care was to be delivered in the new model.

Structural and Process Changes

The new model involved a reduction in physical therapy staff and an increase in nonlicensed caregivers on the unit. Physical therapy committed to two consistent licensed therapists on the thirty-two-bed unit, seven days a week. This represented a decrease of about five PT full time equivalents (two licensed therapists and three PT aides), considering the seven-day coverage. The expectation was that with the education provided, the improved communication and documentation, and physical renovations on the unit (desks at each four-bed quad area with order entry terminals, telephones, and the medical records for those four patients), routine activities would be performed by the "care team." Also built into the new model was a daily morning meeting involving all nursing and therapy staff on the unit. The meetings were to take no more than fifteen minutes and were intended to be used for planning the day's activities. All patients were to be briefly reviewed. Tests, procedures, and new surgeries were to be identified, and therapists were to delegate exercise and ambulation activities to nursing staff for each of their patients.

Morning Rounds. The morning rounds occur at 7:45 a.m. each day, and all caregivers participate. Each registered nurse (RN) reviews her patients, any changes over the last twenty-four hours, expected tests or procedures for the day, and any discharge planning issues that may be emerging. Therapists report the patient's functional status and coordinate the exercise, ambulation, and other activities which are to take place that day with nursing. New patients coming out of surgery or from other units are identified and scheduled. This meeting has proven to be extremely valuable to the team in assuring that patients receive appropriate services and that delays in start of treatment and wasted staff time are reduced. Currently this morning meeting, which eliminates many scheduling and coordinating difficulties, occurs only on the orthopedic unit, but similar forums for information exchange are planned for other areas of the medical center.

Communication with Nursing. Therapists have learned to work more closely with nursing staff, and have developed a greater appreciation for their skills and the demands placed upon them throughout the workday. Therapists have also assumed more responsibility for basic tasks such as assisting patients with bedpans, telephones, and meals. They have also learned to communicate more consistently with the unit manager in resolving problems and improving unit operations. Therapists still meet with their own department managers and refer larger operational problems to them. This has led to more frequent and better communication between the therapy managers and the unit managers as well.

Physical Renovations. The benefits of the physical renovations on the unit (see Chapters 11 and 12) should not be understated. With the installation of a desk at each quad (four patient rooms), additional computer terminals and telephones, and the relocation of the medical records from the central desk to the quad, valuable staff time is saved. Time is no longer wasted searching for charts; receipt and relay of information is often immediate; and communication between physicians, therapists, and other caregivers happens more easily. Family members can also more readily identify and speak to their caregivers, since they are likely to be in the immediate area.

Documentation. Revised evaluation and progress note forms (see Chapter 10) are easier to use and provide physicians and caregivers with clear, readily available information about the patient's functional status. Since therapy evaluations are now integrated into the progress notes section of the chart, some therapists feel that physicians are more likely to see and read their findings and recommendations. While theoretically this should eliminate the need for therapists to make calls to physicians requesting orders, which often delays treatment, objective data are not yet available to substantiate this improvement. Also not yet substantiated is the very strong feeling that therapists do, in fact, spend less time documenting and are therefore spending more time with their patients.

Role Evolution. One of the most significant changes experienced by the therapists has been the evolution of their role. Therapists are now assuming greater responsibility for the overall management of the patient's functional progress. This includes the delegation of activities to others who may also need coaching and education at the time of the delegation. It also means that therapists need to ensure more active follow-up of the activities in which their patients participate each day, rather than being physically present for each of the activities. Therapists must identify, very early in the patient's stay, the most appropriate equipment to be used, how to educate the patient and family members in carrying out specific home programs, and the best setting for the patient to continue recovery upon discharge from the acute setting. Patients are now leaving while still requiring physical assistance for most self care and functional activities. They are not independent. At times, therapists' evaluative, problem solving, and leadership skills are in greater demand than are their actual hands-on treatment skills. Their decisions have far reaching effects on the lives of their patients and must be made with wisdom and compassion. Many new therapists may be unprepared for this new responsibility and must rely upon the guidance and direction of their clinical supervisors and senior staff.

Team Building. An important key to the success of this kind of structure is team building. All members need to view their own roles on the team in a new way. They may also need periodic reinforcement of appropriate team behaviors as well as reminders when old habits reappear. Some members of the care team accept the delegation of activities from therapists less readily than others. This has resulted, at times, in the therapists becoming reluctant to delegate and slipping back to their old, more comfortable role and performing all aspects of the program themselves.

The role of the therapist on the team is still evolving. For team members to experience success in the new model, regular and consistent team meetings need to take place. Communication skills need to be developed and strongly emphasized both in the initial education and in ongoing team meetings. Individual roles and specific job expectations need to be frequently repeated and reinforced until the team demonstrates consistently high cooperation, coordination, communication, and follow through. Team building requires strong managerial commitment and a major investment of time and energy.

Departmental Reorganization. Lastly, with the implementation of patient-focused care and other simultaneous budget reductions, the PM&R department experienced an overall decrease in both staff and managerial positions. This led to a reorganization within

Figure 8.2: Physical Medicine and Rehabilitation After PFC Implementation

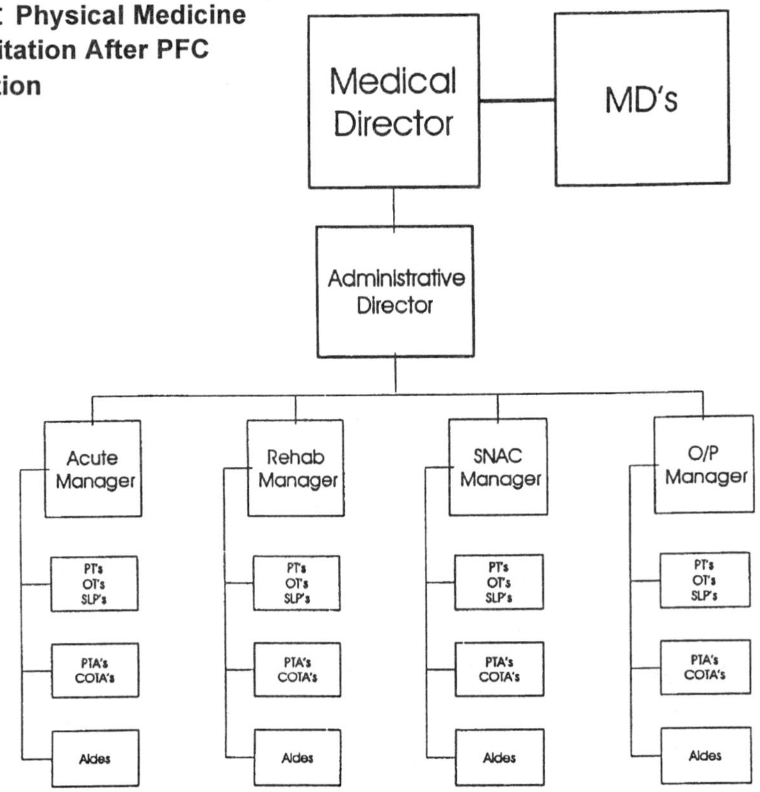

the department (see **Figure 8.2**) to streamline services, eliminate any remaining duplication, and continue to provide superior care with declining resources. The staff to supervisor ratio increased, management layers were removed, and the productivity expectation for each service area increased.

Challenges and Lessons Learned

Changes in the delivery of health care over the past fifteen years have been extensively documented in professional journals and newsletters and a broad understanding has been reached about the many factors contributing to the high cost and inaccessibility of care (see Chapter 1 for an overview). No manual has been produced, however, to guide the front line provider and his/her manager in making services more efficient, effective, and available within the current system. Many rehabilitation professionals are working with physicians, nurses, social workers, and others within their institutions to develop systems for care delivery that will result in better outcomes, reduced cost, and improved satisfaction. Seeking answers to problems facing the industry as a whole, they frequently contact colleagues at other facilities and their professional associations. Often, however, the needed information is not available. This chapter has been written to provide some insight, direction, and practical advice to physical, occupational, and speech therapists contributing to the change process within their institutions and their professions. The following sections summarize some of the challenges and lessons learned during the change process at Cedars-Sinai.

Role Changes

All therapy staff are working on developing a better understanding of their changing role on the care team. They are learning to become better decisionmakers, delegators, and communicators. They are becoming more accountable to nurse managers and accepting that their clinical background may not always be the same as their immediate supervisor. Therapy and nursing managers are becoming more accountable to each other as they recognize the unique contribution each brings to the team effort.

Educating New Staff Members

As attrition occurs, most newly hired staff (therapists as well as nurses and care partners) will not have been cross prepared in the skills they will be expected to perform. Thus, a new ongoing education program has been established which, in contrast to the initial PFC education, assigns the practical component and competency check outs to the individual care units. This structure places new demands on the department. As new care partner staff are hired for the orthopedic unit, for example, the two core therapists on that unit will assume responsibility for overseeing the hands-on therapy activities of those new staff until they have achieved competency. This responsibility has created scheduling and productivity difficulties for the therapies. Also to be dealt with is the need to educate new therapy staff to the specific operations and expectations on each unit, since procedures can vary considerably from unit to unit.

Rotation of Therapy Staff

The department has long acknowledged the need for rehabilitation professionals to rotate among the various service areas. The availability of rotations is an attractive part of the department's staff recruitment program. It is considered to be very important in developing well rounded professionals with the versatility and skills to evaluate and treat a variety of patient problems. This need becomes even more apparent from an organizational standpoint when employees take vacation and sick time and backup coverage must be assigned. The PFC structure imposes limits and special considerations when planning staff rotations. Therapists must remain on a given unit for longer periods (four to six months) in order to establish effective team relationships. The clinical experiences offered by that unit then become unavailable to other therapists. The potential also exists for a therapist to burn out and to lose skills if he/she is not challenged by a wider variety of patient problems.

Student Programs in Physical and Occupational Therapy

The clinical education programs in PT and OT at Cedars-Sinai Medical Center are well known in the professional community for their commitment to quality and comprehensive experiences for students. This comprehensive experience becomes more difficult to arrange, however, when the assigned clinical instructor is the primary therapist on a specialized clinical unit such as orthopedics. The student acquires a great deal of knowledge about the management of hip fracture and multitrauma patients, but the student will have little understanding of the rehabilitation issues for the liver transplant patient. Also of concern are issues relating to productivity. As the student becomes more independent, decreasing the work volume for the student's clinical instructor (the primary therapist on the unit), what does the primary therapist do while the student is safely performing assigned duties?

Seven-Day Coverage

With improvements in systems and operations and a continuing trend toward reducing lengths of stay in acute care, more discussion is taking place concerning providing full hospital services seven days a week. For therapy services, this presents considerable challenges. The department currently provides full service five days, with reduced coverage on weekends. Efforts to supplement weekend therapy coverage with per diem staff have been only minimally successful, and the ability to achieve full seven-day staffing and service has been severely limited by budgetary and human resource constraints. Recognizing that delays in therapy can extend the patient's hospital stay, the department is continuing to look for creative ways to address these issues.

Multidisciplinary Quality Improvement

Despite the notable improvement in communication and collaboration between nursing and therapy, consistency in quality monitoring systems is still a challenge. The approach remains department-oriented (i.e., therapy looks at patients' functional gains during the hospitalization while nursing monitors such items as infection rates and acquisition of decubitus ulcers). Increasing collaboration in multidisciplinary quality improvement measures provides an opportunity for further improvement.

Reporting Structure

The matrix management structure continues to pose challenges. In this change process, differences in the cultures of the nursing department and the PM&R department have become evident. Therapy departments have historically operated with a participatory team-oriented philosophy. Clinical education programs are centered around the team concept and, after graduating and entering the work force, therapists bring this focus (and expectation) into the work place. There is a great deal of collaboration and group discussion when engaged in problem solving or program planning. Therapists want, and expect, to have a voice, to make contributions to changes in the department. Therapists on the unit have also noted the importance of their participation in unit staff meetings and inservices and having access to the information regarding changes on the unit that is available to the nursing staff.

Recommendations for PFC Restructuring

The following recommendations are designed to help other institutions as they embark on their own PFC planning processes.

1) Allow ample time for the planning phase of the project, including time for an adequate examination, understanding, and interpretation of all data used for decision making. If the project is identified as a priority by the executive management group, it will consume a great deal of time and it may be wise to delay other projects and departmental changes until involvement in the restructuring project has decreased.

2) Quickly identify all agendas, realizing that the desired outcomes are improvements in quality as well as a reduction in costs.

3) Know the state laws governing your professional practice and that of others. Model design includes identifying services that can only be provided by licensed professionals, as well as those activities currently performed by licensed staff that do not require their level of education, skill, or cost. Current responsibilities of aides or technicians will be closely examined and staff changes will be negotiated, particularly with respect to the volume of work that can be performed by non-licensed caregivers.

4) Be aware of what colleagues are doing at other facilities—standard of practice in the community is a powerful persuader.

5) Allow adequate time for education—both for nursing and for therapy staff. It is especially important to build in adequate time for the hands-on practice component. Allowances must be made in the schedule for learners who may need more time. There is no substitute for providing the time and resources for newly educated staff to apply these skills with actual patients while a skilled clinician observes and coaches. If not incorporated in the education program, these education activities cannot easily be absorbed into routine work and will require additional therapy staff to effectively assist unit staff in achieving competency in their new duties.

6) Build in the cost of back-up coverage to provide patient care when therapy staff is participating in the education program. This coverage will probably be necessary for several months depending on the number of staff needing education.

7) Build in an ongoing structure for team development after PFC has been implemented. It may not happen automatically and people may slip back into their old, comfortable behavior patterns.

8) Provide education to therapy staff in the areas of delegation, communication, and team building. Most therapists are not automatically comfortable with these new responsibilities. They should also be given time for discussion regarding the changing role of the therapist in health care and the need to begin viewing themselves differently in order to function most effectively in the new structure.

9) Plan for, and provide time for communication between all disciplines, departments, and levels of staff. Lack of information and/or misinformation can be detrimental to the success of the project.

10) Recognize that time is needed to change behaviors as well as underlying attitudes.

Most professionals in the industry will agree that restructuring or reengineering the delivery of care is necessary. A project of this scope and complexity should only be undertaken, however, after research, analysis, and discussion with all involved players. Its impact is far reaching, and Cedars-Sinai is only beginning to realize the benefits of this work. The basic concepts and principles of PFC are good—to take care of patients better, more efficiently, and at less cost. PFC comprises one aspect of a continuous and comprehensive effort to achieve these goals.

Chapter 9

Patient-Focused Care Model For Social Work and Utilization Management

Sharon Mass, PhD, LCSW
David Esquith, LCSW, MPA
Betty Johnson, RN

Many dramatic and sudden changes in the patient census and the financial reimbursement structure of health care in Southern California mandated that local hospitals reexamine and redesign their methods of patient care. This chapter presents social work, discharge planning, and utilization management at Cedars-Sinai Medical Center as it was prior to the patient-focused care redesign; and how, with the redesign, a different model of delivery emerged. This new model integrates elements of social work, discharge planning, and utilization management into a case management approach to patients.

Historical Perspective

Prior to patient-focused care, the Department of Medical Social Work and the Department of Utilization Management, while linked as parts of the entire Cedars-Sinai hospital system, functioned as two separate and distinct departments. The social work staff (all master's-prepared social workers) were members of a centralized department who were assigned to specific services and had direct patient care responsibilities for psychosocial assessment, support, and intervention. They provided community resource referrals and transacted all placements of patients to alternate levels of care (rehabilitation, sub-acute, skilled nursing, board and care, etc.). Social workers did not treat every patient on the unit, instead they were referred to specific patients by physicians and other health care professionals (utilization management coordinators, RNs, PTs, etc.), or patients or patients' families. Although social workers collaborated with the patient caregivers as needed, the social workers' function was autonomous and independent of the unit.

SHARON MASS, PHD, LCSW — Director, Medical Social Work/Utilization Management, Cedars-Sinai Medical Center.

DAVID ESQUITH, LCSW, MPA — Associate Director, Medical Social Work, Cedars-Sinai Medical Center.

BETTY JOHNSON, RN — Associate Director, Utilization Management, Cedars-Sinai Medical Center.

Similar to the social work department, the utilization management coordinators were members of a centralized department who were assigned to specific units. Their responsibilities included the following: concurrent reviewing of charts for appropriateness/timeliness of care, initiating discharge planning referrals to social work and home care departments, collecting data regarding quality issues and health services research, and acting as primary contact for payer information and other related but non-direct patient care contacts. The utilization management coordinator reviewed all patients' charts, provided specific information to all payers, and communicated with physicians about specific care issues. Like social workers, the utilization management coordinator functioned autonomously on the unit.

These two disciplines met daily on the patient unit (with the unit nursing manager and home care coordinator as available) to review patients' status for post-hospital needs. At these meetings, a tentative plan for discharge would be proposed. Other than this information exchange, the social work and utilization management functions were separate in role and department. Occasionally, a patient disposition problem would arise which would necessitate a consultation between the two disciplines, but the respective roles were clearly maintained. When the patient-focused care planning process began, the directors of social work and utilization management participated in the development of the patient-focused care design principles.

After Implementation of Patient-Focused Care

At the patient-focused care design meetings, several model key principles were identified. The design principles of managed demand, redesigned work, and empowered employees predicated the decision that social work would remain a centralized department with oversight for staffing, supervision, and education. Additionally, as a discipline it would be minimally cross-trained. On a daily basis, the individual social worker would be considered a member of the multidisciplinary group of caregivers and would participate in daily meetings with the nurse manager as well as any unit specific clinical services. The nurse manager would provide input to the social worker's performance appraisal. This matrix accountability to the unit allowed for increased team work and more efficient service. In subsequent performance evaluations, all team members were given an opportunity to provide feedback on the social worker's performance. The team completed a form measuring the attitude, quality, quantity, and communication skill of the social worker.

Outcomes

The move to patient-focused care has resulted in several positive consequences for the social worker. Social workers are more integrated as team members on the unit. The function's visibility as a discipline has increased. Social work has become an integral component of orientation and education services for cross-trained personnel, and the unit now has a greater understanding of the social worker's role in patient care. This is evident for referrals for discharge planning are made earlier in a patient's stay. Patient-focused care has enhanced the visibility of social work and opened access for participation on other committees and activities throughout the medical center.

Not viewed as a direct caregiver, the utilization management coordinator has remained peripheral to the unit. Part of his/her function in recent years, however, has been data collection on orthopedic patients for several focused studies conducted by the hospital's Health Services Research Department. With concurrent development of clinical pathways and guidelines for patients on the orthopedic unit, medical social work and utilization management directors determined that a collaborative approach would yield a more coordinated level of post-hospital care planning. The social worker and the utilization management coordinator on the orthopedic unit were partnered to cover certain tasks, to conduct quality assurance reviews, and to identify and discharge patients more efficiently. The average length of stay on this unit dropped significantly, from 7.0 days before patient-focused care redesign to 4.9 days ($F[1,309]=12.10$, $p < 0.001$) after the redesign, with no significant change in the severity of patients for these two time frames. The coordinated social worker/utilization management dyad initiating discharge planning from the point of admission was an important factor contributing to this shortened length of stay.

Patient-Focused Care as a Rationale for Case Management

Patient-focused care represented a major restructuring effort in response to the changing health care climate at Cedars-Sinai. Patients were being admitted more acutely ill and discharged with more acute care needs. Payer requirements were changing daily. A more coordinated approach to the social work, discharge planning, and utilization management function was needed. To further the concept of cross training and integration of these functions, a Quality Action Team was created to develop a model of service delivery that would achieve a seamless level of case management. The goal was to implement a reorganization of social work, discharge planning, and the utilization management function, and to integrate cross training with the two disciplines.

This work group began much like the patient-focused care implementation group. It was comprised of social workers, utilization management coordinators, and the managers from each department. The group developed a list of all the tasks and functions each service provided. They then reviewed each function to ascertain the feasibility of cross training. The finished document required seven months to finalize (see **Table 10.1**). During that time the position of director of utilization management was eliminated and both functions were assigned to report to the director of medical social work. It was planned that each dyad would be housed in an office on their respective nursing unit and function as a case management team. The management/supervisory/support staff would be centrally located in a common area to facilitate ease of communication and operations. This physical relocation/dyad redesign was halted with the infamous Northridge earthquake in January 1994. Several buildings were destroyed, and a space large enough to accommodate all staff was no longer available.

Concomitant with the earthquake was a sudden and unexpected drop in patient census and a drastic decrease in patient reimbursement. In response to these developments a hospital-wide case management initiative was developed. A work group was formed including members from every department interacting in the preadmission, hospital, and post-hospital process. This group developed a vision, job description, and reporting structure for case management for the hospital. (See **Figure 9.1** for the job description.) The initial focus was inpatient admissions and the development process took four months.

Cross Preparation of Staff

The goal was to utilize existing personnel and not hire additional staff. The utilization management coordinator was proficient in many of the case management functions and so the decision was made to expand the role of the utilization management coordinator into a case management position. The work redesign allowed the case managers to be actively involved in developing, coordinating, and directly influencing the care process. They would no longer perform 100% chart reviews. Instead the utilization management coordinators would be assigned to specific services/units, working with those patients targeted as high risk for resource utilization or discharge delays. The new role required that the utilization management coordinators interview patients, communicate with physicians and members of the care team, and follow patients through their hospital stay. They were still responsible for payer information and the data collection for specific studies conducted by the Health Services Research Department.

A ten hour educational program was designed to provide each of the utilization management coordinators with appropriate content to assist in the integration of utilization management and case management (see **Table 9.2**). With the change of role mandating the interviewing of patients and their families, and formally coordinating team conferences, the topic of communication/teambuilding skills was a significant issue as it represented a new and unfamiliar role. Currently, all but one (certified record technician) case manager are registered nurses; however, the social workers' role on the skilled nursing assessment and rehabilitation units is 50% case management content. Thus on these units the social worker is the designated case manager. It is possible that in the future social workers will assume the title of case manager.

Conclusion

Patient-focused care has served as an impetus to force Cedars-Sinai to look what specific services are delivered, and how and by whom they are delivered. The outcome has been the development of a new and different approach to providing these services. Plans include continued monitoring and evaluation to refine this new service delivery. The objectives/outcomes of the model include the following:

- High quality care on a continuum
- Decreased fragmentation of stay
- Decreased readmission rates
- Decreased length of stay

- Appropriate use of resources
- Patient, family physician, and staff satisfaction

Present plans include resuming the original intent to house case managers and social workers together in one office to facilitate collaborative communication for a more seamless delivery of case management. Future areas to explore will be the consideration of case managers effecting simple discharge plans where appropriate and moving toward the integration of the discipline of social work, discharge planning, and case management functions. Cedars-Sinai's experience in transitioning to case management is new and still evolving. The literature suggests that with a single case management process, coordination and discharge planning becomes more efficient and results in greater patient satisfaction. That is Cedars-Sinai's goal.

Patient-focused care is a planned, systematic approach which is clinically driven and patient centered. Case management provides a process which facilitates and coordinates patient care in a seamless manner across the continuum from preadmission through post-hospitalization.

Table 9.1

DEPARTMENT OF
MEDICAL SOCIAL WORK / UTILIZATION MANAGEMENT
CASE MANAGEMENT SERVICES

FUNCTION / TASK	PRIMARY DISCIPLINE			CROSS TRAIN		RANK
	RN	SW	BOTH	YES	NO	
PREADMISSION PLANNING						
•Counseling with patient/family when questions are raised (e.g., by MD) related to planningand arranging hospital admission		SW		YES		3
Confers with patients/ family to discuss needs ranging from care of dependents (including elderly) during hospitalization to housing for out-of-town visitors						
•Preadmission discharge planning		SW		YES		3
Initiate planning for post-hospital care needs (e.g., home health attendant care, nutrition, transportation, housing)						
•In discussion with MD, rechanneling patients to more appropriate care sites			BOTH	YES		3

Table 9.1 (cont.)

FUNCTION / TASK	PRIMARY DISCIPLINE			CROSS TRAIN		RANK
	RN	SW	BOTH	YES	NO	
Patients in need of skilled-nursing care (whose MDs may be planning acute admission) can be assisted with direct SNF admit						
FINANCIAL ASSISTANCE						
•Identify payor class code, admit facesheet, and META worksheet			BOTH	YES		1B
Review insurance information to identify benefits/ limitations of a particular payor						
•Interface with Patient Accounting Representative regardinginsurance, cash, Medicare Part B, etc.			BOTH	YES		1B
Discussions concerning insurance benefits/ limitations as well as to initiate arrangements for financial assistance needs identified						
•Transfer issues: cash account, MediCal accounts, out-of-network cases, etc.		UM		YES		1B

Table 9.1 (cont.)

FUNCTION / TASK	PRIMARY DISCIPLINE (RN / SW / BOTH)	CROSS TRAIN (YES / NO)	RANK
•Advocacy with payors regarding patient eligibility and requirements PRN	BOTH	YES	1B
Discussion with third party payors concerning patient need for a particular service; advocacy for out-of-benefit services as a cost-effective alternative to prolonged hospitalization			
•Financial counseling	SW	YES	3
Discussion with patient/family around options available to them given fiscal constraints; facilitate the optimal use of limited resources			
•Facilitating access to entitlement programs	SW	YES	3
Arrange access for patients to financial/service programs to augment their care needs following discharge			
•Prior authorization issues: MediCal accounts, Blue Cross Prudent Buyer, etc.	UM	YES	3

Table 9.1 (cont.)

FUNCTION / TASK	PRIMARY DISCIPLINE			CROSS TRAIN		RANK
	RN	SW	BOTH	YES	NO	
CLINICAL ASSESSMENT						
•Physical functioning			BOTH	YES		1C
Identify the patients' current (and pre-morbid) level of activity including ambulation, self-care, transfers, community functioning, etc.						
•Emotional/cognitive/mental health			BOTH	YES		1C
Assessment of a patients' current (and pre-morbid) level of functioning; identifying any issues/problems that could impact on his/her (post)hospitalization period						
•Substance abuse/Mental illness			BOTH	YES		1C
Assess for, identify, and address issues related to mental illness and/or substance abuse; history, treatment, and current needs						
•Social supports			BOTH	YES		1C
Assess for patients' connection with family, friends, social organizations; who is available for emotional support, planning for care and/or providing physical care						

Table 9.1 (cont.)

FUNCTION / TASK	PRIMARY DISCIPLINE			CROSS TRAIN		RANK
	RN	SW	BOTH	YES	NO	
•Abuse/neglect		BOTH		YES		1C
Assess for issues of abuse/neglect (for all ages) including high-risk factors that may be flags						
• Crisis intervention		BOTH		YES		1C
Determine the impact of the current reason for hospitalization on patient/family and identify stressors and how well the patient/family is coping						
• High risk screening		BOTH		YES		1C
Identify factors that may place patient at risk for physical/emotional problems						
•Appropriateness of plan/level of care Admission review Level of care Plan of careContinued stay review		UM		YES		3
•Timeliness of care Sequence of care Provision of care		UM		YES **		3
•Quality of care/medical management		UM			NO	

Table 9.1 (cont.)

FUNCTION / TASK	PRIMARY DISCIPLINE			CROSS TRAIN		RANK
	RN	SW	BOTH	YES	NO	
CONTINUITY OF CARE / DISCHARGE PLANNING / MANAGEMENT OF RESOURCES						
• **Assessment of needs**		BOTH		YES		1A
Identification of the patients' limitations and what will be needed at discharge to address these issues						
• **Referral process: internal**		BOTH		YES		1A
To identify the people/services that would benefit the patient and ensure that they are implemented						
• **Discharge Planning Rounds**		BOTH		YES		1A
Attend both daily and weekly rounds prepared to discuss the patients on the floor with an understanding of their needs and the plans being developed for their post-hospital care needs						
• **Discharge location**		BOTH		YES		1A
Identification of the setting at which patient will receive whatever post-hospital needs he/she requires						

Table 9.1 (cont.)

FUNCTION / TASK	PRIMARY DISCIPLINE RN	SW	BOTH	CROSS TRAIN YES	NO	RANK
•Achieve timely discharge to the least restrictive environment		BOTH		YES		1A
Through early intervention, ensure that the identified discharge site is equipped to provide for the patient and able to accommodate those needs on the day the patient is ready for discharge; to also ensure that the patient receives only that care which he/she requires						
•Establish treatment plan/plan of care for discharge		BOTH		YES		1A
Identify all of the issues that need to be and will be addressed during hospitalization and create plan for attending to these issues						
•Long term care/early interventionand planning to facilitate timely discharge		BOTH		YES		1A
Ensure social work involvement early in the hospital course to allow for maximum time for intervention; look towards the patients' long term needs so that the discharge plan, ideally, addresses both the needs immediately following discharge and for the period beyond the transitional period						
•Monitoring/intervening with patients whose utilization patterns relative to discharge planning are inappropriate		BOTH		YES		1A

Table 9.1 (cont.)

FUNCTION / TASK	PRIMARY DISCIPLINE			CROSS TRAIN		RANK
	RN	SW	BOTH	YES	NO	
Actively work with patients who present as potential discharge problems (both from a current and historical perspective) to identify impediments to discharge and develop, in concertwith patient/family/AHPs, strategies to remediate the problem(s)						
•Insure-post hospital care/services are arranged **Facilitate discharge education and teaching** **Facilitate referrals to community agencies**		BOTH		YES		2B
Develop and document appropriate post-hospital setting and services; ensure that any education/teaching/training t hat has been identified as necessary has been provided, and coordinate plans for appropriate community based services						
•Management of length of stay		BOTH		YES		2B
In concert with physician and AHPs work with patient/family towards ensuring implementation of discharge plan within time constraints of need for acute care hospitalization						
•Third party reviews: Blue Cross Prudent Buyer, and other agencies/payors		UM		YES		3

Table 9.1 (cont.)

FUNCTION / TASK	PRIMARY DISCIPLINE RN	SW	BOTH	CROSS TRAIN YES	NO	RANK
•Planning/managing the movement of high utilization of resources patients		BOT H		YES		1C
Working with appropriate physician/hospital staff to allow patient to be managed at the lowest appropriate care level in the hospital and to facilitate the movement from acute (discharge)						
•Advocacy for appropriate use of resources		BOTH		YES		1C
Work towards appropriate plans being in place to minimize discharge delays and the unnecessary use of acute care resources						
•Information		SW/BOTH		YES		1C
Fully communicate (verbally and in the medical record) all plans being developed and implemented						
•Transportation		SW/BOTH		YES		1C
Ensure that the patients' needs to access necessary post-discharge services is in place (e.g., family, medi-van, other community service)						

Table 9.1 (cont.)

FUNCTION / TASK	PRIMARY DISCIPLINE			CROSS TRAIN		RANK
	RN	SW	BOTH	YES	NO	
EDUCATION						
•Health/wellness promotion/prevention		SW		YES		3
In concert with patient/family/AHPs, ensure that the patient has knowledge and awareness of and access to services that will maintain and/or improve health						
•Working with patients/families to encourage patients' optimal use of hospital resources		SW		YES		3
To facilitate the patient/family understanding of the levels of care and the appropriate access to the continuum of care						
•Teach consumer advocacy skills		SW		YES		3
Help the patient/family understand available community resources and how to obtain						
COUNSELING						
•Grief and bereavement work		SW			NO **	3
Provide patient/family with an outlet for his/her emotional response to illness/hospitalization and facilitate the development of appropriate coping strategies						

Table 9.1 (cont.)

FUNCTION / TASK	PRIMARY DISCIPLINE RN	SW	BOTH	CROSS TRAIN YES	NO	RANK
•Manage psychosocial crises to optimize medical interventions		SW			NO ***	3
Help patients/families cope with response to illness as a means of facilitating their acceptance of the need (or the acceptance of a need not existing) for a given treatment						
•Short-term supportive treatment(coping with chronic illness, managing crises of care taking, placement, and so forth)		SW			NO ***	3
Provide a supportive environment for ventilation and dialogue						
•Management of the risks associated with hospitalization			BOTH	YES		2A
Working with patients/families to defuse potentially volatile situations by fostering an understanding of factors affecting health care, interpreting occurrences in lay language, and facilitating communication						
•Adaptation to illness counseling		SW			NO	
Providing an atmosphere conducive to an open discussionto facilitate the patient and family understanding of lifestyle changes while exploring						

Table 9.1 (cont.)

FUNCTION / TASK	PRIMARY DISCIPLINE			CROSS TRAIN		RANK
	RN	SW	BOTH	YES	NO	
means for coping with them; exhibit emphatic understanding of how patient and/or family feel about their own situation—freedom to express sadness, anger, etc.						
RESEARCH						
•**Health services research guidelines**		UM		YES **		3
•**SF-36**		SW		BOTH		3
Administer the questionnaire to patients who are prescreened before admission to obtain pre-morbid lifestyle data						
•**Adverse drug reaction program**		UM		NO		
PROGRAM CONSULTATION TO HOSPITAL STAFF						
•**Risk management**		BOTH		YES		2A
Coordinate patient "risk" issues to help identify such problems before becoming "crises" and to help manage the response to such problems						

Table 9.1 (cont.)

FUNCTION / TASK	PRIMARY DISCIPLINE RN	SW	BOTH	CROSS TRAIN YES	NO	RANK
•**Bioethics**		BOTH		YES		2A
Serve as advocates for patients and families in the decision making process; help patients/families understand options while fostering communication						
•**Case consultation**		BOTH		YES		2A
Provide information and support to hospital staff regarding patient care issues						
•**Interdisciplinary education and collaborati**		BOTH		YES		3
Offer in-services and other consultation to improve the delivery of service through a better understanding of issues affecting the patient						
•**Educational forums**		BOTH		YES		3
Participate on Cedars-Sinai programs designed to improve the delivery of services through an increased understanding of the unique needs of specific patient populations						
•**Participation on hospital committees**		BOTH		YES		3
Regular and ad-hoc participation on committees designed to promote programs to enhance delivery of care						

* SITUATIONAL
** DIAGNOSTIC AND AREA SPECIFIC
*** DEVELOP INCREASED A WARENESS OF NEED/ ABILITY TO IDENTIFY

LEGEND:
1A-C Education
2A: Education without intervention
2B: Change job
– Education/Intervention/ Implementation

FIGURE 9.2

DEPARTMENT: MEDICAL AFFAIRS AND PATIENT CARE SERVICES PAGE:
APPROVED: DATE: 11/7/94
SUBJECT: JOB DESCRIPTION - CASE MANAGER
TITLE CODE: XXXX
REPORTS TO: Director, Medical Social Work/Utilization Management
SUMMARY: ______________________________

Under the direction of Medical Affairs and Patient Care Services, in a matrix reporting relationship, reach and maintain outcomes, including cost per case or per covered life, for a designated patient population as specified in the Cedars-Sinai Medical Center Business Plan. Assesses, plans, implements, coordinates, monitors, and evaluates options and services to meet an individuals' health needs through communication and available resources to promote quality, cost-effective outcomes.

RESPONSIBILITIES:
Routine
Through daily rounds on the patient care units, ensure that the right care is provided in the right place, by the right provider, at the right time, and at the most appropriate cost.

Follow-up on referrals to conduct comprehensive assessments/planning within twelve hours.

Manage in a case management system using ongoing interaction with patients, physicians, and other health providers to meet designated clinical, operational, and financial outcomes for aggregate patient populations.

Assist physicians, patients and their families, staff and payors in providing care for patient populations that is appropriate, effective, and efficient.

Facilitate frequent team "Case Conferences."

Act as a support in case management for staff whose focus are clinical issues.

Manage the processes of care of complex patients and patient populations across the continuum. Facilitate appropriate aftercare activities as defined by service line population needs. Coordinate education for patients and families.
Function as a liason with all departments at Cedars-Sinai and with the community to address concerns regarding the care of patients on a global perspective.

Communicate to third party payers related patient condition, needs, and benefits.

Ensure, negotiate, procure, and obtain insurance authorization where indicated.

Facilitate design and implementation of clinical practice guidelines and pathways; assists other professional disciplines in effectively developing and integrating support modalities into the guidelines and pathways to ensure than an efficient, comprehensive plan of care is established.

Special projects as identified in conjunction with multidisciplinary groups examining care processes at Cedars-Sinai.

Figure 9.2 (cont.)

Additional Duties

Identify quality and efficiency issues in the provision of care.

Interface with the Quality Management Department in concurrent and retrospective monitoring of compliance with clinical guidelines and pathways.

Promotes the role of Case Management within the hospital by effective liason with departments and physicians.

Attend and coordinate with necessary and appropriate multidisciplinary Medical Staff and Medical Center committees.

Assure that aspects of the Case Management system are consistent with regulations affecting the Cedars-Sinai (i.e., JCAHO standards; federal, state and local laws; Medicare and other third party requirements).

Develops and maintains a positive work climate and the overall team effort of the medical center.

Performs related responsibilities as required or directed.

KNOWLEDGE/EDUCATION

Demonstrated expertise in management, problem solving, critical thinking, and data management.

Willingness to advocate and to initiate communication with patients and members of the care team.

R.N. or applicable clinical licensure required. Bachelors preferred. Experience and certification in case management preferred.

Recent sound clinical knowledge. Must have experience in a particular patient population.

Knowledge of medical literature, research methodology, health care delivery systems, financial/reimbursement issues and Medical Center/Medical Staff organizations.

Computer skills (knowledge of spreadsheet analysis, statistical functions, and word processing on a microcomputer and ability to understand larger scope of hospital-wide information systems).

INTERPERSONAL REQUIREMENTS

Excellent written and verbal communication skills. Ability to influence decisions, gain cooperation, and facilitate change with physicians, all levels of management, employees and supervisors of other hospital departments on a continual basis.

Table 9.3: CASE MANAGEMENT EDUCATIONAL PROGRAM

I. CASE MANAGEMENT: THE BIG PICTURE

- A. The Future of Case Management
  1. Changes in the Health Care Market
  2. Strategies for High Performance Organizations
- B. Current Health Care Systems and Financing
  1. Cedars-Sinai Health System
  2. Other Systems, Payment Structures and Their Impact on Provision of Services
- C. Case Studies

II. IMPLEMENTATION OF CASE MANAGEMENT AT CEDARS-SINAI

- A. Introduction to Case Management
  1. Definition and Goals
  2. Case Management Process
     - General Concepts
     - Levels of Involvement
     - Case Finding
     - Key Responsibilities
  3. Case Studies—To Case Manage or Not
- B. Facilitation and Coordination of Patient Care Services
  1. Interface With Patient Care Service
     - Nurse Manager, Clinical Nurse Specialist, Direct Patient Care Providers, and Other Health Care Disciplines
  2. Interface with Patient/Family
     - How to Provide Information
     - How to Get the Information You Need
  3. Interface with MD and Payers

III. RESOURCES AND TOOLS IN CASE MANAGEMENT

- A. Evidence Based Medicine
  1. What is It?
  2. Why is It Important?
- B. Analyzing Effects of Case Management and Identifying Opportunities for Improvement

IV. INTERDISCIPLINARY COLLABORATION

Team Building: Communication, Collaboration, and Negotiation with

- Health Care Team
- Patients
- Families
- Physicians

V. SUMMARY/EVALUATION

- A. Summary Remarks
- B. The Next Steps

For Further Reading:

Bower K. Case Management by Nurses. Missouri: American Nurses Publishing, 1992.

Clancy C. "Patient-Focused Care: Danger or Opportunity." *Social Work Administration* 20(4) 1994: pgs. 1-11

Cohen E and T Cesta. *Nursing Case Management: From Concept to Evaluation.* St. Louis: Mosby, 1993.

Colone M. "Case Management and Managed Care." *Social Work Administration* 19(3) 1993: pgs 1-10

Del Togno-Armanasco V et al. *Collaborative Nursing Case Management: A Handbook for Development and Implementation.* Springer Verlag New York, 1993.

Mc Donagh K. *Patient-Centered Hospital Care.* Michigan: American College Healthcare Executives, 1993.

Parsons ML and CL Murdaugh. *Patient Focused Care: A Model for Restructuring.* Maryland: Aspen, 1994.

Quick B. "Integrating Case Management and Utilization Management." Nursing Management 25(11) 1994:52-56.

Section II

Redesigning Organizational Systems To Support Patient-Focused Care Models

This section details the redesign of organizational systems necessary to support the patient-focused care models described in Section I. Chapter 10 describes the concepts and forms developed for the new PFC documentation system, as well as how the system provides the institution's caregivers with a smooth transition from paper-based to future automated systems. The following chapter details the information systems environment at Cedars-Sinai, an environment that is similar to that present in many comparable institutions, and the steps being taken to provide technology enablers for patient-focused care within current fiscal constraints. Chapter 12 provides information on materials management and environmental services support for PFC. Materials management functions remain centralized and the department has assumed additional tasks, while housekeeping functions have been moved to patient care units. Chapter 13 provides a detailed description of the PFC education program, including curriculum materials and sample class schedules. Chapter 14 presents the human resources perspective, with details on developing job classifications, compensation, recruitment, and a section on team building and staff involvement in a patient-focused care environment. Finally, Chapter 15 presents the detailed evaluation plan, including methods and tools for PFC evaluation, while Chapter 16 presents evaluation findings for the Cedars-Sinai PFC effort to date.

Chapter 10

Documentation: A Clinical Application in Transition

Terry Chamorro, RN, MSN

Enablers of Patient-Focused Care

An "enabler" is an entity that must be developed or in place for a paradigm shift, such as a new operational model to occur. Ideas that result from the paradigm shift itself are also identified as enablers when they serve to further enhance the power of that change.[1] Well-designed documentation systems are clearly enablers of both types. Documentation initially serves as a potent tool to save time and improve efficiency in redesigning processes of clinical care. Later, because charting occurs on tangible and consistent forms, documentation becomes a powerful reinforcer of the new conceptual thinking. In addition, the improved management of information not only facilitates better patient outcomes, but can also enhance regulatory and risk management outcomes for the institution.

Automating documentation using computerized systems, particularly point-of-care clinical systems, is one of the most important enablers to support patient-focused care (PFC). Much time and effort must be expended, however, before the complete migration to the computerized patient records (CPR) defined in the 1991 National Academy of Science's Institute of Medicine report is accomplished.[2] Design, development, and cost issues have prevented deployment of clinical information systems in many institutions undergoing restructuring and the new operations must be advanced without this valuable tool. Furthermore, even if the institution were able to implement such systems, the steep learning curve and cultural impact of a massive conversion to automated clinical documentation would threaten to overwhelm a staff already undergoing rapid and unsettling change due to the re-engineering process.

Although the accelerated PFC implementation schedule at Cedars-Sinai precluded the immediate implementation of extensive new automated systems (see Chapter 11 for details), the documentation system developed for PFC employed a conceptual framework which organized data in a manner similar to computerized clinical systems. Designing paper documents to match the flow of computerized data increases the clinician's sophistication and helps break down user barriers prior to implementation of

TERRY CHAMORRO, RN, MSN—Project Manager, Nursing Research and Development, Cedars-Sinai Medical Center.

fully-automated systems. The new paper-based system allows for stepwise change and provides a transition period to facilitate the shift to a computerized patient record.

General principles of information management were useful in guiding the reconstruction of paper-based patient care documentation and resulted in a documentation matrix that had the potential of improving efficiency for the multidisciplinary care providers and benefiting operational change. The following sections detail specific information management concepts to consider when designing documentation systems, whether paper-based or automated, to support PFC.

Information Management Concepts

Information management concepts such as accessing information, creating a shared vocabulary, and controlling redundancy can be thought of as general goals that guide the development of new documentation systems, whether paper-based or automated. The following sections detail these concepts, along with some of the specific strategies used by Cedars-Sinai to realize these goals when implementing a new paper-based documentation system.

Information Access

Improved storage and accessibility of patient information is the primary incentive for computerized patient records. Although many financial and management benefits alone will be derived from computerized records, it is physicians, nurses, and other providers who will be most supported because instant accessibility to patient information at the time of encounter will allow them to make immediate and appropriate health care decisions for the patient.

Access to patient information on manual systems is often a problem for clinicians. Information should be ready and visible at the point-of-care, no less so when paper-based than electronic. Reengineering paper documentation offers an opportunity to position and display patient data in a less scattered, more user-friendly manner, significantly increasing accessibility to the clinician. Redesigned work resulting from the patient-focused implementation may mean that data and information are needed at different places and different intervals in the workflow. A "managed" approach that provides accessibility to information is important, even in the microsystems of daily patient care.

Shared Vocabulary for the Multidisciplinary Team

The patient-centered approach to care emphasizes that all providers must be moving on a single track in helping the patient achieve defined outcomes. This multidisciplinary goal-orientation offers the opportunity to develop new, interrelated methods of charting among team members, and to consolidate and predefine data previously reported in uncontrolled narrative form. Similar to computerized records, this change will result in a different kind of medical record, one that is very structured, encoded, and less "chatty," in contrast to today's unstructured, duplicative notes found in the paper record.[3]

The sharing of information among clinical team members is awkward in paper-based systems. Clinicians not only need to exchange information between one another but must abide by regulatory requirements that mandate clearly operational multi- or interdisciplinary documentation. In fact, the rigidity of paper forms appears to eliminate or significantly reduce the opportunity for true multidisciplinary charting because two or more team members may need to access the form and enter data simultaneously.

These issues have resulted in documentation that has generally remained compartmentalized by individual specialties. With this long standing isolation, different disciplines have developed their own vocabularies or workplace terminology. Restructuring the paper record brings with it the opportunity to build a common language for the total team which will migrate easily to electronic databases, overcoming one hurdle in implementing a facility-wide automated clinical system in the future.

Because the relationship between health care disciplines must become more closely aligned, the terminology used throughout the medical record must be universal and acceptable to all providers. This suggests that discipline-specific language such as "nursing diagnoses" may no longer be appropriate in documentation. Nursing diagnoses are noted to facilitate the planning process for nurses and provide a focus for relating interventions, outcomes, and evaluation.[4] They are also a means for holding nursing accountable.[5] Patient-focused, rather than discipline-focused, decisions must now be made in the workplace.

While prior to PFC implementation Cedars-Sinai had promoted nursing diagnoses as an excellent vehicle to communicate, organize work, and focus nursing research, the PFC documentation team felt that this singular vocabulary did not lend itself to the unified, interdisciplinary plan for patient care and integrated charting required by PFC. Others have also noted that nursing diagnoses tend to place limits upon multidisciplinary teamwork, creating a parallel system which isolates nurses from the treatment team.[6] What was needed to unify the disciplines was a problem list, using diagnostic terms acceptable to the full complement of providers including nursing. Although a few nursing diagnostic terms were acceptable to other providers at Cedars-Sinai as useful problem statements, in general, the diagnoses list was not appropriate as a multidisciplinary problem list.

To date, no national consensus on a standardized patient health care problem list exists. In fact, the lack of universal problem definitions and standardized vocabulary is identified by medical informaticists as a serious impediment to the immediate development of the computer-based patient record (CPR).[7] Without national standards to draw upon, current efforts are underway at Cedars-Sinai to refine appropriate problem lists using a single vocabulary acceptable to multiple providers as the vehicle for revised internal documentation systems.

Controlling Redundancy

Reducing Documentation Time. The most important goal for any documentation re-engineering project is to reduce the amount of time required for charting. The time spent by a nurse in manual charting of patient care has been estimated to be from 15% to as high as 40% of the work shift. Time spent in documentation by other providers may not be as well chronicled, but it is widely accepted that a significant percentage of any health care professional's workday is spent in writing lengthy, narrative notes describing consults, evaluations, and treatments.

Creating a quick, uncomplicated data entry method on paper for the clinician is one step in curtailing time expenditure. Reducing the number of pieces of paper on which data must be entered is clearly another. Other controls on time expenditure can be found in reducing the vast redundancy in manual documentation systems where the same facts are written numerous times in different places.

Individual professionals frequently identify redundancy as a major issue within their own documentation set, and the problem is compounded when the collective charting of multiple disciplines such as nursing, social services, and physical medicine therapies are taken together. Redundancy is initiated in the medical record when clinicians of different disciplines work separately with forms in different sections of the chart. It will occur as well when new forms are initiated in a patchwork response to newly-defined needs, demands, or regulations. Redundancy also becomes a problem when one discipline, lacking access to the collection and recording of information completed earlier by another health care provider, obtains and records identical data. Not only does this consume productive provider time better allocated to other tasks, but is also a frequent source of annoyance to the patient who must again recount his history.

Attributes of a Model Documentation System

There are many authorities that command attention when striving to build superior clinical documentation systems. Listing the parameters and influences acting upon the record and its content was an early step in the Cedars-Sinai documentation project. Awareness of these concepts not only aids the construction of a good record, but is important in building the educational processes for the implementation phase which follows. The following sections detail the attributes of a model documentation system and provide specific examples from the paper-based system developed at Cedars-Sinai.

Maintaining the Patient Perspective

The primary premise governing any good record is that it must reflect an accurate and concise picture of the patient at any given moment in the continuum of care. Without shuffling among multiple pages, it is important for a clinician reviewing records to find information in an orderly, sequential progression. Current paper-based records are often scattered, requiring a search across several sections of the chart to determine the status of the patient.[8]

Figure 10.1: Generic Patient Data for Team Care

CEDARS-SINAI MEDICAL CENTER

C S

PATIENT PROFILE

MEDICAL - SURGICAL

DATE ADMITTED	TIME ADMITTED	AGE	SEX ☐ M ☐ F	MARITAL STATUS ☐ S ☐ M ☐ Sep ☐ W
HEIGHT	WEIGHT	SPECIAL DIET		
OCCUPATION		LANGUAGE SPOKEN	INTERPRETER NEEDED ☐ Yes ☐ No	
RELIGION			DESIRES TO SEE CLERGY ☐ Yes ☐ No	

PATIENT I.D.

RELIGIOUS / CULTURAL / SPIRITUAL ACTIVITIES DURING HOSPITALIZATION

ALLERGIES / SENSITIVITIES: MEDICATIONS:	REACTION
CONTRAST MEDIA / DYE:	
FOODS:	
OTHER:	

ADMITTING DIAGNOSIS:

SYMPTOMS NECESSITATING HOSPITALIZATION:

GOAL(S) FOR THIS HOSPITALIZATION

Patient has Advance Directive ☐ Yes ☐ No ☐ In Chart ☐ CSMC Brochure Given

MEDICATIONS REGULARLY TAKEN	DOSE	FREQ	TIME LAST DOSE TAKEN

☐ Brought medication(s) to the hospital ☐ Vitamin /Mineral Supplements
☐ Medications sent home with family ☐ Nutritional Supplement
☐ Patient has difficulty taking medications

MEDICAL HISTORY	Date		Date
☐ Heart Disease		☐ Bleeding Disorder	
☐ Stroke/Vascular Disease		☐ Hepatitis / Liver Disease	
☐ Hypertension		☐ Diabetes	
☐ Pulmonary Disease		☐ Arthritis/Rheumatic Disease	
☐ GI Problems		☐ Musculoskeletal / Back Injury	
☐ GU/Renal Disease		☐ Seizures	
☐ Gynecologic Problems		☐ Psychiatric Illness	
☐ Cancer: Define Type			
Other			
Surgeries			

EXPLANATION OF SERVICES TO PATIENT / FAMILY

☐ Nurse Call System ☐ TV
☐ Bathroom Emergency Cord ☐ Education Channels
☐ Bed Control ☐ Fall Information Sheet
☐ Phone ☐ Meal Service Orientation
☐ Desires Phone Blocked ☐ Desires Menu Selection by Phone
☐ Volunteer Services ☐ Hospitality Center X4444
☐ Social Services ☐ Interpreter Services

☐ Instructed on Safekeeping of Valuables
☐ Refused Safekeeping of Valuables

Signature	Title	Signature	Title	Signature	Title

PATIENT PROFILE PATIENT PROFILE PATIENT PROFILE

Summarizing the Patient's Progress. Assigning one section of the records exclusively to chronological summary statements on the patient's progress is one way to provide all team members with essential information necessary to continue or advance to the next step in care. The patient's status as well as ongoing plan of care should be apparent from information contained in just a few summaries. Confining one's review to this section should provide the clinician with a vignette of the patient.

Department- or Function-Specific Sections. The remaining sections of the record may be left as discrete compartments for department- or function-specific records, much of it comprised of flow sheets and graphics that detail routine or repetitive procedures and activities. These are primarily intradisciplinary communication instruments, nurse-to-nurse or therapist-to-therapist worksheets, and are reviewed by providers from other disciplines only when there is a special interest in detailed data about periodic activities, monitoring, or treatments. When a phase of treatments or a subset of activities is completed, a brief note, structured or narrative, on the outcome is brought forward into the multidisciplinary progress section as an "executive summary" for the whole team.

Primary and Secondary Levels of Information

Sharing Baseline Data. Although constrained by a paper system, it is possible to collect baseline data on a single occasion that will serve all disciplines as the primary level of information throughout the patient stay. These data profile the patient, delineating meaningful information on the health history as well as current symptoms, medications, and concerns. The information is usually obtained by nursing personnel, since the patient's initial clinical encounter in the hospital setting is the nurse. However, the information is primary to every provider. If each new provider entering the case re-acquires the same information, the insidious process of redundancy within the medical record has begun.

Positioning Baseline Data. Positioning this baseline information in the medical record so that it is conveniently accessible to all reinforces the "write once, read many" concept promoted in the Cedars-Sinai documentation re-engineering process. Generic data are recorded in a structured, predefined format, keeping the focus on material relevant to the hospital stay, rather than an all-inclusive history which provides little added benefit. The Patient Profile for the adult medical-surgical patient, **Figure 10.1**, provides an example of primary data important to all providers on the team. The section labeled "Medical History" also provides an example of one method to remain focused and control the recording of superfluous information. This grouping is tightly edited to achieve a representative core of diseases or events which have the potential to significantly impact the current hospital stay of a typical medical-surgical patient. The list was restricted with the knowledge that other facts in the medical history, while interesting, probably have little influence on the present patient management.

Adding Discipline-Specific Information. The Patient Profile from is referenced by each clinical discipline on the care team before proceeding to a more detailed evaluation specific to the therapy or monitoring that they will provide. One section of the Profile, shown in **Figure 10.2**, also contains information which flags potential risks and indicates if another therapist should be consulted. As other health care providers enter the care team, microsystems of information gathering and documentation are activated. An example of a second level of information, obtained by the activities therapists in the psychiatric setting and building upon or "exploding" from the initial psychiatric Patient Profile, is provided in **Figure 10.3**.

Figure 10.2: Risk Factors Serve as Flags for Clinical Consults

MEDICAL - SURGICAL PATIENT PROFILE

DISCHARGE PLANNING HIGH RISK CRITERIA

Age: ☐ 0-5 ☐ 6-17 ☐ 18-44 ☐ 45-64 ☐ 65-74 ☐ 75+

Pre-Admission Living Status

- ☐ Apartment
- ☐ House — Easily Accessibility? yes ☐ no ☐
- ☐ Condo/Townhouse
  - ☐ Alone: self care
  - ☐ Alone: intermittant care available
  - ☐ Alone: family/friend full time care available
  - ☐ Alone: unable to care for self
  - ☐ Lives with family/friend, full time care available
  - ☐ Lives with family/friend, intermittant care
  - ☐ Lives with attendant
  - ☐ Home Health Care
  - ☐ Homeless Shelter
  - ☐ Group Home
  - ☐ Board and Care________
  - ☐ SNF / ECF________
  - ☐ Other Hospital
  - ☐ Is primary caregiver to another
  - ☐ Not available

Mobility Aids

- ☐ Collar ☐ Brace
- ☐ Cane ☐ Crutches
- ☐ Walker

Skin Condition: ________

Special

- ☐ Tracheostomy/Ventilator
- ☐ Trauma Service
- ☐ Multiple E R Admissions
- ☐ History of Discharge Problems
- ☐ High Risk Pregnancy/Low Birth Weight
- ☐ "J" Doe Admission
- ☐ Unfunded Patient
- ☐ Guardianship Issues
- ☐ Chronic/Catastrophic Illness
- ☐ Terminal/Pre-terminal Illness
- ☐ Disfigurement

Suspected Pre-admission Abuse/Neg________

Current Mental / Behavior Status:

- ☐ Mental Status Deficits
- ☐ Suicidal
- ☐ Depressed
- ☐ History of Non-Compliance
- ☐ Smoker (Amt / Day)________
- ☐ ETOH (Amt / Freq)________

Special Problems or Concerns________

Patient's Perception of Current Functional Ability

- ☐ Angina / Chest Pain
- ☐ Respiratory Problems with: ☐ Activity ☐ Rest
- ☐ Mobility Problems
- ☐ Incontinent of: ☐ Stool ☐ Urine
- ☐ Nutritional Problems
- ☐ Difficulty with: ☐ Chewing ☐ Swallowing
- ☐ Recent Weight: ☐ Loss ☐ Gain
- ☐ Activities of Daily Living/Self Care Restrictions
- ☐ Communication Deficits/Disorders

Usual Coping Mechanisms: ________

Sensory Deficits

- ☐ Sight ☐ Hearing ☐ Taste
- ☐ Touch ☐ Smell

Family / Self Participation in Care / Recovery

- ☐ Desires to be Active in Planning Care
- ☐ Family / Friends Supportive
- ☐ Family / Friends Active / Involved in Care

Learning Needs for Discharge: ________

Figure 10.4 is an example of a structured summary relating the patient's progress following a week or series of physical therapy treatments. Not only is it valuable communication from one physical therapist to another, the information is of special interest to the physician ordering therapy. It also informs nursing and social service of the patient's progress, which will be incorporated it into plans for discharge.

Each ancillary health care discipline has developed similar structured evaluations to capture the definitive data set required to initiate therapeutic work. To tailor the information more specifically to a particular patient population, several departments have developed unique evaluation forms for each setting (e.g., pediatric, acute medical-surgical, or acute rehabilitation). An automated clinical charting system would easily manage the duplicity of customization and microsystems, and the benefits to the clinician are apparent. Although, cumbersome in a paper system, multiple customized forms are feasible with personal computers, graphics software, and today's desk-top publishing capabilities.

Aggregating Data

Reconstruction of the paper record also affords the chance to aggregate data in a more logical sequence to truly contribute to information products or summaries.[9] In the same manner as customization for electronic charting, data entry is structured so that the user is led through a series of specifically-chosen data elements until a data set is complete. This results in choice, high-quality data that more appropriately and efficiently reflect the processes of a patient encounter.

Figure 10.3: Second Level Data Are Discipline Specific

CEDARS-SINAI MEDICAL CENTER
DEPARTMENT OF PSYCHIATRY
ADMISSION ASSESSMENT: ACTIVITIES THERAPY

INTERVIEW DATE__________

LIMITATION ON ACTIVITIES:__________

PATIENT I.D.

SELF CARE HISTORY:

	INDEPENDENT	VARIABLE	HAS DIFFICULTY
MEAL PLANNING & PREPARATION:	☐	☐	☐
APPEARANCE / GROOMING:	☐	☐	☐
USE OF TRANSPORTATION:	☐	☐	☐

COMMENT:__________

LEISURE / RECREATIONAL HISTORY:

LEISURE ACTIVITIES CURRENTLY PARTICIPATING IN:

SOCIAL__________

CREATIVE__________

PHYSICAL / EXERCISE__________

SPECTATOR__________

INTELLECTUAL__________

SOLITARY/ RELAXATION__________

VOLUNTEER / SUPPORT SELF-HELP GROUPS__________

COMMENT:__________

OCCUPATIONAL HISTORY:

☐ PATIENT EXPECTS TO RETURN TO CURRENT JOB DOING __________ AND RESPONSIBILITIES INCLUDE__________

☐ PATIENT HAS WORKED ______ YEARS.

☐ PATIENT EXPRESSES INTEREST IN VOCATIONAL REFERRALS

TASK PERFORMANCE SKILLS (ASSESSED BY OBSERVATION IN SHORT TERM STRUCTURED TASK)

ENGAGEMENT:
- ☐ NEEDS NO ENCOURAGEMENT TO BEGIN TASKS
- ☐ NEEDS SOME ENCOURAGEMENT
- ☐ DOES NOT ENGAGE IN ACTIVITY

CONCENTRATION:
- ☐ NO DIFFICULTY FULL SESSION
- ☐ ABLE TO CONCENTRATE ON TASK______MINUTES
- ☐ UNABLE TO CONCENTRATE

FOLLOW DIRECTIONS:
- ☐ CARRIES OUT DIRECTIONS W / O PROBLEMS
- ☐ CARRIES OUT DIRECTIONS: TROUBLE WITH > 2 STEP DIRECTIONS
- ☐ UNABLE TO CARRY OUT DIRECTIONS

ATTENTION TO DETAIL
- ☐ PAYS ATTENTION APPROPRIATELY
- ☐ MORE ATTENTION TO DETAIL THAN IS REQUIRED
- ☐ SO CONCERNED PROJECT WILL NOT BE FINISHED

PROBLEM SOLVING
- ☐ SOLVES PROBLEMS WITHOUT ASSISTANCE
- ☐ CAN SOLVE AFTER ASSIST IS GIVEN
- ☐ UNABLE TO RECOGNIZE OR SOLVE A PROBLEM

DECISION MAKING
- ☐ MAKE OWN DECISIONS
- ☐ MAKES DECISION BUT SEEKS THERAPIST APPROVAL
- ☐ CANNOT MAKE ANY DECISIONS TO REFUSES TO MAKE DECISIONS

FRUSTRATION TOLERANCE
- ☐ HANDLES TASKS WITHOUT BECOMING OVERLY FRUSTRATED
- ☐ BECOMES FRUSTRATED WITH COMPLEX TASK BUT ABLE TO HANDLE SIMPLE TASKS
- ☐ BECOMES FRUSTRATED WITH SIMPLE TASK/ REFUSES OR IS UNABLE TO FUNCTION

MOTOR FUNCTIONING	INDEPENDENT	VARIABLE	HAS DIFFICULTY
GROSS:	☐	☐	☐
FINE	☐	☐	☐

COMMENT:__________

RECOMMENDATIONS:

☐ ACTIVITIES THERAPY WILL BE DEFERRED UNTIL IT IS FELT PATIENT MAY BENEFIT

☐ IT IS FELT THAT __________ IS APPROPRIATE FOR & WOULD BENEFIT FROM THE ACTIVITIES THERAPY TREATMENT PROGRAM. THE PATIENT WILL BE TREATED IN SMALL GROUPS AND UNIT ACTIVITIES AS TOLERATED. TREATMENT WILL CONTINUE FOR THE DURATION OF HOSPITALIZATION UNLESS OTHERWISE INDICATED BY A PHYSICIAN'S ORDER. TREATMENT GOALS & PROGRESS WILL BE ASSESSED WEEKLY AND REPORTED IN THE CHART AND DURING MULTIDISCIPLINARY TREATMENT PLANNING SESSIONS.

TREATMENT PLAN:

DISCHARGE PLAN::

SIGNATURE OF ACTIVITY THERAPIST DATE

INPATIENT ADMISSION ASSESSMENT: ACTIVITIES THERAPY

Organized, clustered data allow quick review of information and give the clinician tools to make prompt decisions and initiate the next health care intervention. An example of a cluster of predefined data which lends itself to rapid entry and provides easy assimilation of a large amount of information is demonstrated in **Figure 10.5**. Converting to predominantly structured data also reduces the tortuous deciphering task as well as the inaccuracies that can occur from misreading handwritten notes.

Figure 10.4: The Structured Summary for the Multidiciplinary Progress Notes

PHYSICAL THERAPY TREATMENT SUMMARY

DATE TIME ______DAYS ☐ WEEKLY ☐ DISCHARGE PATIENT NAME______

PATIENT PROGRESS:

BED MOBILITY
IMPROVED FROM______TO______

TRANSFER
IMPROVED FROM______TO______

AMBULATION
IMPROVED FROM______TO______

BALANCE
IMPROVED FROM______TO______

COORDINATION
IMPROVED FROM______TO______

MOTOR CONTROL
IMPROVED FROM______TO______

R O M INCREASED FROM______TO______

MUSCLE STRENGTH
INCREASED FROM______TO______

WOUND CONDITION
IMPROVED BY______

COGNITION IMPROVED FROM______TO______

PAIN DECREASED FROM______TO______

OTHER______

PATIENT VERBALIZES
PRECAUTIONS / LIMITATIONS ☐ YES ☐ NO

GOALS ACHIEVED ☐ YES ☐ NO EXPLAIN:______

SHORT TERM GOALS: TIME FRAME______

IMPROVE BED MOBILITY TO______

IMPROVE TRANSFER TO______

IMPROVE AMBULATION TO______

IMPROVE BALANCE TO______

IMPROVE MOTOR CONTROL TO______

IMPROVE COGNITION TO______

INCREASE R O M TO______

INCREASE MUSCLE STRENGTH TO______

IMPROVE WOUND CONDITION BY______

DECREASE PAIN TO ______ON SCALE OF 0__10

PATIENT ABLE TO VERBALIZE
PRECAUTIONS / LIMITATIONS BY______

OTHER______

OTHER______

OTHER______

D / C PLANNING:
☐ ECF ☐ HOME ☐ BOARD & CARE ☐ REHAB ☐ HOME c̄ HOME HEALTH ☐ HOME c̄ O.P. ☐______

EQUIPMENT ORDERED / RECEIVED:______

FOLLOW-UP:______

HOME PROGRAM: ☐ YES ☐ NO

FAMILY / CAREGIVER INSTRUCTION: ☐ YES ☐ NO

THERAPIST SIGNATURE

PHYSICAL THERAPY TREATMENT SUMMARY

PHYSICAL THERAPY TREATMENT SUMMARY

Clinical Prompts

Quality of clinical care is defined as the degree of adherence to generally recognized standards of good practice and the achievement of anticipated outcomes.[10] Paper documents are poor at supporting quality measurement and comparison because the labor expenditure involved in extraction of indicators or individual data elements is unrealistic. Patient care documentation tools composed of predictive, structured data, however, do have the potential to improve quality of care because the configured data serve as "prompts" to the clinician. Structuring the data on a charting form encourages better performance by clinicians by delineating essential data elements, such as in the assessment of a specific physiologic system or actions circumscribed by standards of practice. **Figure 10.6** demonstrates documentation that prompts nursing staff to carry out standard practice activities on the orthopedic unit.

Exception Charting

The medical record is an important repository of sequential patient encounters. Often, the change in patient status is minimal throughout the progression of encounters, but this fact is difficult to discern in the typical descriptive charting format. "Charting by

Figure 10.5: Clustered Data Allows Rapid Entry and Easy Assimilation

CEDARS-SINAI MEDICAL CENTER

OCCUPATIONAL THERAPY EVALUATION PROFILE

OCCUPATIONAL THERAPY EVALUATION

RANGE OF MOTION	RIGHT ACTIVE/PASSIVE 1/4	1/2	3/4	WNL	LEFT ACTIVE/PASSIVE 1/4	1/2	3/4	WNL
SHOULDER								
ELBOW								
WRIST								
HAND								

STRENGTH (KEY: 0=Zero T=Trace P=Poor F=Fair G=Good N=Normal)	RIGHT	LEFT
SHOULDER		
ELBOW		
WRIST		
HAND		

TONE	RIGHT WNL	HYPER TONIC	HYPO TONIC		LEFT WNL	HYPER TONIC	HYPO TONIC
NECK				NECK			
SCAPULA				SCAPULA			
SHOULDER				SHOULDER			
ELBOW				ELBOW			
FOREARM				FOREARM			
WRIST				WRIST			
HAND				HAND			
TRUNK				TRUNK			
PELVIS				PELVIS			
L.E.				L.E.			

EQUIPMENT HAS	NEEDS

U E FUNCTIONAL USE	RIGHT WFL	WITH DIFFICULTY	UNABLE	LEFT WFL	WITH DIFFICULTY	UNABLE
HAND FROM LAP TO:						
OPPOSITE KNEE						
MOUTH						
OPPOSITE SHOULDER						
FOREHEAD						
TOP OF HEAD						
BEHIND HEAD						
LOW BACK						
PROXIMAL PLACING						
GRASP						
RELEASE						
LATERAL PINCH						
PALMER PINCH						
OPPOSITION						
COORDINATION:						
FINGER TO NOSE						
DIADOCHOKINESIA						
GRAPHICS						
MANIPULATION						
OTHER:						

RIGHT/LEFT UE USED AS ☐ STABILIZER ☐ GROSS ASSIST ☐ FUNCTIONAL ASSIST *BILATERAL INTEGRATION:* ☐ YES ☐ NO

Figure 10.6: Structured Data Prompts Clinical Performance

ACTIVITIES AND INTERVENTIONS

ORTHOPEDICS

PROCEDURES, ACTIVITIES

SPECIALIZED CARE	PROCEDURE, TREATMENT, ACTIVITY TIME →	7 0700	8 0800	9 0900	10 1000	11 1100	12 1200	1 1300	2 1400	3 1500
	WEIGHT BEARING PRECAUTIONS									
	NEURO - VASCULAR CHECKS									
	BUCK'S TRACTION (A = APPLIED C = CHECKED)									
	ABDUCTION DEVICE (O = ON X = OFF)									
	PELVIC TRACTION (O = ON X = OFF)									
	CERVICAL TRACTION (O = ON X = OFF)									
	IMMOBILIZER: LOCATION___________									
	SLINGS: EXTREMITY_____________									
	EXTREMITY ELEVATION									
	CAST CHECKS									

exception" is a system that has gained acceptance in the last decade as an efficient documentation method that facilitates the recording of pertinent information and reduces lengthy, unnecessary wording. The decision was made to endorse "exception" charting on both structured forms and in narrative charting at Cedars-Sinai. This strategy has been accepted by others as a cost-effective measure having the potential to significantly reduce the volume of documentation without sacrificing quality.[11, 12]

Since exception charting implies a stripped down version of charting, it has been subjected to legal challenge when not used in an suitable manner or backed by appropriate written policy.[13, 14] Conceptually, exception charting focuses attention on the truly rele-

Figure 10.7: Charting by Exception After Initial Comprehensive Assessment

CEDARS-SINAI MEDICAL CENTER

PATIENT ASSESSMENT

DEPARTMENT OF PSYCHIATRY

PATIENT I.D.

ASSESSMENT DATE ____ TIME ____ □ Initial □ Weekly □ Transfer □ Discharge | ASSESSMENT DATE ____ TIME ____ | ASSESSMENT DATE ____ TIME ____

PSYCHOMOTOR APPEARANCE GAIT

APPEARANCE: □ Clean & Neat □ Disheveled □ Unbathed □ Odorous □ ____

PSYCHOMOTOR BEHAVIOR □ Normal □ Retarded □ Agitated □ Restless □ Clumsy □ Tics □ Tremors □ Gestures □ Hyperactive □ Catatonic □ Waxy Flexibility □ Compulsive Repetitive Acts □ ____

GAIT □ Steady □ Unsteady □ Limp □ Shuffle □ Stagger □ List □ Unable to Ambulate □ Ambulates with Assistance □ Ambulates with Assistive Device____

WNL - CLEAN, NEAT APPEARANCE; NORMAL BEHAVIOR; STEADY GAIT.
WNL □ UNCHANGED □ EXCEPTION: | WNL □ UNCHANGED □ EXCEPTION:

L O C SPEECH

LEVEL OF CONSCOUSNESS □ Awake & Alert □ Drowsy □ Groggy □ Stuporous □ Hyperalert □ Responsive to Voice □ Unresponsive □ ____

SPEECH □ Conversational □ Normal Rate □ Normal Flow □ Verbose □ Pressured □ Slurred □ Rapid □ Slow Rate of Speech □ Rhyming □ Mute □ Aphasic □ ____

WNL - AWAKE & ALERT; CONVERSATIONAL, SPEECH HAS NORMAL RATE & FLOW
WNL □ UNCHANGED □ EXCEPTION: | WNL □ UNCHANGED □ EXCEPTION:

ORIENTATION ATTENTION MEMORY

ORIENTATION □ Oriented to Person □ Oriented to Place □ Disoriented X 4 □ Oriented to Time □ Oriented to Role

MEMORY Short Term: □ Intact □ Impaired □ ____ Long Term: □ Intact □ Impaired

ATTENTION SPAN □ Satisfactory □ Focused □ Distractable □ Poor □ ____

WNL - ORIENTED TO PERSON, PLACE, TIME & ROLE; SHORT & LONG TERM MEMORY INTACT; ATTENTION SATISFACTORY & FOCUSED
WNL □ UNCHANGED □ EXCEPTION: | WNL □ UNCHANGED □ EXCEPTION:

MOOD AFFECT

MOOD □ Relaxed □ Happy □ Anxious □ Angry □ Irritable □ Labile □ Euphoric □ Suspicious □ Depressed □ Fearful □ Agitated □ Apathetic ____

AFFECT □ Full Ranged □ Appropriate to Content □ Blunted □ Flat □ Inappropriate to Content □ ____

WNL - HAPPY, RELAXED MOOD; AFFECT HAS FULL RANGE, APPROPRIATE TO CONTENT
WNL □ UNCHANGED □ EXCEPTION: | WNL □ UNCHANGED □ EXCEPTION:

JUDGEMENT INSIGHT

JUDGEMENT □ Appropriate □ Impaired □ ____

INSIGHT □ Appropriate / Intact □ Limited □ Absent □ ____

WNL - JUDGEMENT AND INSIGHT APPROPRIATE / INTACT
WNL □ UNCHANGED □ EXCEPTION: | WNL □ UNCHANGED □ EXCEPTION:

THOUGHT PROCESS THOUGHT CONTENT

THOUGHT PROCESS □ Appropriate / Logical □ Slow □ Rapid / Fast □ Blocking □ Concrete □ Loose □ Flight of Ideas □ Tangential □ Thought Broadcasting □ Ideas of Reference □ ____

THOUGHT CONTENT □ Normal / Appropriate
Delusions of □ Persecution □ Grandeur □ ____
??? Hallucinations □ Auditory □ Visual □ ____
□ Phobias re:____ □ Obsessions re:____
□ Sucidal □ Thoughts □ Plan □ Recent Attempt
□ Homicidal Towards____ □ Thoughts □ Plan □ Recent Attempt

WNL - LOGICAL & APPROPRIATE THOUGHT; CONTENT NORMAL, APPROPRIATE
WNL □ UNCHANGED □ EXCEPTION: | WNL □ UNCHANGED □ EXCEPTION:

RELATIONS TO STAFF

MANNER ATTITUDE IN RELATING TO STAFF □ Friendly □ Cooperative □ Uncooperative □ Guarded □ Evasive □ Hostile □ Seductive □ Childlike/Dependent □ Suspicious □ Indifferent □ Antagonistic □ Sarcastic □ Argumentative □ Provacative □ ____

WNL - COOPERATIVE & FRIENDLY WITH STAFF
WNL □ UNCHANGED □ EXCEPTION: | WNL □ UNCHANGED □ EXCEPTION:

SIGNATURE & TITLE | SIGNATURE & TITLE | SIGNATURE & TITLE

vant issues in the patient's care, issues in which the caregiver has the opportunity to make positive differences. Charting by exception alerts the clinician to concentrate on communication of abnormal findings or changing status without repetition of the normal or that which is unchanged.

In the Cedars-Sinai interpretation of exception charting, documentation of the initial assessment or evaluation of the patient is thorough and comprehensive, establishing the baseline for reflecting abnormalities or exceptions as they occur. While documentation by exception formed the basis for some Cedars-Sinai nursing forms in the past, the concept was introduced to the other clinical departments and inaugurated throughout the total documentation system with patient-focused restructuring. With the recent introduction of collaborative clinical pathways for patient care, the concept also forms the basis for documentation, and the progress note is composed entirely of the outcome-oriented exception analyses. **Figure 10.7** is an example of exception charting built upon a detailed baseline assessment.

Flow Data and Graphics

Repeat transcription of information from sequential observations or monitoring lends itself to flow charts and graphic records, documentation tools long accepted in health care. Trends are easily noted in vital signs, weight, fluid intake and output, and so forth when displayed in a flow data fashion. Repetitive tasks such as turning the patient in bed, releasing restraints, and patient ambulation are also optimally documented on flow-type worksheets. With the redesigned PFC skill mix, it was also necessary to create easy, straightforward documentation for the Clinical Partner. In the design of new forms, physiologic parameters and repetitive tasks were transferred to flow charts. Work is also underway to combine several flow sheets into a single form to further reduce the paper shuffle. Cedars-Sinai's other clinical departments (e.g., respiratory services, physical therapy, etc.) have also reviewed their required data, adapting to the flow data concept. **Figure 10.8** provides an example of respiratory treatment managed via flow charting.

Regulatory Requirements and Standards of Care

Regulations and standards influence clinical charting. Much of the data contained in an institution's records result from regulations imposed by governmental or voluntary agencies. Additions are often made to documents following a facility's experience with agency surveys and written evaluations. Regulatory language differs considerably among care settings and, therefore, shapes their record keeping. For example, some settings such as obstetrics require reports at certain intervals and demand inclusion of specific data elements in the clinical documents.

The fact that patient care is a multidisciplinary effort is also reinforced by regulatory language. The care team's ongoing plan for the patient should be evident in a good documentation system. Despite such regulatory mandates, the care plan, with singular goals and synchronized interventions reflecting continuity among all team members, is seldom achieved in the paper-based record. The usual practice of dedicating discrete sections of the medical record to various disciplines may promote adequate intra-disciplinary comunication, but fails in the promotion of the inter-disciplinary thrust and planning.

The Cedars-Sinai documentation restructuring gave particular attention to the interdisciplinary approach and set about to promote a parallel approach and continuity in patient care through the Patient Progress section discussed earlier. Regulations speak to a number of activities undertaken in the course of patient care, for example, the condi-

Figure 10.8: Flow-Type Data: Respiratory Treatment

CEDARS-SINAI MEDICAL CENTER

INPATIENT TREATMENT RECORD
RESPIRATORY TREATMENT

THERAPY

--- CODES ---

BREATH SOUNDS	EVALUATION	COUGH CHARACTERISTICS	SPUTUM CHARACTERISTICS	AEROSOL METHOD OF DELIVERY
Cl = Clear	R = L	None = No Cough	Cl = Clear	MT = Mist Tent
S = Stridor	R > L	Dry = Dry Cough	W = White	OH = Oxy Hood
R = Rhonchi	R < L	Prod = Productive	Y = Yellow	AM = Aero Mask
W = Wheezes		N P = Non-Productive	G = Green	TC = Trach Collar
Crack = Crackles			BS = Bloody	TT = Trach Tee
Rub = Rub				FT = Face Tent
				ISO = Isolette

PATIENT I.D.

DATE / TIME →						
TREATMENTS / PROCEDURES						
AEROSOL THERAPY (C = CONT, I = INTERM / METHOD SEE CODES)	/	/	/	/	/	/
TEMPERATURE (C = COOL, W = WARM / TEMP °)	/T °	/T °	/T °	/T °	/T °	/T °
FIO_2 SET						
FIO_2 ANALYZED						
HAND HELD NEBULIZER						
MEDICATION USED						
DOSE (DESIGNATE IN CC OF % SOLN OR IN MG)						
POSTURAL DRAINAGE (P = PERCUSSION, V = VIBRATION)						
RIGHT LUNG (DESIGNATE UL, ML, LL, ALL)						
LEFT LUNG (DESIGNATE UL, LING, LL, ALL)						
PHYSIOLOGIC SIGNS BEFORE TREATMENT						
PULSE						
RESPIRATORY RATE						
BREATH SOUNDS (REFER TO CODES)						
PHYSIOLOGIC SIGNS AFTER TREATMENT						
PULSE						
RESPIRATORY RATE						
BREATH SOUNDS (REFER TO CODES)						
COUGH CHARACTERISTICS (REFER TO CODES)						
SPUTUM CHARACTERISTICS (REFER TO CODES)						
POST TX BREATHING (ACCORDING TO PATIENT) (I = IMPROVED, W = WORSE, U = UNCHANGED)						
M.D.I. INSTRUCTION						
MEDICATION USED						
DOSE (DESIGNATE IN # OF PUFFS)						
S.M.I. INSTRUCTION						
EQUIPMENT						
APPLICATION (S = SET-UP, C = CHANGE)						
O_2 DEVICE REAPPLIED						
NASAL CANNULA (DESIGNATE LITERS / MIN)	L/M	L/M	L/M	L/M	L/M	L/M
O_2 MASK (DESIGNATE LITERS / MIN)	L/M	L/M	L/M	L/M	L/M	L/M
VENTI MASK (DESIGNATE FIO2 SET / ANALYZED)	/	/	/	/	/	/
IF TREATMENT NOT GIVEN: DESCRIBE (R = REFUSED, U = UNABLE, O = OCCUPIED)						
INITIALS →						

COMMENTS:

TIME →	7 0700	8 0800	9 0900	10 1000	11 1100	12 1200	1 1300	2 1400	3 1500	4 1600	5 1700	6 1800	7 1900	8 2000	9 2100	10 2200	11 2300	12 2400	1 0100	2 0200	3 0300	4 0400	5 0500	6 0600
CONTINUOUS O_2 HOURS OF USE ←→																								
O_2 SAT % PULSE OX. (✓ = SPOT CHECK, ←→ = CONTINUOUS)																								
INITIALS →																								

SIGNATURE	INIT.	SIGNATURE	INIT.	SIGNATURE	INIT.	SIGNATURE	INIT.

tions for use of patient restraints. Many regulatory-demanded tasks are best managed in the flow-data format. Prior to implementation, the Cedars-Sinai documentation systems were carefully cross-checked to assure that any care component specifically addressed in regulatory language was positioned in a form.

Aside from regulatory mandates, nationally accepted standards of care influence clinical documentation. Diversity does exist in the care of the different populations. Psychiatric care of patients differs significantly from that of medical or surgical patients. In recent decades, professional societies have been formed to express special interests and address appropriate quality care for specific patient populations. Within nursing, cancer care and pediatric care are just two examples of such professional societies. Other professional groups represent specific health care disciplines such as occupational therapy. As gate-keepers for quality within the specialty, it is natural for these societies to develop "Standards of Care." These standards provide another potential influence upon documentation. Hospitals eager to demonstrate that they are "state-of the art" sometimes adapt professional standards and incorporate them into portions of the patient care records.

The Chart as a Legal Document

Documentation of clinical events and therapeutic maneuvers, communication between team members, and evaluation of care through research and review are three long-accepted functions of the medical record.[15] In addition to these roles, the medical record is seen by most clinicians as a legal document in that it delineates the care upon which medical treatment decisions are based.[16] Many believe that quality documentation is a reflection of quality care. If so, well-disciplined documentation has the potential to assist in loss prevention if one assumes that structured writing tends to inspire structured, comprehensive performance.

The revision of documentation requires an assurance that the composition of the forms is comprehensive enough for clinical charting and can withstand the scrutiny of the courts. This is particularly important when there is a movement to reduce and refocus content of the records. Many clinicians feel secure in detailed descriptions, vast word pictures describing the patient or encounter. They are concerned when any attempt is made to strip away the bulk of verbiage and reduce records to terse descriptors of the abnormal or the exception.

Structured data entry in which the user enters data in response to predefined prompts on the form represents a cultural shift requiring clinicians to learn new ways to synthesize information. Well designed documents constructed to reflect the clinical decisionmaking process, as well as the powerful regulatory requirements, have the capability of serving the clinician and the facility well should the challenge of litigation occur.

The Patient-Focused Documentation System

Systems Architecture

An early goal in PFC work redesign was to construct a single documentation system that would apply to all patients in the acute care facility. Cross preparation and the movement of personnel between settings is among the hallmarks in efficient use of a labor force. Therefore, it was thought that documentation forms should be consistent across all settings to ease staff adaptation when working temporarily in a new or unfamiliar care setting. Post acute care areas such as skilled nursing and acute rehabilitation were recognized as probable exceptions since these arenas are bound by a number of regulations and unique reporting criteria that influence the character of their charting systems.

Workflow Analyses. Early in the documentation restructuring process, workflow analyses were undertaken in the various settings, primarily to assure that information would be at the right place at the right time. Discussions about the work, however, highlighted the realization that the differences between patient populations were too significant to further pursue the single-system concept. Not only was there a different emphasis on the data elements relevant to caring for a specific patient group, but the nature of patient observations and encounters differed. It became apparent that retaining multiple systems using the historical groupings already in existence benefited patient-focused care and efforts to consolidate several charting systems into a single "one size fits all" system were abandoned.

Customizing Systems. Based upon this decision, documentation development moved to customize and refine individual systems as the best means of maximizing efficiency for providers. Each system was then enhanced by as much structuring or pre-defining of appropriate data elements as practical. Seven systems were developed, clustered in the following dimensions: adult intensive care, medical-surgical general care, intensive and general pediatric care, obstetrics, psychiatric care, acute rehabilitative care, and acute skilled nursing care. A similar "look and feel" was preserved among the systems, however, to diminish confusion for physicians and staff moving between settings.

Continuity

Each system is initiated by the patient profile, the baseline data form described above (**Figure 10.1**). Succeeding forms expand upon that baseline data and migrate toward discipline-specific forms that are retained in their own discrete sections of the record. The patient progress section, outlining the ongoing plan for care and the progress summaries, returns to the multidisciplinary perspective.

Problem-Focused Narrative Notes. Problem definition directs the cognitive care planning process and forms the basis for projecting logical and appropriate outcomes for the patient. The task force had a two-fold purpose in adopting the problem-focused narrative note. The note reports the continuum of progress made by the patient towards selected outcomes and, at the same time, conveys the plan of care by outlining the next logical step to be taken. Since the notes are in sequence, the last note communicates the latest actions and plan to the next provider.

PIP Charting. An acronym, "PIP," was devised for the structure of the handwritten notes. "PIP" stands for "problem," "intervention and response," and "plan." The acronym was selected both to prompt the written structure of the note and to facilitate education of staff in using the note. These individualized notes, meant to be brief, succinct, and sequential, have been adopted by nursing and the ancillary providers and are

Figure 10.9: Overlay for Home Care Follow-Up

HOME HEALTH CARE FOLLOW-UP PLAN

DATE REVIEWED: HOME CARE FOLLOW-UP PLAN PATIENT'S NAME:

FOLLOW-UP

MD ORDERS FOR HOME HEALTH SERVICES
☐ RECEIVED ☐ PENDING ☐ DECLINED

SERVICES ORDERED FOR ☐ SN ☐ PT ☐ OT ☐ ST
☐ ET ☐ HHA ☐ MSW ☐ HOSPICE ☐ INFUSION THERAPY

AGENCY TO PROVIDE CARE____________

PHONE______ CONTACT____________

☐ PATIENT INFORMED OF HOME CARE PLAN
ANTICIPATED START DATE FOR CARE ____/____/____

☐ PATIENT NOT TO RECEIVE HOME CARE:
☐ NO NEEDS PER M.D. ☐ NO SKILLED NEEDS ☐ PATIENT/FAMILY REFUSES

☐ PATIENT DISCHARGED TO SNAC / REHAB / ECF / ______ (OTHER)

COMMENTS

FORM 10151 1/95

EQUIPMENT ARRANGEMENTS

ITEM	DELIVERY DATE	ROOM	HOME	AGENCY PHONE	CON-TACT
WALKER					
WALKER W/ WHEEL					
BSC					
B. BENCH					
HOSPITAL BED					
WHEELCHAIR					
O_2 PORTABLE					
O_2 STATIONARY					
HHN					
ORAL SUCTION					
GASTRIC SUCTION					
APNEA MONITOR					

COMMENTS

SIGNATURE

congruent with the physician note and accompanying orders. Thus, rather than having a separate plan of care buried in obscurity on some page of the medical record, the care plan is dynamic and relevant to the patient's current circumstances.

Preprinted Labels. In instances where data were usually repetitive among patients, some disciplines took the summary note a step further by structuring these summary notes and preprinting them on label stock for overlay in the appropriate sequence in the patient progress section. One such overlay, the "Home Care Follow-Up Plan," is shown in **Figure 10.9**. Capitalizing upon predictive data, these preprinted overlays save time and avoid the difficult-to-read handwritten entry. Although the printed "label" is more costly, this cost is negligible when minutes of clinical time can be saved. During the planning phase, the cost of one minute of nursing time was calculated to equal the printing and processing of three to five of these labels, a fact that influenced the decision to use overlays.

The Transition

It is apparent that many elements influence the design of documentation systems. A model system should allow quick data entry, reducing time expenditure by the clinician to a minimum. The plan of care for the patient should be obvious and the status of the patient easily interpreted at random points in the record. Patient care should reflect the efforts of the team in concert with one another. Regulatory and reporting requirements for the setting should be evident and the documents, if properly completed, must be convincing and without potential challenge in a court of law. Although there are limitations to a paper-based system, challenges and opportunities exist to improve charting for the clinician through a systems approach. The system must match the workflow of its seting, however, and be responsive to a myriad of external influences while still demonstrating a clear perspective of the patient.

Health care professionals, like others, are rapidly adapting to new environments as the business world moves from the Information Technology Era of the last decade into the Networking Era projected for the forthcoming decade.[17] Remaining on a manual system during the facility's restructuring processes gives time for individuals to assimilate the newer concepts in data flow so that when automated systems arrive, customization to fit the workflow will be handled expeditiously and the introduction of computer systems will be less disruptive to the culture of the workplace.

The Cedars-Sinai documentation project was viewed as a valuable transition time to organize and manage clinical information under newer concepts while the institution positioned itself to implement automated clinical systems appropriate to the evolving enterprise. Data acquisition for future automated systems is expected to come principally from the manual clinical system.[18] A further benefit gained from this period is time for adaptation to the re-engineered operations of the patient-focused care. Automated clinical information systems, when introduced, will then prove to be a true enabler, further enhancing the power of patient-focused restructuring.

References

1 Lathrop JP. "Enablers for Change". *In Restructuring Health Care: The Patient-Focused Paradigm,* Lathrop PJ, Ed. San Francisco, CA: Jossey - Bass Publishers, 1993.

2 Institute of Medicine, Committee on Improving the Patient Record. The Computer-Based Patient Record: *An Essential Technology for Health Care,* Dick RS and EB Steen, Eds. Washington, D.C: Academy Press, 1991.

3 Appleby C. "Retrotech." *Hospitals & Health Networks* 69(5) 1995: 40-42.

4 Worthy MK, L Siegrist-Mueller, "Integrating a "Plan of Care Into Documentation Systems", *Nursing Management* 23(10) 1992: 68-72.

5 Krenz M, B Karlik, S Kiniry. "A Nursing Diagnosis Based Model: Guiding Nursing Practice" *Journal of Nursing Administration* 19(5) 1989:32 - 36.

6 Scahill L. "Nursing Diagnosis vs Goal-oriented Treatment Planning in Inpatient Child Psychiatry". Image: *Journal of Nursing Scholarship.* 23(2) 1991: 95 - 98.

7 Gibson RF, Blackford M. "Health Care Information Management Systems to Support CPI." *In Clinical Practice Improvement: A New Technology for Developing Cost-Effective Quality Health Care.* Horn SD and DSP Hopkins (Eds), New York, NY: Faulkner & Gray, 1994.

8 Burke LJ, J Murphy. *Charting by Exception: A Cost-Effective, Quality Approach,* Somerset, NJ: Wiley, 1988.

9 Hannah KJ. "Transforming Information: Data Management Support of Health Care Reorganization." *Journal of American Medical Informatics Association* 2(3)1995:147-155.

10 Krenz M, B Karlik, S Kiniry. "A Nursing Diagnosis Based Model: Guiding Nursing Practice" *Journal of Nursing Administration* 19(5) 1989:32 - 36.

11 Comstock LG, TE Moff. "Cost-effective, Time-efficient Charting". *Nursing Management* 22(7) 1991:44 - 48.

12 Burke LJ, J Murphy. *Charting by Exception: A Cost-Effective, Quality Approach,* Somerset, NJ: Wiley, 1988.

13 Tammelleo AD. "*Charting By Exception: There Are Perils*". RN 57(10) 1994: 71-2.

14 Tammelleo AD. "Court Holds "Charting By Exception" Policy Negligent". *Regan Report on Nursing Law* 34(12) 1994:2.

15 Weed L. *Medical Education and Patient Care*. Clevelan, OH: Case Western Reserve Press, 1969.

16 Fiesta J. "QA and Risk Management: Reducing Liability Exposure." *Nursing Management* 22(2) 1991: 14 - 5.

17 Suszkowski GJ. "Information Technology and Personal Transformation." *HIMSS News: Healthcare Information and Management Systems Society* 4(9) 1993: 6-7.

18 Levy AH, DP Lawrance. "Data Acquisition and the Computer-based Patient Record". In *Aspects of the Computer-based Patient Record.* Ball MJ and MF Collen, Eds. New York, NY: Springer-Verlag, 1992.

Chapter 11

Technology To Support Patient-Focused Care

Maggie Stempson, RN, BSN
Jeanette Polaschek, RN, MBA

As restructuring occurs throughout the health care industry, the demand for information and information services is increasing. The information services department no longer merely provides the data processing functions of financial and volume reporting. A paradigm shift has occurred in which information and information processing tools have become as vital to the delivery of patient care as the spyhmomanometer and stethoscope. The patient-focused care movement stresses broadening the skills of caregivers and bringing the care team closer to the patient. These fundamental design principles cannot be realized when caregivers do not have the "tools of the trade," at the point of care. Information and information processing tools, like medical tools, are requisite enablers to allow the caregiver to give care in a patient-focused environment.

Evolution of Information Services

Over the past ten to fifteen years, the role of technology and the Department of Information Services has changed dramatically. This is true of the information services (IS) role in the health care industry in general and at Cedars-Sinai Medical Center specifically. The IS focus has changed from traditional data processing functions, primarily supporting finance functions, to information processing and providing information to the clinical practice arena.

Changes in Technology

Early generation systems ran on mainframe computers. Mainframe computers are large workhorse machines, which are centrally located and maintained. The mainframe requires its own special physical environment and is, therefore, usually remotely located and inaccessible to the user. User access to the mainframe computer was via a "dumb" terminal. These terminals had a display device and a keyboard and lite pen as input devices, but no intelligence of their own. The high maintenance requirements of these

MAGGIE STEMPSON, RN, BSN—Project Manager, Information Systems Services, Cedars-Sinai Medical Center.

JEANETTE POLASCHEK, RN, MBA—Associate Director, User Support Services, Information Systems Services, Cedars-Sinai Medical Center.

mainframe computers made them unavailable to users during these maintenance, or "downtimes."

The mainframe applications, or systems, accessed by the users were not designed to bring information to the clinician. The emphasis was on capturing patient charges that fed financial systems which generated patient bills. Many of these systems were borrowed and adapted from the banking and manufacturing industries. The applications evolved into admissions, discharge, and transfer (ADT), and order entry and charge capture systems. These transaction-based systems did an adequate job of meeting the limited demands of the fee-for-service environment. Statistics and trends regarding revenue generation and volumes of services were obtainable.

The second generation in "clinical" systems coincided with the maturation of the minicomputer. The minicomputer was smaller and less costly. Although it still required a special physical environment, the smaller size allowed decentralization to a department -specific computer room. Thus, a proliferation in departmental systems was seen. Departments, such as the laboratory and radiology, were producing revenue and were viewed as funding the business of the hospital. As a result, minicomputer-based departmental systems for processing orders, capturing and generating department specific charges, and reporting on department specific revenue generation and product volumes blossomed. The focus of these systems was on automating the functions of the ancillary department, thereby maximizing the efficiency of the department, not on getting information to the clinician. Because it was justifiable based on revenue generation, institutions invested capital money in these systems.

The minicomputer technology offered more flexibility than mainframe technology in that it was less centralized and required less overhead. The user, however, was still restricted by the same "dumb" terminal access, and it was generally not possible to transmit information from one system to another. In addition, the user was still mystified by the technology and at the mercy of a system that could produce only certain types of information at certain times of the day.

Software development was also in a state of transition. Minicomputer software was meant to be "user" maintained. Programmers were still required to maintain operating systems, but the new generation systems were meant to be "turnkey" systems. That is, an expert user, usually within the department, was responsible for maintaining the application part of the system.

Hospitals across the country, which had already invested in mainframe technology, invested in minicomputer technology. And, hospitals across the country live with those investments today. Cedars-Sinai is one of those institutions. These systems and the computers on which they live are lovingly call our "legacy" systems.

As the evolution of mainframe to minicomputers was taking place, an evolution in communication technology was also occurring. In the mainframe world, computers could not communicate with one another. As a result, users often had to use multiple "dumb" devices to access different systems. The minicomputer era, and its software technology, led to the interface revolution. Complex communication technology evolved to transmit basic information, such as patient name and identification number, from one system to another.

The new generation of computers revolutionized the world of health care information processing. Chip technology came into maturity and personal desktop computers became affordable. Once desktop "smart" devices were affordable, the demand to provide systems utilizing this technology was extraordinary. Further, communication technology, which allows the transmission of large volumes of data over very fast and reliable networks, is now available. These networks not only allow computers to talk with one another, but computers can now interact with one another. The intelligent desk top device allows the user to access information from different systems via a single device. The user is able to bring the information from many systems to the desktop for use in clinical decisionmaking.

New Functions and Skills

Other factors, besides technology, also come into play when reviewing the new generation of information processing tools. The users of information systems are more computer literate than ever before. As the cost of computer technology becomes affordable and home computers are becoming as commonplace as VCRs, users demand that this technology be available in the patient care arena as well.

A shift in the reimbursement structure is also driving information processing requirements. In the fee-for-service environment, capturing charges so as to generate patient bills and revenue was the priority. The shift to Diagnosis Related Group (DRG) payment and capitated or contracted payment schedules, regardless of the volume and type of services rendered, has created a demand for systems which support decisionmaking and assist in the management of resources. The overall decrease in revenue flow resulting from the new payment systems has forced organizations to become "lean and mean." With fewer human resources available to gather and analyze information, information systems and tools have become fundamental to survival.

One final evolutionary phenomenon has occurred in the realm of health care information services. There has been shift in the skills required of staff in the IS department. Traditional systems and technology required frequent maintenance and, therefore, IS departments were staffed with technical experts. The need for clinical representation in IS was identified when the shift in focus from financial to clinical systems occurred. The new generation of information services requires still another new set of skills. The IS staff member must still understand the technology, but it is equally important to understand the shifts in the health care industry as payment systems change and restructuring evolves.

In addition to meeting these new skills requirements, IS departments are also called upon to assist user departments, which have fewer resources than in the past, to assist in defining requirements for new systems as well as system related project management. IS staff members are viewed as experts in planning for new systems and technology. Further, the expectation is that IS staff will manage the project plan, implementation, education, and support for new systems. Implicit in this expectation is the assumption that the IS staff member will be knowledgeable about intra- and interdepartmental operations and understand the impact of restructuring and reengineering. Ten years ago, IS departments were viewed as support departments that provided data processing services. Today, IS staff are involved in all levels of health system decisionmaking and operations.

Cedars-Sinai's Information Systems Services Evolution

Executive management in the IS department at Cedars-Sinai began planning for the new generation of information processing tools prior to the patient-focused care revolution. Strategic plans supporting the long term direction of the health system, under new payment guidelines and positioning the department to make use of leading-edge technology, were developed.

When the generation of minicomputers revolutionized the world of hospital departmental information processing, many institutions invested large amounts of capital in these systems. Although the architecture of these systems is archaic, these investments have to be protected while planning for migration to the new generation of systems. Cedars-Sinai is a classic example of this situation. Planning at Cedars-Sinai focused on three main areas:

- Communication technology,
- New generation systems, and
- Information systems support staff.

Communication Technology

Tactical planning to migrate from a traditional communication infrastructure to the new high speed, highly integrated network technology began in 1991. This new infrastructure planning and implementation was critical to supporting new systems and distributed processing requirements, no small task at Cedars-Sinai. The infrastructure had to be implemented in two eight-story patient care towers, an eight story professional and ancillary tower, and five multistory remote buildings, an effort that took place over several years. **Figure 11.1** illustrates this fiber infrastructure.

Figure 11.1: Fiber Infrastructure Schematic

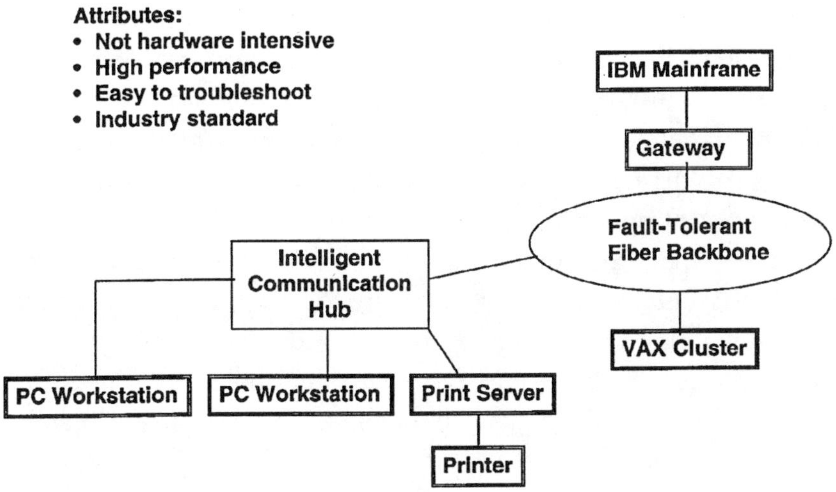

New Generation Systems

At the same time, planning for the acquisition of new generation systems began. Requirements for these systems focused on open architecture; that is, the ability to coexist with any other system, client technology where information and processing is available on a desk top device, and functionality which would support the new payment schemes and the management of patient care and resource utilization. It soon became evident that the vendors supplying health care systems had not yet caught up with the requirements of the industry. Development was underway, but systems to replace the existing patient management and order processing systems were several years away. Therefore, planning focused on maintaining these "legacy" systems while positioning the hospital for state of the art systems of the future. The demands for user friendly single device access to all of the legacy systems was so great that this also became a planning priority. Finally, planning focused on supporting departments which would eventually be faced with downsizing to meet the efficiency needs required to survive in a environment of diminishing revenues.

Information Systems Support Staff

Strategic and tactical plans were also put in place to develop the skill component in the Department of Information Systems Services (ISS). In 1993, the division of User Support Services was established in the ISS Department. Since the inception of the division, the staff complement has increased from four to seventeen. Clinical expertise also has a high profile, with four registered nurses in the department. At the same time, the technical staff complement has decreased and moved from mainframe expertise to the world of new technologies.

Pre-PFC Environment

Existing Systems

Prior to the patient-focused care movement, the technology environment at Cedars-Sinai was not unlike other health care institutions, and much of this environment still exists today. The patient management admission, discharge and transfer system, and the order processing system run on an IBM mainframe computer. In addition, this computer supports the patient accounting system, home grown radiology film tracking and pharmacy systems, and the materials management system. The clinical laboratory system resides on a DEC VAX cluster of computers. In addition, a results database containing laboratory, anatomic pathology, imaging and pulmonary results; a cardiovascular database; a drug information database; and the electronic mail system reside on this cluster. Interfaces exist between the IBM patient management and order processing systems and the VAX cluster to transmit data between the two computers. A critical care documentation system, residing on Hewlett-Packard minicomputer is in place in two of ten intensive care areas. An operating room scheduling and documentation system, residing on a PC-based Local Area Network (LAN) is also in place. (See **Figure 11.2**)

Figure 11.2: Current Information Systems

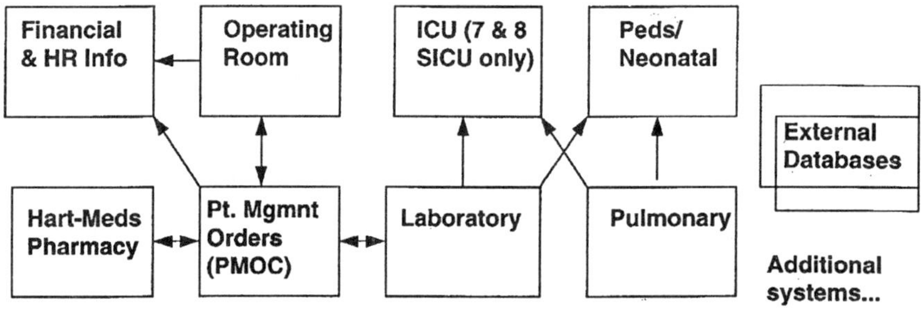

Data Entry and Retrieval

Data entry and retrieval was accomplished via IBM and DEC dumb terminals. IBM devices had lite pens to assist with data entry and retrieval. A menu application, residing on the IBM mainframe, allowed users to access both IBM and VAX applications from a single IBM device. Terminals were centrally located at the nurse station in patient care areas and in central locations in ancillary departments. Data communication took place over slow inflexible lines with "dumb" terminal and controller communication servers. Voice devices were centralized at the nurse station in patient care areas as well as in departments. Communication between care providers often occurred via the patient call system. **Figure 11.3** shows the nursing station prior to PFC implementation.

Figure 11.3: Diagram of Nurse Station

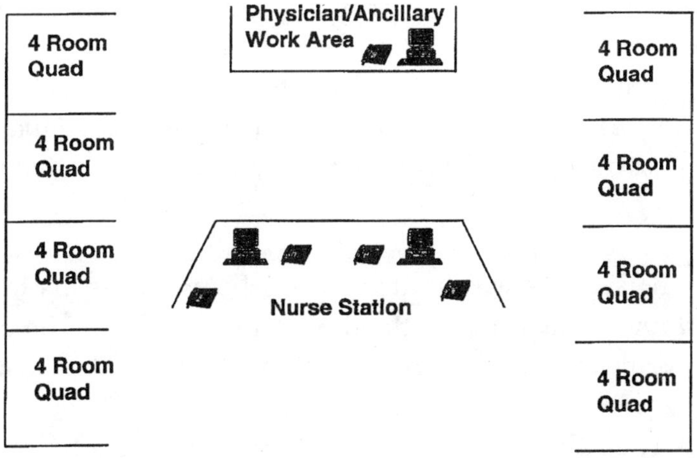

Access to system functionality was also departmentalized. Inpatient admission, discharge, and transfer functions were accessed only by staff in the Department of Admissions. Order entry access was limited to nursing or the specific ordering department. Although all nursing personnel were educated in the use of the order entry system, this function was primarily accomplished by clerical support staff because of the central location of the input devices. Order processing functions were accessed in the respective departments. **Figure 11.4** illustrates this order entry process.

Figure 11.4: Order Entry Process

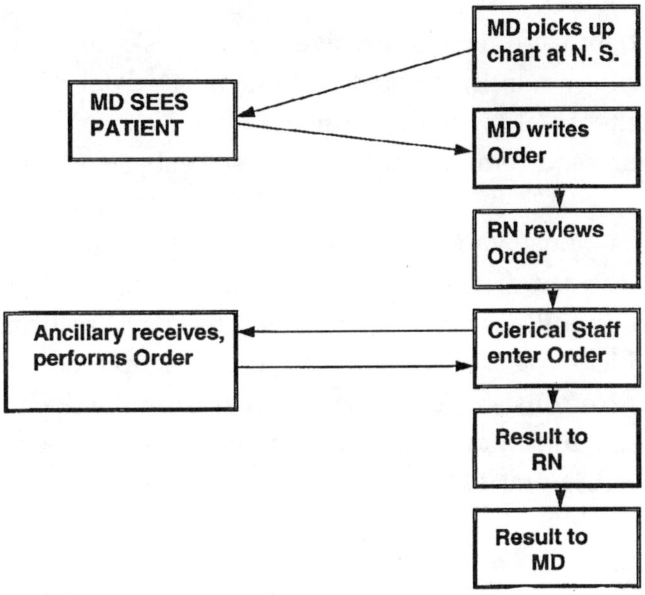

Results inquiry to the clinical laboratory system was available in patient care areas and some departments. This results inquiry was primarily used by on-campus users, although remote access was possible. The clinical results database containing laboratory, imaging, and pulmonary results was primarily accessed remotely by physician office.

Although inquiry to the pharmacy system was available via nurse station terminals, the use of the system was primarily by staff in the pharmacy services department. The imaging film tracking and operating room systems were used exclusively by staff in each department.

Physicians' use of the systems was limited. The laboratory results inquiry system was used by housestaff and some private attending staff members. The one exception was the critical care information system. As a documentation system with data entry and retrieval devices placed proximal to the point of service, the critical care information system has always been heavily used by nursing and physician staff members.

ISS Involvement in PFC Planning and Implementation

IS executive management participated in the Cedars-Sinai patient-focused care process almost from its inception. As the movement became defined and specific task forces were formed, clinical staff members from User Support Services became active participants. The importance of clinical representation from IS, as well as the participation of clinicians from other departments in the planning of IS strategy to support PFC, cannot be overemphasized. Patient-focused care is a redefinition of a clinical care model and demands a clinical background to translate the design principles into systems requirements and implementation strategies for traditional technical information services department.

ISS staff members were heavily involved in the task forces focusing on the admissions process, technology requirements definition, and model development. In addition, ISS staff worked extensively with departments, such as imaging, pharmacy, and emergency, to define system requirements and lead the systems acquisition process.

As planning for housewide implementation of PFC progressed, a specific technology task force was formed. This task force, initially chaired by the nurse manager of the PFC pilot orthopedics unit, was charged with defining and prioritizing the technology related enablers which would eventually support the implementation of the new care models. The task force consisted of representatives from the departments of nursing, materials management, and information systems services. PFC enablers were identified and prioritized. (See Chapter 10 for more information.) The priorities focused on the following:

1. Renovate the physical environment at the point of patient care.
2. Provide data and voice devices at the point of patient care.
3. Streamline current system functionality by both decreasing the length of time

required to execute a function and removing the traditional departmental boundaries to system functionality.
4. When possible, deploy the system to the customer rather than the other way around.
5. Provide easier access to hospital systems.
6. Implement order entry between the patient care area and those departments not yet automated.
7. Provide leading edge technology and systems to support patient care.
8. Begin planning for the replacement of current legacy systems.

Once the priorities were defined, the leadership of the technology task force moved from the nurse manager to the clinical IS representative and the charge of the task force became the planning and implementation of the defined enablers.

In addition to participation in institution wide task forces, the IS PFC project leader began building teams internal to the Information Systems Services Department. These teams were to be responsible for the deliverables as defined by the users. Countless hours were spend by ISS staff in these efforts. The PFC initiative, superimposed on an internal downsizing effort, created a true challenge for the ISS Department.

Technology Implementation and Outcomes

Implementation of the technology recommendations described below was embedded in the overall PFC plan to restructure the delivery of care and bring caregivers closer to the patient. This plan included minor remodeling of each existing quad (i.e., four patient rooms opening onto a common alcove off the main corridor) to install a modular desk with appropriate work space, provision for the storage of patient charts, and improved communications technologies. Thus caregivers would perform communications tasks (i.e., order entry, documentation, consultation with medical record and/or other caregivers) just outside the patient room rather than in a central area such as the nursing station. (See Chapter 12 for additional information on the remodeling effort.) The expected impacts of these enabling initiatives on the PFC service standards included the following:

- Timely transmission of test results,
- Decreased time spent in documentation,
- Improved coordination of care,
- Improved response time to patient call lights,
- Reduced lost charges,
- Improved physician satisfaction, and
- Facilitation of clinical pathway management.

The technology task force's specific recommendations are discussed in detail below. The recommendations are listed in priority order. In many cases, however, implementation occurred concurrently.

Intelligent Work Stations at Quads

The task force recommended providing data entry and retrieval ability closer to the point of patient care. IS recognized that the new generation of systems made use of personal computer (PC) technology and graphical user interfaces, thus the proliferation of dumb terminals to the point of service was not considered. To help meet the service standards listed above, the task force recommended the placement of a PC in each quad area. Before the devices could be installed, however, the communication infrastructure had to be completed. In May 1994, requirements for location and numbers of devices were completed. The fiber backbone had been implemented during 1992 and 1993. Between June 1994 and February 1995, seventeen horizontal fiber cable runs and four hundred data and voice cable runs were completed. The cabling was coordinated with the remodeling of the quad areas and the implementation of the modular documentation desks.

Concurrent with work on the communication infrastructure, IS began a design effort to provide PC software which would give the user single sign-on access to the multiple hospital systems, thereby giving the illusion of a single system. The design requirements for this sign-on application were:

1. Accommodate existing and future "dumb" terminal applications that run on the mainframe and minicomputers.
2. Accommodate newer client-server software such as a new Sybase-based radiology scheduling system.
3. Avoid making code changes to existing applications.
4. Give users a single log-on name and password across all applications, regardless of the operating system or hardware platform.
5. Provide automatic password synchronization among all applications.
6. Provide user-specific profiles so that the same workstation can be used by different clinical specialists.
7. Allow transfer of key information such as the medical record number and patient name between applications.
8. Use Microsoft Windows.

Support and maintenance for the PCs were a major concern for the IS department. Recognizing that many clinicians are uncomfortable with PC computer functions, and that IS did not have the support personnel to constantly restore files and configurations to individual PCs, a decision was made to "user proof" the devices as much as possible. The single sign-on applications locks out the traditional Windows functionality. Further, floppy disk locks were inserted to prevent the loading of software on the PCs. "Remote control" support, and automated, centralized software distribution were also design requirements.

The VAX computer is used as an access server. A profile for each user is maintained on the server. When a user signs on to the PC in a quad, the PC software transmits a message to the server which transmits information regarding the applications that the user

Figure 11.5: Cedars-Sinai's Clinician Documentation Desk

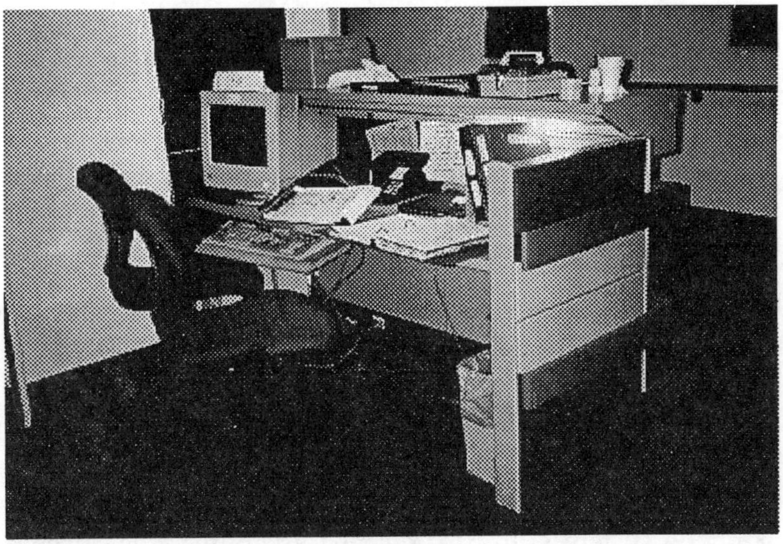

may access back to the PC. The user then accesses the desired application by clicking on the desired button. The PC software signs the user on to the application without further action from the user.

In November 1994, PCs were installed on the pilot nursing floor. Pilot operations continued until January 1995, when the housewide rollout began. By June 1995, 125 computers had been installed in the quad and nurse station areas. At lease one dumb terminal was left at each nurse station for users who either do not have access to, or have not been educated, on the new device. These terminals will be replaced once education is complete. **Figure 11.5** shows the modular desk with the PC and telephone, as well as workspace and storage for patient records that were installed in each quad.

Outcomes. Satisfaction with the new devices and sign-on application is mixed. Many staff members were dependent upon the lite pen for data entry. Although the same functionality is available with a track ball built into the keyboard, the transition has been difficult. Most staff are not computer literate and have some degree of difficulty mastering the mouse-like device. Further, although the systems accessed are the same as were accessed via the dumb terminals, the look and feel is different because of the Windows presentation.

Although the professional nursing staff had been educated in order entry many years ago, most did not use the order entry system because of the central location of the input devices. Further, the professional staff did not inquire for test results for the same reasons. With the deployment of PC devices to the quads, the expectation is that the caregiver will enter the orders. In addition to education regarding the new sign-on procedure, much re-education in the use of the legacy systems was required.

New Telephone System

Improving communications between staff at the central nurse station and the patient care staff was expected to impact the following service standards:

- Improved response time
- Improved coordination of care
- Improved service quality

In defining specific technology recommendations, the technology task force investigated telephone system replacement as well as other communication strategies such as beepers and locator systems. Beeper and locator systems were found to be very costly, however, and the task force recommended replacing the telephone system with additional systems to be recommended in future fiscal years.

A new modular phone system with user defined attributes was selected. The fact that the system is modular allows for future expansion. The user defined characteristics allow intercom and ring/no ring options as well as other amenities such as preprogrammed dialing and redial. Voice devices were installed in each remodeled quad area as well as at the central nurse station and in conference rooms and nurse manager offices. **Figure 11.6** illustrates the PFC configured nurse station.

Outcomes. Response to the new phone system has been very positive. Particularly appreciated is the intercom functionality. A staff member answering the phone in the central nurse station can use the intercom to communicate with the caregiver in the quad. The caregiver can then respond to the phone call without leaving the quad area. The fact that the ring option can be disabled in the quad area minimizes the disruption to the care giver and the patient.

Figure 11.6: PFC Configured Nurse Station

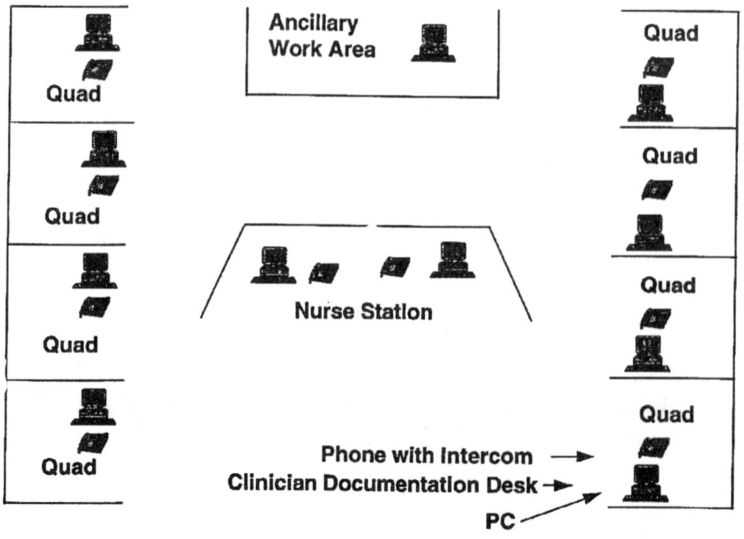

Fully Integrated Order Entry in Remaining Departments

Although order entry is implemented between the nurse stations and the majority of ancillary departments at Cedars-Sinai, departments such as the noninvasive vascular laboratory, food and nutrition services, and pulmonary services are still processing orders manually. Automation of the order processing functions to these departments will provide consistency in the ordering process, since all orders will be placed from the patient care quad rather than relying on manual orders being placed from the central nurse station. Further, order processing time will be reduced because the order can be placed immediately after the physician writes the order, rather than having to "walk" the order to a central location for entry. The number of staff members and steps involved in the order entry process are both reduced. **Figure 11.7** shows the post-PFC order entry process.

Figure 11.7: PFC Order Entry Process

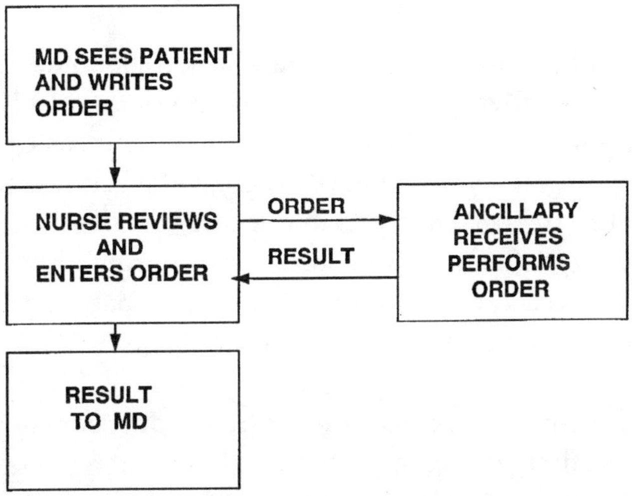

As available human resources were limited, the process for expanding the current order entry system did not begin until March 1995. Design efforts to support order entry between food and nutrition services and nursing are actively underway. Food and nutrition services is also actively pursuing the acquisition of a patient menuing system, and it is hoped that an interface between the order entry system and the new system will be implemented. Efforts to automate order entry between nursing and the noninvasive vascular laboratory and pulmonary services are scheduled for the end of 1995.

New Ancillary Department Information Systems

Cedars-Sinai purchased a new pharmacy information system in July 1994, with "go-live" planned for September 1995. Although the new system does not provide order entry functions that are significantly different from the previous system, the management-functionality is greatly enhanced. Therapeutic drug monitoring and clinical alerts are inherent in the new system. Drug utilization monitoring and reporting are also present in the new system as well as other enhanced reporting capabilities. This enhanced monitoring functionality has the potential to help reduce patient length of stay.

Efforts are currently underway to expand the critical care documentation system from the two ICUs currently installed to the remaining six ICUs. The first expansion will be to the pediatric ICU. Planning for new system acquisition to support departmental requirements are also underway in the departments of imaging and obstetrics.

Streamline Admission, Discharge, and Transfer System Functionality

Recognizing that the current patient management admission, discharge, and transfer system was not going to be replaced in the near future, the technology task force recommended streamlining the functionality of the current system. Further, in support of the PFC design principle to move services closer to the patient, a function that would allow the admissions process to take place at the patient bedside was recommended. In addition, the new function had to be fast in order to get the patient into the system and allow the delivery of care to commence.

The technology task force formed a secondary task force to design this new "fast path" admit function. Essentially, the new function mimics the old function, but redundant data is eliminated and the entry of information other than basic patient demographics is optional. An entry on a dynamic worklist is created each time the function is executed to enable admissions/financial analysts to track these patients and follow up on the collection of the necessary financial and insurance information. Performance standards assure that the information required for creation of a patient bill will be collected in a timely fashion if not collected at the time of admission.

Laptop computers were also purchased to facilitate admission done at the location of the patient. Communication technology, however, is still an open issue in full implementation of the bedside admission process. Currently, telephone lines in patient rooms are being used to dial in to the hospital ADT system. The recommendation is to have a data port in every room, and the IS strategic plan includes using wireless technology for this communication. Although cost is still a barrier to housewide implementation, a pilot is planned for the women's health area.

Prior to PFC implementation, staff in the admissions department was responsible for transferring and discharging patients in the ADT system. Because of fluctuating work volumes, delays in execution of the functions sometimes occur. The result is that the computer system does not show a patient who has actually been transferred in the new bed on the new nurse station immediately, potentially causing a delay in getting services to the patient. With the implementation of PFC, nursing staff are being given access to the transfer and discharge functions. These functions can be done via the PC in the patient care quad by the staff member caring for the patient. Again, the information is more timely, with fewer steps in the process and a reduction in the number of staff members involved in the transaction is reduced.

Future Plans

Single Log-on

The single log-on application is a focal point for future planning efforts. Plans are underway to provide access to the new pharmacy system, a clinical guideline database, the surgery schedule, and a database of clinical pathways. The single log-on application will be implemented in other departments as dumb terminals continue to be replaced with desktop intelligent devices.

Clinical Pathways

The implementation of clinical pathways also demands a documentation and tracking system which specifically accommodates the pathways. (See Chapter 10 for details on documentation and Part III of the book for information on clinical pathways.) A review of vendor-supported systems available in this marketplace is underway. This new system will be accessed from the quad PC by caregivers in all disciplines, as well as physicians and nurses.

ADT Streamlining

Further streamlining of the current admissions, discharge and transfer system will be considered and efforts to acquire a new ADT system may occur in 1996-97.

Lessons Learned

There are lessons to be learned from the implementation of any major organizational change effort. Some of the more significant lessons will be discussed here.

Synchronization of Timelines

The importance of implementation sequencing cannot be overemphasized. Budget concerns dictated the rapid implementation of the PFC care models housewide, but the implementation of the technology enablers required a longer timeline. Thus the PFC models were implemented in each patient care area prior to the promised enablers. IS could not provide the infrastructure and the single sign-on access to current systems via PC technology in the time frames set forth for the implementation of the models. As a result, the caregivers were faced with the challenge of providing care according to PFC models, but the tools to enable that care were not fully available.

Education of Staff

Once the devices were implemented, education was slow. A decision was made to do on-the-job education. With very limited resources (two people), much of the education was done one-on-one. As stated earlier, much re-education in the use of current systems also took place, lengthening the anticipated education time.

Plan for Physician Education

IS and the PFC task forces recognized that the physicians would want to access information from the new devices. However, because of limited resources, education for physicians was given a lower priority than education for the other caregivers. Physicians must be included in planning process and receive information in a timely fashion, even if education is not to take place immediately. Every effort was made to provide requesting physicians with access and education, but the effort was not adequate to prevent physicians from complaining of poor communication.

Intense Project Planning and Management

The time commitment to project planning and management was extraordinary. Because of the numbers of people from various disciplines involved in the implementation of the technology recommendations, it was a constant challenge to keep the projects moving forward. Implementation of the recommendations involving the departments of admissions, nursing, and information systems services required frequent meetings to achieve buy-in from all parties and to assure that the projects remained at the top of each department's priority list. Further, it was a challenge to keep PFC-related projects at the top of the IS priority lists. As nursing already had data input and retrieval devices located centrally in the patient care areas, it was occasionally difficult for IS staff not directly involved in PFC planning to understand the urgency associated with the quad implementation of the PCs. Again, clinical presence in information systems is invaluable. The design principles and goals of PFC must be translated repeatedly. The IS clinical project leader must communicate to colleagues that PFC is not just a "nursing" project, but rather a new way of delivering care and that IS is as much a part of the effort as every other department.

Conclusion

In summary, the Cedars-Sinai PFC effort has been supported by a variety of technology strategies. Decisions to acquire and/or adapt existing systems reflect the current fiscal concerns faced by most health care institutions today. In some instances, acquisition of new enablers (e.g., beeper and locator systems, new ADT system) has been deferred because of budget constraints. Other, less costly solutions have been found (i.e., the new telephone system, streamlining the existing ADT system), however, to support the patient-focused care models in the interim period.

Outcome measures also show success, including a decrease in time spent documenting (see Chapter 16) as a result of the new documentation system (Chapter 10) and accompanying technological enablers. The remodeling effort to put desks and PCs in the quads is particularly well-liked by physicians, as evidenced by survey responses and physician complaints when the implementation timeline was delayed in some areas. Response time to patient call lights also shows improvement in preliminary evaluation findings. Overall, Cedars-Sinai's outcomes reflect an ongoing change process in which models of patient care are continuously evaluated and improvements continue to be made to enable caregivers to provide high quality, cost-efficient care and service to patients.

Chapter 12

Materials Management and Environmental Services For Patient-Focused Care

Melanie Miller, RN, MN
Brian Williams

The Materials Management Services Department and Environmental Services Department at Cedars-Sinai Medical Center were both integrally involved in the planning and implementation of patient-focused care (PFC). Implementing the care model described in Chapter 5 involved moving both housekeeping and transportation services to the patient care unit, while materials management support remained centralized in Materials Management Services Department. Both materials management and environmental services experienced substantial reductions in staff with the implementation of new care models (i.e., transporters and housekeepers), but the departments remained supportive of the process and the PFC principles. This chapter describes the details of the changes in the delivery of patient support services, including the challenges encountered during the implementation process and recommendations for similar projects at other institutions.

Materials Management Services

Melanie Miller, RN, MN

Materials management services positioned itself to support patient care services during the implementation of PFC by focusing on providing quality service in the most cost efficient manner. Representatives from materials management were members of each of the divisional task forces developing PFC care delivery models. Materials management tasks were inventoried along with all other tasks required to provide care and service to patients. The following sections describe the analyses used to develop a more cost efficient system for handling materials for patient care.

Changes in Materials Management Structure and Processes

Structural Changes. The materials management division of support services was formerly composed of thirteen departmental units, each with an individual mission, an individual statement of goals, and individual department procedures. After PFC implementation, materials management services streamlined its organizational structure. The departmental units (e.g., central issues, central processing, linen and distribution, etc.)

MELANIE MILLER, RN, MN—Director, Support Services/Materials Management, Cedars-Sinai Medical Center.
BRIAN WILLIAMS—Director, Environmental Services, Cedars-Sinai Medical Center.

chose to remain centralized, after reviewing studies of staff time and motion, productivity, and work shadowing. Materials management services became a division with fewer units whose goal is to provide seamless, quality service to all PFC patient care areas. Patient transportation, one of the former departments, was functionally redeployed to each PFC team in order to reduce nonproductive time spend by transporters waiting for work. By redeploying transportation tasks to the patient care unit, patients are transported more efficiently by members of the unit PFC team. This change resulted in a reduction of seventy-nine full time positions, which were transferred to patient care units. Patient transports and discharges are presently built into the PFC unit daily scheduling model.

Process Changes. Prior to PFC, patient care unit staff had inventoried and stocked both chargeable and non-chargeable supplies at the unit level. This process resulted in staff duplication, rework, and supply overstock and hoarding practices. Materials management managers and staff evaluated the approaches of other health care facilities to streamline supply management and proposed that materials management take on responsibility for supplies for each patient care unit.

The materials management department also adopted the concept of the service wheel in which the customer, or patient, is at the center or hub, and all services performed for the customer comprise the spokes of the wheel. This concept assisted the department in developing services to augment and complement the PFC team, rather than complicate or circumvent teamwork at the unit level.

Service contracting was an integral part of the materials management proposal to take responsibility for supplies at the unit level. In developing a service contract, each party (i.e., materials management and the individual patient care unit) agrees to assume responsibility for specific aspects of the work to be done. (The specific service contract is described in further detail in the section on physical restructuring.) The materials management department realized that success would hinge on buy-in on both sides. The PFC goal to maximize the caregiver time spent with patients versus problem solving supply management issues provided an impetus to design a new system of materials management.

Work Redesign in Materials Management

Work Shadowing. The department began its involvement in PFC by conducting work shadowing studies to provide detailed information on job design. Additionally, the studies would help to determine whether materials management would be able to perform the tasks required to assume responsibility for supplies on patient care units without additional full time personnel. Work shadowing entails close review of each team member's time for all tasks completed in a two-, four- or eight-hour time period. Work shadowing observations can be recorded in fifteen, thirty, forty-five, or sixty minute increments. The department's technical staff decided to record tasks performed in fifteen minute increments to more closely reflect the number of staff hours needed to complete a task. The staff was concerned that incremental process steps would be lost without such frequent recordings.

The staff also wanted to ensure that the work shadowing findings actually reflected how well each staff member was assessing and prioritizing the tasks within their control. Individuals received assignments in specific areas, but staff were allowed to prioritize their own work steps. Customers on the patient care units were satisfied with the staff assigned to their units and were confident that the defined work would be completed.

Work shadowing provided empirical data and graphs to help management define ready and waiting, transport, actual tasks, break, lunch, and meeting time. Work shadowing results for logistics technicians showed that opportunities for improving work productivity were to be found in reducing ready and waiting time and consolidating similar tasks (see **Figures 12.1**). Opportunities were also available through reducing the number of trips per each staff person and ensuring that all trips resulted in a "full" return trip (i.e., accomplished a task on the return trip as well). On the third shift, for example, transport consumed 24% of the work time. These analyses resulted in the supervisory staff scrutinizing the current schedules for improved productivity opportunities. The supervisory staff also determined that added tasks could be completed without requesting additional full time equivalents (FTEs), except in Central Issues Department where additional staff would be required to meet the new quality and customer service standards.

Figure 12.1 Logistics Technicians 1st Shift

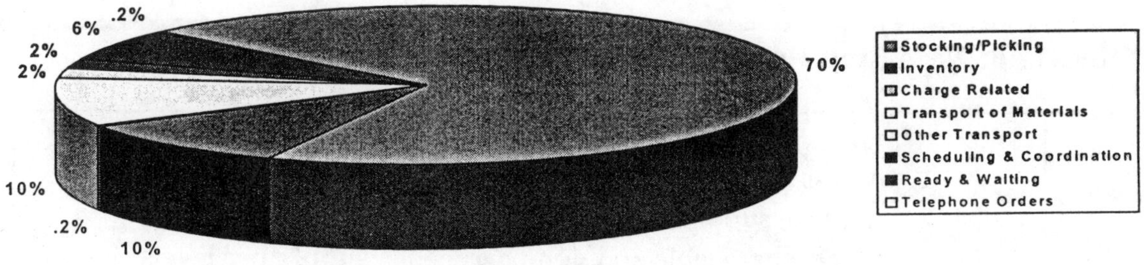

Logistics Technicians 3rd Shift

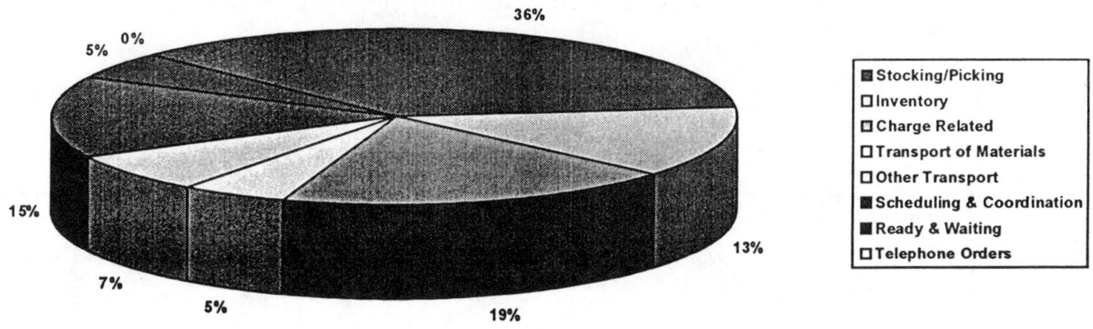

The process of work shadowing also provided renewed confidence on the part of management staff that the department would be able to provide added service for the PFC project and meet the design goal to remove the materials management responsibility from the PFC team and enable them to spend their time more efficiently in patient care. If materials management could provide a fail safe, cost-efficient supply replenishment process for caregivers, staff satisfaction should also be positively affected.

Physical Restructuring Process Improvements

Materials management also championed physical restructuring on the care unit to complement the PFC model. The goal of restructuring was to improve team efficiency by providing patient rooms with access to supplies, equipment, medical records, and information systems. Data analyses from work sampling showed that physical modification for linen and supplies would reduce caregivers steps by 50%. On average caregivers made nine trips per patient per day. Improving supply and linen accessibility would be a boon to staff satisfaction.

The service contract developed by materials management consisted of nine preliminary steps required of nurse managers and their staff in conjunction with materials management. The nine steps guided both departments in planning a modestly priced, modular storage renovation project to support a redesigned work plan (see **Table 12.1**). A philosophical change related to actually stocking more supplies rather than fewer was also adopted by Materials Management Services. While the cost of additional supplies might be questioned in a managed care environment, actually placing more supplies at the bedside resulted in less hoarding in the clean utility room and reduced costs per nursing unit of an average of $2,000 - $5,000 (one time savings).

Table 12.1: Nine Step Program for Storage Renovation

1. Assess unit supply needs.
2. Analyze supply usage.
3. Create chargeable and non-chargeable supply par levels.
4. Evaluate space efficiency.
5. Determine economical storage layout.
6. Build storage according to plan.
7. Label storage containers with supply par level information.
8. Bin locate all supplies.
9. Design requisition to follow supply plan.

Table 12.2: Materials and Service Benefits

- Concentrated patient supplies and linens in the quad for the caregivers.
- Maximizes quad storage capacity.
- Fewer steps for the care team—on average reduced trips per patient by 50%.
- Minimal central inventory in the clean utility area.
- Improved productivity—minimizes inventory and replenishment time.
- Modular supply storage allows unit by unit standardization.
- Standard design templates in tandem with modular storage provide flexibility for growth and service need modifications.

Table 12.2 details the benefits of the new system. Nurse managers are only responsible for monitoring supply expenses, rather than having direct responsibility for ordering and replenishing chargeable and non-chargeable supplies. The department also took a closer look at linen distribution and consolidated linen in each quad. A quad consists of four patient rooms with doors opening into an alcove on the hallway. Nurservers outside patient rooms support each suite. Nurservers are decentralized storage areas designed to house linens, supplies, and medications close to each patient room based upon par levels for that patient population. They also provide for separation between clean supplies and soiled linen and equipment. The result was readily available linen for all patients in the quad. Linen was labeled by type and located in the center of the quad for easy access.

Support departments also suggested that a desk be placed in the alcove outside each quad to allow caregivers to work closer to their patients. The desk would also facilitate communication, documentation, care networking, and reduce steps and confusion. The desk design required a lot of thought and discussion. Two caregivers required appropriate work space. The desk needed to include space for a computer, telephone, patient records, as well as surface work space. The physician required a separate area, which became the transaction counter, for physician and ancillary staff documentation. The transaction counter and desk allowed the caregiver to document in view of all patients but with confidentiality intact. The desks with counters attached were purchased and installed as modular units at a price within the PFC budget.

In summary, a materials management services department that understands the value of providing a seamless, total quality approach to supply management becomes integral to the patient focused process. Materials management managers were encouraged to evaluate current functions with the patient and caregiver in mind. Each task in the department needed to be studied to determine methods of reducing steps, minimizing duplication, and restructuring tasks to service the customer most effectively. The department had to stretch and look inside itself as well as at patient care services to understand the opportunity presented by PFC. Mortar and plaster notwithstanding, both physical and philosophical changes were required on all department levels to ensure success. Post-implementation staff satisfaction results from the patient care units indicate, however, that the transport and management of linens and supplies no longer detract caregivers from focusing on patient care. The materials management service contract has met its goal in supporting the delivery of patient care.

Environmental Services

Brian Williams

Like materials management, Environmental Services Department (EVS) tasks and functions, as well as the potential redeployment of those functions to the patient care areas, were reviewed during the PFC design process along with all clinical and support tasks required to provide patient care. The care model task force for the pilot orthopedic unit, as well as each of the subsequent divisional care model task forces, included representatives from the Environmental Services Department. Each task force inventoried all functions required to support patient care in their division/level of care and then discussed the feasibility of decentralization—item by item. **Table 12.3** gives examples of the types of environmental services functions discussed The goal of the environmental services redesign was to improve operational efficiency and patient satisfaction. There was significant discussion on the advantages of each unit having their "own" cleaning staff and the potential for improving quality and consistency.

Table 12.3: Examples of Environmental Services Department Functions

1. vent cleaning
2. high ledge and surface dusting
3. window cleaning
4. curtain/cubicle cleaning
5. sanitizing (room and restroom)
6. bed sanitizing (after discharge)
7. bed making (after discharge)
8. wall cleaning
9. trash removal
10. hallway cleaning
11. public restroom and area cleaning
12. cleaning of ancillary rooms (utility, nurses station, etc.)
13. carpet shampooing
14. floor refinishing
15. stairwells

Detailed information on the time required to perform each task was provided to the task forces to enable managers to estimate the number of staff hours needed to perform environmental services functions. Environmental services also provided the task forces with a current listing of the number of full-time equivalents EVS personnel required to perform specific environmental services functions. These estimates varied by unit, taking into account the average daily census, type of patient population, and number of admissions and discharges per day. For consistency, the task forces decided that Cedars-Sinai as a whole would restructure the cleaning roles directly related to patient care areas into the support partner responsibilities to improve operational efficiency, enhance teamwork, and meet customer needs. The environmental services FTEs required to perform these functions in the past were transferred to the patient care unit to be incorporated into unit staffing as support partners. The functions that fell outside of patient care (carpet shampooing, floor refinishing, public areas, and ancillary departments) remained centralized. Each unit determined the number of support partners required to perform both cleaning and other support partner functions (e.g., transportation) on that particular unit and established staffing needs for the individual unit. Cost savings as well as improved service were anticipated from eliminating travel time from unit to unit and because support partners would also be able to perform other functions such as patient transportation, resulting in more flexible and efficient use of employee time.

Selection of Support Partners

Although support partners were actually selected and hired by nurse managers, the Environmental Services Department played a key role in the support partner selection process. In the beginning, the selection process consisted of panel interviews which, although very useful, were overly time consuming. The process was replaced by a screening procedure conducted by the Human Resources Department, an interview with an EVS manager, and then an interview with the nurse manager. Reliable candidates from the EVS department were encouraged and supported by the EVS managers throughout the process. This support included assistance with previous job performance data. The time and attention committed to this process resulted in sixty candidates being selected from the EVS department out of the seventy-two positions being transferred to patient care services.

Educating Unit-Based Staff

Although housekeeping tasks are primarily performed by support and clinical partners, licensed staff were also required to attend the environmental and other support services classes. (See Chapter 13 for a detailed description of the PFC educational program.) Environmental services representatives were members of the education and training task force and worked with the task force to develop and implement the education program. For the PFC environmental classes, the EVS department used its existing program and then designed a training manual tailor made for patient-focused care. It contained cleaning processes, chemical usage, and safety, with a section that would address the specific needs of specialty areas. The manual was also designed to serve as a resource to the nurse manager and other team members. The training was provided by EVS management staff. Environmental services furnished the patient care area with cleaning staff during the training sessions (two weeks), at times making it difficult to meet other ongoing EVS responsibilities. This strain was corrected by ensuring an adequate supply of per diem cleaning staff based on the projected training schedules for each unit.

It was also important that the clinical partners (CPs), as well as support partners (SPs), understood and practiced proper cleaning techniques. Occasional resistance was encountered from the clinical partners, who perhaps thought they would be routinely used for cleaning needs for which they may have felt over-qualified. This resistance was generally isolated to a few CPs and it was not always verbalized. Both EVS trainers and nursing had to reinforce the fact that having CPs available to help the SPs when needed was vital to the success of the team. Once the training was completed, a competency checklist ensured that each person trained could practice proper cleaning techniques and infection control (see **Table 12.4**). In the event that an individual failed to pass the competency review, EVS provided retraining. There were no cases of failure after the second session.

The Implementation Process—Facing Change

Implementation was the next step—a time of both fear and excitement for individuals experiencing major changes in their own roles and in their work environment. For those cleaning technicians looking optimistically toward the future, it was a chance to work closer to the patient and to learn new skills. For those who were unsure of their ability to learn, it was a time of anxiety and apprehension. It was also a time of rapid change for the department and hospital as a whole. At the end of the implementation process, the EVS management team was also to undergo significant changes and reductions. It was difficult at times to keep the managers focused on the future, for the future was very uncertain for them personally. Managers, who were effectively eliminated, needed support and direction in determining how they could fit into other areas of the organization or how to look at outside options. After PFC was completely implemented, six management positions were eliminated.

Details for Successful Implementation

Attention to details was essential for a smooth and successful implementation. Many small items may be overlooked prior to implementation leading to major problems later. Prior to PFC, the EVS department had been using one cleaning cart equipped with a bucket, wringer, and cleaning supplies for approximately thirty rooms. The SPs were going to be responsible for approximately fifteen rooms each, necessitating two to three additional carts for each area. Even if equipment needs were anticipated in advance, delivery of equipment may not be timely. For instance, additional vacuums were needed for staff to clean patient rooms. They arrived late and caused inefficiencies due to staff borrowing equipment from one another.

The supply distribution system also needed to be reconfigured, as there had been only three major supply distribution closets, and there were now more than thirty closets.

Table 12.4
ENVIRONMENTAL SERVICES - COMPETENCY ASSURANCE BASED ON TRAINING MODULES & ONE-ON-ONE MENTORING

NAME: ________________________ DATE: ____________

TRAINER: _____________________ SP INITIAL: ________________

The above person has demonstrated the ability to perform the following tasks:

SESSION 1	YES	NO
Cart items are placed on proper shelf.	____	____
Cart is kept clean and organized.	____	____
Environmental Control closet is kept clean and organized.	____	____
Knows where to take soiled mops.	____	____
Is aware of Safety Guidelines where children are present.	____	____
Understands and can demonstrate basic upright vacuum maintenance, i.e. replace bag/filter, and unclog neck and head of machine.	____	____
SESSION 2		
Clean cloths are used in each room.	____	____
Seven steps are used correctly and in order.	____	____
Sanitation of occupied room completed correctly.	____	____
Restroom is cleaned correctly including the toilet, shower/tub, sink and fixtures.	____	____
SESSION 3		
All bottles have correct labels.	____	____
Understands use of each chemical.	____	____
Understands use and location of MSDS and product safety labels.	____	____
Demonstrates proper mixing techniques (use of dilution rate and adding chemical to water to avoid splashing of undiluted solution.	____	____

SESSION 4	YES	NO
Wet mopping is completed by drawing the mop parallel to the baseboards and furnishings to avoid splashing these items before mopping open area.	____	____
Wet floor signs are used and placed properly at entrances and corners.	____	____
Mop water is changed in hard surface rooms after every three rooms or more often if soiled or directly after cleaning an isolation room.	____	____
Mop water is changed after 10 - 15 uses in rooms with carpeting or more often if soiled or directly after cleaning an isolation room.	____	____
SESSION 5		
All soiled items and equipment (as required by area) are removed from the room prior to cleaning discharge.	____	____
Sanitation of discharge room completed, including high dusting, complete cleaning of bed and mattress, inside of cabinets and overbed trays, and all other cleanable items.	____	____
Linen is placed on completely sanitized bed and bed is made correctly based on unit specific procedures.	____	____
SESSION 6		
Universal precautions are used at times when cleaning and handling soiled material.	____	____
Proper gloves are used when cleaning and handling soiled material.	____	____
Handwashing is completed after cleaning patient room.	____	____
The following items are handled correctly, including the proper bag and the sealing of bag with tape:		
1. Medical or Potentially Infectious Material (red).	____	____
2. Soiled Linen (yellow bag).	____	____
3. Sharps (clear) - separate from all waste.	____	____
OTHER UNIT SPECIFIC ITEMS (PLEASE LIST)		
1. ________________________________	____	____
2. ________________________________	____	____

Other small, but potentially important, concerns included having enough keys for the toilet paper and paper towel dispensers, enough clean mops for the additional users, and making sure that the cleaning chemicals were properly diluted. To meet these challenges in the details of change, hundreds of keys were ordered, EVS made a schedule for the support partners to obtain their supplies from the EVS storeroom at designated days and times, and EVS purchased a chemical dilution system that would refill five gallon dispensers. EVS continues to look at ways in which to improve the system, which may in the future include a joint venture with materials management.

Lessons Learned

Incorporating the following strategies into the PFC design process can help smooth the change process and improve communication between the EVS department and patient care units:

1. Make sure that the areas of responsibility are clearly defined prior to the determination of the FTE resources to be allocated to the unit. It may be helpful to use a "floor plan" that would designate by color the areas of responsibility for both the EVS staff and the support partners.
2. Include a mechanism for providing cleaning staff on a per diem basis throughout the training process and after implementation.
3. Develop a mutual process by which projects and daily cleaning of hard and soft surfaces (carpets and tile floor) can be maintained in a preventive system.
4. Form a working partnership that clearly defines current and future plans for inspections, annual training and competency, and joint responsibilities for ensuring all areas are a source of pride in terms of cleanliness.

In conclusion, it is important that the redesign of EVS functions into SP responsibilities be carefully considered. The decision on decentralization should be determined based on the needs of the individual institution. Cedars-Sinai's experience thus far indicates that those EVS technicians who became support partners have had an excellent learning and development opportunity, resulting in higher morale and job satisfaction. Program evaluation findings (see also Chapter 16) also show improvements in customer satisfaction. The training and implementation steps are also essential to a positive outcome. Time is needed to ensure adequate attention to detail and open lines of communication to resolve those small items that "fall through the cracks," but have the potential to become a source of significant disagreement. The institution's principle quality improvement processes should then continue to fine tune the program on an ongoing basis.

Conclusion

In summary, the restructuring of materials management and housekeeping functions is key to a successful redesign effort. Representatives from the central departments must fully participate in the design, staff preparation, and implementation phases of the project. In addition, post-implementation evaluation data validate the need for ongoing interactive planning. A monthly PFC supportive services team meeting is held to address supply distribution and equipment issues. The team has successfully employed the ongoing Cedars-Sinai quality improvement process, resulting in decreased processing time for supply/equipment requests, improved access to stock, and cleaner patient care units.

Chapter 13

Patient-Focused Care Educational Program: Cross Preparing Health Care Personnel To Meet Work Redesign Goals

JoAnn Whitaker, RN, MS
Deborah Wilson, BA

Implementing patient-focused care (PFC) requires a cross-prepared, multiskilled staff capable of meeting increased demands for service and continuous quality improvement. Few hospitals are prepared, however, to educate staff for cross-prepared, multiskilled positions. Traditionally education has been discipline-specific. The laboratory, for example, may educate and supervise phlebotomists, and the pulmonary division provides education for respiratory care. Developing an education program to prepare staff for multiskilled jobs requires an integration of these educational efforts. In addition, it requires establishing linkages between clinical services, education, and quality improvement efforts. This chapter provides health care organizations with an outline of the educational processes initiated to prepare health care personnel for redesigned roles.

The structure of the PFC housewide implementation effort at Cedars-Sinai (see Chapter 3) included a multidisciplinary education task force and multidisciplinary task forces charged with adapting the generic PFC care model to meet the needs of each division (e.g., medicine, surgery, pediatrics) and/or level of care (e.g., critical care, post-acute care). Early in the planning process, a PFC education program that included modules specific to orthopedics was developed. Following implementation of PFC on the orthopedic pilot unit, the education task force initiated work with divisional task forces to refine the program and develop division-specific modules for housewide implementation. The resulting program consisted of a series of generic PFC education modules with additional modules created to meet specific divisional requirements. The education program for surgical unit personnel, for example, included modules designed to prepare them for the redesigned roles. The Surgery Care Model is detailed in **Table 13.1.** The

JOANN WHITAKER, RN, MS—Education Program Coordinator, Nursing Research and Development, Cedars-Sinai Medical Center.

DEBORAH F WILSON, BA—Director, Employee Development and Opportunity, Human Resources Cedars-Sinai Medical Center.

Acknowledgment: Please refer to the appendix of this chapter for a list of the Faculty for Cedars-Sinai's educational program. Without the help of these individuals, this multidisciplinary effort would not have been possible.

Table 13.1: Surgery Care Model

Unit-Based Care Giver Roles

POSITION	PRINCIPAL ACCOUNTABILITY EXAMPLES	
RN	• Assessments • Care Planning • Evaluation • Supervision • Patient Education • Discharge Planning • Order Entry • Medication Administration	• Assists with: – Simple RT – Simple PT – Simple OT – Phlebotomy
LVN II	• Simple Respiratory Therapy • Med administration: PO, IM, SC, eye/ear drops • IV starts • Trach suctioning/care • Central line care • Transfusions • Order Entry	• Bladder irrigation/catheterization • Dressing/wound care • Chest tube care • Neuro/vasc checks • Invasive specimen collection • Phlebotomy • Simple PT • Glucose and guiaic testing
Clinical Partner	• Simple Physical Therapy • Simple Occupational Therapy • EKG • ADL • Vital signs	• Basic patient care tasks • Transportation • Simple food and nutrition • Order Entry • Assist MDs with procedures
Support Partner	• Transportation • Simple Food and Nutrition • Daily Environmental Service • ADL	

Care Giver Roles

POSITION	PRINCIPAL ACCOUNTABILITY EXAMPLES
Respiratory Care Practitioners	• Complex RT procedures • Attempt to "dedicate" personnel by service • ADL
Physical, Occupational, and Speech Therapists	• Current role plus cross-prepared ADL and order entry
Laboratory	• Current role for A.M. blood draws and routine requests
Material Management	• All supplies, linen, and equipment
Pharmacist	• Current role • ADL (transplant pharmacist)
Medical Social Worker	• Current role plus cross-prepared ADL
Imaging	• Current role
Clinical Dieticians	• Current role plus cross-prepared ADL • Dedicated clinical dietician for transplants on 6N
Dietary Stewards	• Current role
Volunteers	• ADL • Transportation • Assist with meals

Table 13.1: (cont.) Decentralization Recommendation Summary

DEPARTMENT	ACTIVITIES	UNITS AFFECTED	WHO PERFORMS
Physical Therapy	• Simple: mobility conditioning • Complex	• All • All	• Care Team • PT redeployed to unit
Occupational Therapy	• All	• 6N*	• OT redeployed to unit
Respiratory Therapy	• Simple: HHN, MDI, CPT, Oximetry, Heated Aerosol, SMI, Free flow O_2 delivery	• All	• LVN, RN
Transportation	• To all areas except Radiology, Nuc Med, MRI	• All	• Support Partner
Environmental Services	• Daily cleaning	• All	• Support Partner
EKG	• EKGs	• 6N*	• Clinical Partner

*Cardiovascular Thoracic/Liver Surgery

development of this program embodied the unified effort and participation of staff, managers, educators, and clinical experts from a variety of disciplines. All focused on achieving the following program objectives:

1) implementing educational programs to empower staff, facilitate collegiality, and enhance the quality of patient care provided,
2) enhancing the skills of staff to participate as collaborative patient care team members, and;
3) expanding the technical knowledge base of care team members to facilitate the preparation of multiskilled patient caregivers.

This chapter details the planning, development, and implementation of patient-focused care cross preparation programs at Cedars-Sinai, including the challenges encountered and suggestions for other institutions on strategies to meet those challenges.

Program Planning and Development Process

The patient-focused care education task force consisted of a core group of key personnel representing each discipline involved in patient-focused care. Members of the task force included subject matter experts, experts in program design, managers, and educators. The task force worked with the professional and technical staff who routinely performed the skills to be cross prepared to determine role requirements. Although task force members were content and/or clinical experts, most were not experienced in program development and evaluation. The Nursing Research and Development Department provided guidelines regarding program development and a format to follow in the development of course outlines, script, and evaluation tools. Nursing Research and Development also constructed written objective examinations and conducted examination item analyses to ensure reliability and validity of program pre- and post-tests.

Table 13.2: Education Program Design Principles

- The composition of each education program should consist of staff from the same unit to help foster a team effort.
- Nurse Managers will attend the initial education program scheduled for their unit(s) to facilitate project implementation and to serve as a resource to the staff.
- The total number of staff attending each education session should not exceed thirty employees.
- Select clinical nurses within each unit will attend Respiratory Therapy, Physical Therapy and Occupational Therapy train-the-trainer sessions. These unit-based educators will collaborate with Respiratory, Physical and Occupational Therapists in supervising and evaluating staff during skills labs and clinical competency settings.
- A one-day post program "super clinical day" will be planned to facilitate completion of clinical competencies. Unit based educators will coordinate scheduling with Respiratory, Physical and Occupational Therapists to complete clinical competencies.
- A "Specialty Training Module" will be developed for each division to introduce ancillary care team members to the patient population and to their roles and responsibilities relative to unit based protocols and ADLS.
- Order entry sessions will be scheduled following each education program. Staff should be scheduled by the nurse manager to attend a four-hour course, or a two-hour refresher course, based on the individual's learning needs.
- Educational program evaluation will be conducted by the evaluation committee sixty to ninety days post-completion of each divisional education program.

To design the program, patient-focused care education task force members from specific disciplines formed subgroups that met separately from the core task force group. Each subgroup was charged with the following objectives:

- identifying skills requiring licensure and/or certification
- identifying requirements for job performance
- designing specific modules including the evaluation and assessment methods
- calculating education costs
- identifying potential faculty
- identifying program entry requirements and prerequisites
- designing didactic and experiential components
- developing pre-assessment and clinical evaluation tools

The core task force group reviewed and approved all modules developed by specific subgroups representing each discipline. The task force ensured that the modules submitted by specific disciplines were consistent with adult education principles, were cost-effective, adhered to educational design principles and the implementation timeline, and met the medical center's customer service standards. The task force formulated the design principles listed in **Table 13.2** to facilitate the planning, development, and implementation of the education programs. The task force also researched health and safety codes and professional practice regulations to assure compliance with licensure and/or certification restrictions.

Education task force members were also members of the care model and/or evaluation task forces to assure education program integrity. Chairpersons from care model task forces also participated in the education design process. Managers and chairpersons from divisional care model task forces presented their delivery models to the education task force. Subsequently drafts of divisional education programs were presented to care model task forces prior to implementation. This interactive program design process enhanced communication and resulted in an educational product that met the unique needs of different patient care divisions.

Program Implementation

The patient-focused care education program was initially implemented in August 1993 on the pilot, orthopedic unit. Subsequent education programs were implemented February through September 1994 for medical-surgical, critical care, skilled nursing, rehabilitation, women's health, pediatrics, psychiatry, chemical dependency, and the emergency room. The overall program consisted of the following content:

- a review of the principles and tenets of patient-focused care (i.e., restructuring)
- team building
- organizational skills
- a divisional specialty module, which concentrated on basic patient care issues and activities of daily living (e.g., grooming, ambulation, feeding, etc.) related to the patient population served
- social services
- documentation responsibilities
- delegation and assignment making
- information system order entry
- cross preparation modules for unlicensed staff (dietary, transportation, environmental service, twelve lead EKG, physical and occupational therapy skills)
- Cross preparation modules for licensed staff (respiratory therapy, physical and occupational therapy, twelve lead EKG, and phlebotomy)

A modular educational format provided the flexibility to allow caregivers to attend those modules appropriate to their own roles. Assignment to attend various cross preparation modules was based upon the patient population served, the specific educational needs of the staff, previous patient care experience, and individual job responsibilities. Newly hired staff were required to attend housewide and nursing orientation prior to enrollment into the PFC educational program. They were also required to attend supplemental programs as appropriate, and/or successfully challenge pretests, prior to enrollment into PFC classes.

Table 13.3: Supplementary Education Modules

I. Medical Surgical Program		
	Program Description	A two week program designed to prepare unlicensed staff, with or without previous patient care experience, to assume basic patient care and technical skills. Program content includes: acute health care organizational structure and team responsibilities, patient personal care needs, basic patient care, and skilled nursing care. This course is a pre-requisite for clinical partners.
II. LVN II Program		
	Program Description	A two week program designed to promote the growth and development of licensed vocational nurses. This program is designed to assist LVNs acquire the requisite knowledge and skills to function in an expanded role. Program content includes: an IV certification program, transcription of orders, basic ostomy care, diabetes/blood glucose monitoring, interpretation of laboratory values, patient education, and assertiveness and communication skills. This program is a prerequisite for LVNIIs.

Preparing Unlicensed Personnel

The PFC model included two categories of unlicensed workers—support partners and clinical partners. The support partner role was designed to perform transportation and environmental services functions. The clinical partner role was designed to provide direct patient care and tasks such as dietary, transportation, and environmental services functions. Clinical partners were required to successfully complete the medical surgical technician program as a prerequisite to patient-focused care education. This program was developed at Cedars-Sinai in 1991. Medical surgical technicians were required to successfully complete the program and clinical supervision before assuming direct patient care responsibilities (see **Table 13.3** for a program description and see appendix for a detailed MST Program Schedule).

Implementation of PFC increased the demand for both clinical and support partner roles, and openings were made available to qualified employees. Individuals were encouraged to move into new positions, beginning with the minimally educated support partner. The clerical and secretarial support staff were particularly interested in the clinical partner positions, but most lacked direct patient care experience. In order to facilitate career ladder opportunities, unlicensed staff were encouraged to enroll in the Cedars-Sinai's collaborative nursing assistant, home health aide, and licensed vocational nursing programs. These programs are conducted by local technical and associate of arts degree schools in collaboration with Nursing Research and Development.

The Employee Development and Opportunity Department also conducted informational and educational assessment sessions to address the needs of displaced workers from transportation and environmental services interested in pursuing support partner roles in particular. It was clear, however, that many employees lacked the basic skills to complete the education programs satisfactorily. Many employees who had functioned successfully as environmental services housekeepers were unable to read and comprehend English well enough to pass the written competency examination required for the support partner role. Employees were encouraged to identify their knowledge and skill deficiencies and to attend the existing workplace literacy program prior to applying for a PFC position. Information sessions were held, and individual skills assessment was also available for interested employees. Deficits were identified, tutoring classes (i.e., English as a second language and accent reduction) were provided. All information was presented at the reading level required to pass the PFC education program.

Licensed Vocational Nursing Staff

The PFC delivery model was also designed for the utilization of intravenous therapy certified licensed vocational nursing (LVN) II staff. Upon initiation of patient-focused care education, only 60% of the LVN staff were certified to start and manage peripheral intravenous (IV) lines. Therefore, supplemental LVN II classes were offered concurrently with PFC education so that the remaining 40% of the LVN staff could attend this requisite program (see **Table 13.3**).

Additional Education Strategies

Since PFC is based upon the concept that all caregivers will understand the principles of patient-focused care and be able to respond to basic patient needs, PFC education had to be provided for caregivers in departments that were to remain centralized as well. Some groups of caregivers, however, were unable to attend scheduled PFC education sessions, and special arrangements were needed. Individualized patient-focused care informational sessions, for example, were organized for the pharmacy department, volunteer services, and physicians. The pharmacy department lacked the resources to release staff to attend the regularly scheduled housewide PFC education sessions. To meet pharmacy department needs, nursing services offered an activities of daily living (ADL) program for the pharmacy education coordinator, who subsequently coordinated and taught "ADL Classes" for appropriate pharmacy personnel.

Volunteer services, in collaboration with the education task force, incorporated the principles and tenets of patient-focused care into the monthly volunteer orientation program. Physicians were introduced to the PFC delivery system through informal unit based informational sessions conducted by nurse managers and nursing administrative staff. Physicians also received an orientation to the redesigned roles and responsibilities of patient care staff in each departmental advisory committee (e.g., Medical Advisory, Pediatric Advisory, etc.).

Patient-Focused Care Personnel Preparation Requirements

PFC education was required for all unit-based staff, as well as other staff with patient care responsibilities. The following section, along with the accompanying tables, describes the educational program in greater detail.

Day 1

The first day of the education program, as well as the specialty divisional model on Day 2, focused on the overall philosophy and tenets of the PFC delivery model applicable to all care team members, ancillary, and deployed staff. Ancillary and deployed staff consisted of dietary technicians, nursing communication technicians, medical social workers, pharmacists, respiratory therapists, and physical and occupational therapists. The first day of the PFC education program included patient-focused care and team building, organizational skills, food and nutrition, transportation safety, and environmental services.

Team Building. Team building comprised a critical component of the PFC educational program. It was essential to develop a cohesive team of individuals who understood the principles and tenets of the restructuring process and who would begin to understand each other as colleagues with different backgrounds and to value those differences. The team building class attempted to build successful teams by clarifying work relationships and role delineation. Through discussion and small group activities, licensed and unlicensed personnel established a proactive approach to problem solving by becoming aware of, and sensitive to, individual differences. The team building class was an interactive class that utilized group exercises to encourage collaboration. Each group also constructed a storyboard which illustrated their vision of the new patient care delivery system. (See Chapter 14 for more details.)

Table 13.4: Patient-Focused Care Personnel Education Requirements (Surgical Division)

A. Day 1 and Day 2

Education Modules	Hours	Participants
Day 1		
Patient Focused Care & Team Building Organizational Skills Food & Nutrition Transportation Safety Environmental Services	2 hours 1 1/2 hours 1 hour 1 hour 1 hour	All care team members Ancillary & deployed staff
Day 2		
Surgical Division Specialty Module		
Session I - ADLS	1 hour	Ancillary & deployed staff
Session II Specialty Module Delegation & Assignment Making Support Rounds	1 hour 2 hours 1 hour	All care team members

B. Cross Preparation: Licensed Personnel

Cross Preparation Modules Licensed Care Team Members	Didactic hours
Day 3	
Physical Therapy Cross Preparation Module	8 hours
Day 4	
Physical Therapy Cross Preparation Module & Skills Laboratory	4 hours
12-Lead EKG Cross Preparation Module & Skills Laboratory	3 hours
Day 5	
Occupational Therapy Cross Preparation Module & Skills Laboratory	8 hours
Day 6-9	
Respiratory Therapy Cross Preparation Module & Skills Laboratory	26 hours
Day 8-10	
Phlebotomy Cross Preparation Module & Clinical Practicum	8 hours
Day 10	
Phlebotomy Cross Preparation Modules & Clinical Practicum	5 hours
Documentation	2 hours

A ten day program plus an eighty hour clinical session.

Table 13.4 (cont.)

C. Cross Preparation: Unlicensed Personnel

Cross Preparation Modules Unlicensed Care Team Members	Didactic hours	Participants
Day 3		
Physical Therapy Cross Preparation Module	8 hours	Clinical Partner
Food & Nutrition Cross Preparation Module & on-the-job training	8 hours	Support Partner
Day 4		
Physical Therapy Cross Preparation Module & Skills Laboratory 12-Lead EKG Cross Preparation Module & Skills Laboratory	4 hours 3 hours	Clinical Partner
Environmental Services cross preparation module	8 hour	Support Partners
Day 5		
Occupational Therapy Cross Preparation Module & Skills Laboratory	8 hours	Clinical Partners
Environmental Services on-the-job preparation	8 hours	Support Partners
Day 6		
Transportation Cross Preparation Module	3 hours	Clinical & Support Partners
Environmental Services Cross Preparation Module	5 hours	Clinical Partner
Day 7		
Documentation Class Direct patient care responsibilities	1 1/2 hours 2 hours	Clinical Partners

A seven day program plus an eighty hour clinical and experiental program.

Supportive Services. Although newly assumed dietary, transportation, and environmental services duties were primarily within the clinical and support partners' job descriptions, licensed staff were also assigned to attend these classes. The ultimate goal of utilizing cross-prepared unlicensed staff in these new roles was to enhance patient care and increase patient satisfaction. Because the registered nurse is primarily responsible for patient care, it was important for licensed staff to be cognizant of the new functions and job responsibilities assumed by unlicensed staff. Patient-focused care's team approach also requires that all care team members assume PFC tasks as appropriate.

Day 2

The second day of the program included a specialty division module, delegation and assignment making, and support rounds. A specialty model was incorporated into each divisional PFC education program. The course content was based on the divisional care model design and the specific patient population. **Table 13.4** provides an overview of the surgical division program for both licensed and unlicensed personnel, listing the program modules, hours, and personnel attending each module.

Specialty Modules. The surgical division specialty module on Day 2 provides an example of division specific content. The module consisted of two sessions, and was designed to address patient care needs in the general surgical care areas. Session I, designed for ancillary and deployed staff, included information on how to move patients and equipment, ADLs, safety precautions and the customer service strategy. Session II, designed for both licensed and unlicensed care team members, included postoperative patient care responsibilities, and related equipment. (See Examples of Specialty Modules in this chapter's appendix.)

Delegation and Assignment Making. Professional decisionmaking skills such as delegation and assignment making were an integral part of the education program for licensed staff. The key to a successful restructured patient care delivery system lies in delegating tasks appropriately. The delegation and assignment making class was initially designed for only licensed staff; however, feedback from licensed staff who attended the first class indicated that all care team members would benefit from knowing the roles and expectations of each team member. Consequently, both licensed and unlicensed care team members were immediately assigned to attend the delegation and assignment making class together.

Nurse managers assisted with teaching this component of the program. The delegation and assignment making class, presented by an education program coordinator, consisted of a discussion and small group work regarding the principles of delegation and assignment making, followed by a presentation from the care unit nurse manager. Nurse managers presented their unit's care model, reviewed assignment making guidelines, and reinforced the philosophy and tenets of patient-focused care. Support rounds were conducted by the nursing liaison specialist. Clinical directors and nurse managers attended support rounds, as requested, to answer questions and address concerns expressed by the staff.

Cross Preparation

Following the first two days of the program, classes were geared to meet individual care team members' particular cross preparation needs. The teaching methodology included didactic instruction, laboratory simulation, and actual clinical practice under the supervision of a preceptor. Medical terminology was incorporated into the PFC cross preparation subject matter to facilitate immediate association and understanding of medical terminology by unlicensed staff.

The length of the cross preparation program varied by division. Staff from each nursing division attended predesigned cross preparation modules based on the patient population and the staff's needs. The education task force developed an education calendar and scheduled five to eight sessions per division. The calendar was disseminated housewide to give each division ample time to enroll staff.

Except for the divisional specialty module, the program content on Days 1 and 2 was generic to all divisions. On Day 2 of the program, staff from the various divisions separated to attend their specific divisional specialty module and came together again to attend applicable subject matter (e.g., delegation and assignment making and support rounds). Unlicensed care team members (clinical and support partners) attended the following modules: food and nutrition, transportation, and environmental services. Licensed staff attended the following modules as appropriate: respiratory therapy, twelve lead EKG, phlebotomy, physical therapy, and occupational therapy classes. Clinical partners were also assigned to attend physical therapy and occupational therapy classes along with the licensed staff. Clinical partners assigned to surgical areas also attended the twelve lead EKG class. Specific class attendance was determined based on the unit's care model design and the individual's job description.

Nurse Manager Responsibilities

Nurse managers were responsible for enrolling staff in the PFC education program at least two weeks prior to the program start date. To demonstrate support for the program,

Table 13.5: Patient-Focused Care Education Nurse Manager Responsibilities

- Enroll staff into Patient Focused Care Education Program at least twoweeks prior to program start date.
- Participants must attend every day of the program **No Exceptions.**
- Coordinate staff's completion of the following prerequisites before attending Patient Focused Care Education:

	PREREQUISITES
New Hires	General & Nursing Core Orientation
Clinical Partners	MST course or successful completion of challenge exam.
LVNs	LVN II Program, or successful completion of challenge exam. LVNs with a previously issued IV certificate must successfully complete the challenge exam and IV practicum.

- Assign clinical preceptors to work with:

  Support Partners - 2 1/2 hours of Day 3 and Days 6-10 of the PFC Program.

  Clinical Partners - Days 7-10 of the PFC Program.

- Designate PT/OT and Respiratory Train-the-Trainers for the unit.
- Attend the program with the Nursing Director the last day to answer questions and reinforce the goals of Patient Focused Care.
- Sign-up designated staff members for appropriate clinical competencies (EKG, Phlebotomy, Respiratory and PT/OT).
- Nurse Managers must attend the Patient Focused Care Education Program.

nurse managers attended the first program scheduled for their unit. In addition to presenting their unit's care model design and assignment-making structure in the delegation and assignment making class, nurse managers were also available during support rounds and the last day of the program to answer questions and to reinforce the goals of patient-focused care. They were also responsible for enforcing the requirement that all staff attend the entire PFC education program and ensuring that newly hired staff complete the core orientation and other prerequisite programs prior to enrolling in the PFC education program. In the clinical setting, nurse managers assigned preceptors to monitor and evaluate the performance of clinical and support partners. They also assigned preceptors and/or supertrainers to evaluate and assess the competency of cross-prepared technical and licensed personnel. **Table 13.5** details the nurse managers' responsibilities.

Table 13.6: Physical Therapy Skills-Lab Guidelines for Educators

INSTRUCTIONS FOR LAB INSTRUCTORS:

Thank you for participating in the PT portion of PFC Education.

PROCEDURE:

There will be eleven learners/instructor. The group will remain with the same instructor the duration of the lab (i.e., **No rotations**). Each of you will run the lab and do the competency checkoffs for the following:

Competencies:

1) Bed Mobility - rolling
   - bridging
   - supine to sit
2) Transfers - standing pivot
   - partial stand
3) Walking - sit to stand
   - ambulation
4) Passive range of motion

10:45 - 12:45 lst lab period
12:45 - 13:45 Lunch
13:45 - 14:45 2nd lab period
14:45 - 15:00 Break
15:00 - 16:00 Final lab period

Try to have all learners remain until everyone has been checked off, encouraging them to help each other and continue to learn.

Please: demonstrate the skill:
have them practice
have them perform skill for competency checkoff

Suggestion: given a particular diagnosis that the learner works with, have them do passive range of motion, assist with bed mobility, have them get out of bed, walk, and return to chair or bed.

Suggestion: have the more experienced staff perform first to give the less experienced more time to observe.

Table 13.7: Skills Laboratories

	Staff
I. Respiratory, PT/OT Skills Labs	
• educator to learner ratio range 1:11 • All skills demonstrated at one station under the supervision of one educator • Stations manned by experts and nursing education supertrainers • All skills were demonstrated by the educator with a return demonstration by the learner. • Learners referred to checklists which outlined critical skills trainees needed to perform to successfully pass the station.	RNs LVN IIs Clinical Partners
II. Phlebotomy Clinical Practicum	
• Educator to learner ratio 1:1 • Staff participate in a 3-4 hr clinical practicum with an expert	RNs LVN IIs
III. Twelve Lead EKG	
• Educator to learner ratio 1:6 • Staff participated in a 3 hour skills lab and 3-4 hr clinical practicum with a phlebotomist	RNs LVN IIs Clinical Partners Respiratory Care Partners (as applicable)
IV. Transportation-on-the-Unit-Preparation	
• Educator to learner ratio 1:1 • Staff participated in a 3-4 hr on-the-unit session	Clinical Partners Support Partners
V. Environmental Services	
• Educator to learner ratio 1:1 • Staff participated in an 8-16 hour on-the unit session	Clinical partner Support partners
VI. Food & Nutrition Services	
• Educator to learner ratio 1:2 • Staff participated in a 1-3 hr on-the unit session	Clinical partners Support partners (as applicable, based on unit assignment)

Skill Labs and Competency Assessment

The goal of utilizing multiskilled, cross-prepared staff was to bring as much knowledge and skill to the immediate patient care team as possible. Staff were cross prepared to perform skills with an adequate volume on their unit to maintain competency over time. On units where the volume was inadequate to maintain the staff's competency in a particular skill (e.g., PT/OT or respiratory) deployed central staff were utilized. In this situation, deployed central staff attended the division's specialty ADL module to become familiar with the unit, patient population, and specific patient care responsibilities. Deployed staff were assigned to attend appropriate classes based on the unit in which they worked as well as their job responsibilities.

Skill Labs

At Cedars-Sinai, conducting skills labs required a great deal of coordination, with more than 2,000 staff members being rotated through numerous skill lab settings. Class size was kept to a maximum of thirty to thirty-five people to maintain the actual hands-on practice component at no more than ten to twelve enrollees per educator. The Nursing Research and Development Department organized physical and occupational therapy (PT/OT) and respiratory supertrainer sessions to prepare education program coordinators to assist clinical experts with conducting skills laboratories. Selected Clinical Nurse Threes (CN IIIs) and Clinical Nurse Fours (CN IVs) also attended PT/OT and respiratory train-the-trainer sessions. These nurses became unit-based supertrainers who were utilized to assist with employee orientation and evaluation of clinical competencies. A PT/OT and respiratory skills lab calendar was also prepared to assist with the coordination and scheduling of the many skill labs and to ensure the participation of all appropriate staff.

Each education program coordinator was expected to participate in a specific number of skill labs each month. Several patient rooms on the nursing unit were blocked off and assigned for skill lab use. The skills laboratory instructor to participant ratio was 1:11 for PT/OT licensed skills lab participants and 1:6 for unlicensed skills lab participants; there was a 1:10 ratio for respiratory therapy and twelve lead EKG labs and 1:1 for phlebotomy clinical practicums. Unlicensed staff participated in a 1:2 preceptor to student ratio during transportation and environmental services on-the-job training. Participants remained with the same instructor throughout the entire skills laboratory experience.

Physical therapy skills were videotaped by the primary instructor for later use in the PT skills lab. Participants were allowed to view the videotape prior to performing return demonstrations during the skills lab. This technique was extremely helpful in ensuring consistency in the demonstration of physical therapy techniques. During the skills labs, educators referred to checklists that outlined critical activities and demonstration skills to successfully pass the station. Educators demonstrated skills for the entire group, and each participant was expected to perform a return demonstration. Each participant was presented with a different scenario that could possibly happen in the work environment. The more experienced staff were encouraged to demonstrate first, to allow the less experienced staff additional time to observe. A remedial station was available for employees needing additional instruction and/or practice. **Tables 13.6** and **13.7** detail the skills laboratory requirements.

Performance Checklists

As participants demonstrated skills during the skills labs, educators recorded their performance on the appropriate checklist. The participant's performance would be documented as satisfactory, required cueing, or unsatisfactory. Checklists utilized during the skill labs were forwarded to the nurse managers to inform them of their staffs' skills abilities (i.e., who performed satisfactorily and who was in need of more assistance). Clinical experts, unit based supertrainers, and education program coordinators provided assistance with clinical follow up and in monitoring and evaluating clinical competencies of all care team members. Selected CN IIIs and CN IVs became supertrainers and were utilized in the orientation of cross prepared staff. Staff nurses who demonstrated exem-

Table 13.8: Cedars-Sinai's Assessment Tools and Tests

CEDARS-SINAI MEDICAL CENTER.

PATIENT-FOCUSED CARE
SURGICAL DIVISION
Assessment Tools and Pre-Post Tests

Assessment Tools:

- Dietary Checklist
- Environmental Service
- LVN II Checklist
- LVN II I.V. Therapy/Blood Administration Module
- Medical Surgical Technician Checklist
- Transportation Checklist
- EKG Checklist
- Occupational Therapy Competency Checklist
- Physical Therapy Training Modules
- Respiratory Assessment Tools
    - 0_2/Aerosol Therapy Clinical Assessment Tool
    - HHD./MDI Therapy Clinical Assessment Tools
    - Chest Physiotherapy Clinical Assessment Tool
    - Incentive Spirometry Clinical Assessment Tool
    - Airways, Bags, E-Cylinder Clinical Assessment Tool
    - Pulse Oximetry Clinical Assessment Tool
- Physical/Occupational Therapy & Respiratory Therapy Checklists

Pre-Post Tests: (Pre- and Post-Tests are on File in Nursing Research & Development)

- Food and Nutrition Post-Test
- LVN II I.V. Certification Post-Test
- LVN II Program Post-Test
- Medical Surgical Technician Program Post-Test
- Occupational Therapy Pre- & Post-Test
- Patient Transportation Post-Test
- Physical Therapy Pre- & Post-Test Assessment
- Respiratory Post-Test
    - 0_2/Aerosol Therapy Post-Test
    - Inhalation Pharmacology Post-Test
    - HHN/MDI Therapy Post-Test
    - Chest Physiotherapy Post-Test
    - Incentive Spirometry Post-Test
    - Airways, Bags, E-Cylinder Post-Test
    - Pulse Oximetry Post-Test
- Surgical Division Final Exams for Licensed & Non-Licensed Staff

plary skills during the skills lab setting also received additional preparation to become supertrainers. These unit-based resources assisted colleagues in need of follow-up and more practice.

All cross-prepared skills involved practice in a skills lab with subsequent competency assessment in the clinical setting under the supervision of an expert. Staff who successfully completed cross-preparation programs also demonstrated competency by completing clinical checklists under the supervision of a preceptor in the clinical setting. Clinical checklists correlated with course objectives and included critical cognitive and psychomotor skills that the staff had to demonstrate to successfully complete the program. Assessment tools (i.e., pre- and post-tests) were also developed for each module. To successfully complete the program, staff had to pass an end of program post-test with a score of 80%. (Please refer to this chapter's appendix for the Physical and Occupational Therapy and Respiratory Clinical Checklists.) **Table 13.8** lists all of the assessment tools and tests used for cross preparation.

Challenges and Strategies

Cedars-Sinai's educational program development encountered a number of challenges during the rapid planning and implementation period. These challenges, along with strategies designed to meet these challenges, are described in the following sections. Such "lessons learned" can be helpful to other institutions in their own PFC educational efforts.

Reading and Language Limitations

Assessment of some unlicensed program participants revealed reading problems and/or limitations in comprehending the English language. The Employee Development and Opportunities Department recommended the use of verbal examinations to teach these individuals. This recommendation was inconsistent, however, with Cedars-Sinai's standard that every participant pass an objective written examination with a minimum score of 80%. In addition, all newly hired and reclassified personnel had been informed of the examination requirement during the screening and hiring process. Consequently, the written examination was retained and a few individuals were unable to successfully complete the program. These participants were referred to the workplace literacy program, which provided tutoring in reading, and English as a second language classes. Upon completion of the appropriate program they were eligible to seek another PFC position and re-attend the PFC educational program.

Participant Anxiety

During the program many participants became pre-occupied with, and overly anxious about, successfully passing the post-tests for each module. To lessen student anxiety and hopefully achieve better retention of the subject matter, the exam on Day 2 of the program was deleted. This change was possible because the material presented during the first two days mainly addressed PFC philosophy and cross-preparation concepts, and each participant would complete comprehensive cross-preparation modules and post-tests later in the program. Participants would also complete an end-of-program final examination that consisted of a compilation of test questions from appropriate cross-preparation modules.

Logistical Issues

The large number of employees completing the education program presented a difficult logistical challenge in obtaining adequate classroom space, coordinating multiple skill labs and on-unit experiences, and obtaining replacement clinical staff. Prior to resolving the space issue, the task force considered options such as renting a trailer or converting the cafeteria into a classroom during off hours. Other logistical issues addressed included deciding whether classes should be offered on each shift and defining class size and composition. It was decided to offer only day classes, using patient rooms for skill labs and mixing licensed and unlicensed staff in the same classes whenever appropriate. A great deal of coordination and scheduling was necessary because of the massive numbers of staff needing education and the number of sessions and skill labs offered for each division. When concurrent sessions were initiated, the task force sought the assistance of several education program coordinators from the Nursing Research and Development Department to assist with program coordination and administration of post-tests. Per diem staff were used to replace clinical staff enrolled in classes. Throughout the education program, core nursing personnel (a minimum of 60% of registered nurses) staffed the patient care units.

Program Outcomes

The results of this educational endeavor have been measured in both short and long term outcomes. Short term evaluations summaries were compiled from end of program formative evaluation responses from program participants. Data for each patient care unit was measured by the PFC evaluation task force at three-month, six-month and twelve-month intervals post program implementation. The overall measures included competency assessment, clinical outcomes, service outcomes, customer satisfaction, and financial impact. The evaluation design and findings are described in detail in Chapters 15 and 16.

A twelve month post program competency evaluation tool "Cross Preparation Summative Program Evaluation" was developed with input from each discipline involved in the cross-preparation process. (Please refer to this chapter's appendix for Cedars-Sinai Medical Center Cross Preparation Summative Evaluation forms for licensed and unlicensed personnel.) The initial "cross preparation summative program" evaluation tools were developed and disseminated to the orthopedic unit in January 1995 as part of the twelve month post program evaluation study. The competency assessment is conducted concomitantly with the yearly performance appraisal. After cross-prepared care team members complete a self assessment, they are assigned to a preceptor (i.e., a clinical expert who evaluates the employee's competency).

Summary

Patient-focused care classes have been incorporated into the monthly general and nursing orientation programs. A monthly clinical practicum has also been implemented in collaboration with laboratory medicine, respiratory therapy, and environmental services and materials management. Newly hired and cross-prepared staff in need of additional practice and supervision are assigned to appropriate clinical practicums. This system serves a twofold purpose. It ensures that newly hired care team members are cross prepared in a timely and consistent manner, and it provides a mechanism to evaluate ongoing competency of cross prepared staff.

This educational process is only the beginning of a major culture change involving a newly restructured patient care delivery system. Utilizing multiskilled, cross-prepared staff helps facilitate the initial transition in establishing a culture of clinically competent cross-prepared staff capable of delivering efficient cost-effective, quality-focused patient care.

Appendix: MST Training Program

DAY I

0800-0815	Welcome Introduction & Program Overview *JoAnn Whitaker, RN*
0815-0945	Professional Conduct, Interpersonal and Patient/Family Communications Patient Rights Confidentiality *Marilyn Shirk, R.N., CNS*
0945-1000	Break
1000-1130	Hygienic Care (Bathing & Oral Care) *JoAnn Whitaker, RN*
1130-1230	Lunch
1230-1330	Observation, Reporting and Documenting of Assigned Tasks *Magda Bunoy, RN*
1330-1345	Break
1345-1530	Vital Signs *JoAnn Whitaker, RN*
1530-1630	Specimen Collection *Magda Bunoy, RN*

DAY II

0830-1000	Bedmaking (Occupied & Unoccupied *JoAnn Whitaker, RN*
1000-1015	Break
1015-1100	Heights & Weights *Magda Bunoy, RN*
1100-1215	Universal Isolation Precautions *Elsie Fontanilla, RN*
1215-1315	Lunch
1315-1415	Recording Intake & Output *Mierfe Calica, RN*
1415-1430	Break
1430-1530	Admission Process Securing Patient Valuables *Mierfe Calica, RN*
1530-1630	Post Mortem Care *Magda Bunoy, RN*

DAY III

0830-0930	Safety Measures (Fall precautions, use of Restraints, Patient Rounds) *Debra Tomaschik, RN*
0930-1030	Pre & Post Op Care *Debra Tomashick, RN*
1030-1045	Break
1045-1145	Tap Water Enemas *Nena Villania, RN*
1145-1245	Lunch
1245-1330	Application of Hot & Cold Compresses *Nena Villania, RN*
1330-1430	Diabetic Care *Lisa Wierwille, RN*
1430-1445	Break
1445-1545	Nourishments (Assisting Patients with Meals) *Gail Millan, RN*
1545-1630	Patient Comfort Measures Part II AM/PM Care, Use of Bedpans

Appendix: MST Training Program (cont.)

DAY IV

0800-0900	Patient Comfort Measures (Skin Care, Perineal Care, Care of Incontinent Patients, Foley Catheter Care and Removal) *Jo Martinson, RN, CETN* *Glenda Hamburg, RN. CETN*
0900-1000	Prevention of Dermal Ulcers *Jo Martinson, RN, CETN* *Glenda Hamburg, RN, CETN*
1000-1015	Break
1015-1115	Ostomy & Dermal Ulcer Care *Jo Martinson, RN, CETN* *Glenda Hamburg, RN, CETN*
1115-1200	Discharge & Transfers *Mierfe Calica, RN*
1200-1300	Lunch
1300-1500	BLS Course A *JoAnn Whitaker, RN*
1500-1515	Break
1515-1630	Post Test & Maniken Practice

DAY V

(0700-1445)	Clinical Orientation with a Preceptor
1430-1530	Room 2028 MST Post Test

Appendix: Examples of Specialty Modules

ACTIVITIES OF DAILY LIVING (ADL) MODULE FOR ANCILLARY PERSONNEL (SESSION I)

TARGET AUDIENCE: medical social workers, support partners, speech therapists, respiratory therapists, dieticians and dietary technicians, pharmacists and pharmacy technicians

I. RESOURCES
   A. Appropriate departments
   B. Equipment and supplies
   C. Team members, chain of command

II. DIRECT PATIENT CARE
   A. Assisting patient out of and back to bed
   B. Assisting patient to bathroom
   C. Assisting patient with bedpan, commode, urinals
   D. Moving patient care equipment
   E. Setting patient up for meals
   F. Changing patient gown
   G. Things to notify nurse immediately
   H. Make/assist patient with phone calls
   I. Patient safety issues

III. INDIRECT PATIENT CARE
   A. Infection Control
   B. Specimen handling
   C. General straightening of room
   D. Bag all linens

SURGICAL DIVISION SPECIALTY MODULE (SESSION II)

TARGET AUDIENCE: Clinical partners

I. PRE-OPERATIVE
   A. Care of belongings, glasses, dentures
   B. NPO
   C. Voiding

II. POST-OPERATIVE
   A. Activities
   B. Taking vital signs
   C. Weights/I&O's
   D. Potential post-surgical complications
   E. Post surgical drains
   F. Skin and wound care
   G. Patient safety
   H. Equipment functions

Appendix: Respiratory Clinical Checklist

CEDARS-SINAI MEDICAL CENTER
ORIENTATION: STANDARDS/CRITERIA

UPON COMPLETION PLACE IN EMPLOYEE'S FILE IN NURSING RECORDS

PATIENT FOCUSED CARE CLINICAL CHECKLIST RESPIRATORY COMPETENCY MODULE

INSTRUCTIONS:

1. SKILLS ASSESSMENT - Employee to check appropriate column, & submit to the preceptor within two (2) weeks of orientation.
2. EVALUATION - The preceptor completes the evaluation column utilizing the rating scale after observing the employee demonstrate and/or describe the procedure.
3. Upon completion of this checklist, place in employee's file in Nursing Records.

NAME OF EMPLOYEE	TITLE	UNIT	SHIFT	DATE STARTED

SCALE:

S = Satisfactory: Performs according to policy and procedure, and quality improvement standards
U = Unsatisfactory: Does not perform according to policy and procedure, and quality improvement standards
O = No opportunity to perform
NA = Not applicable

	SKILLS ASSESSMENT TO BE COMPLETED BY THE ORIENTEE AND RETURNED TO THE PRECEPTOR		EVALUATION TO BE COMPLETED BY THE PRECEPTOR		
	NEVER PERFORMED PROCEDURE	PROCEDURE PERFORMED	DATE	RATING	INITIALS
STANDARD: Checks completeness of MD order, verifies medical necessity of therapy, selects appropriate equipment, adheres to personal and patient safety, and follows policy and procedure regarding respiratory treatments.					
I. OXYGEN VENTIMASK (VM SYSTEMS):					
1. Checks physician order for completeness (i.e., Ventimask, oxygen %, duration of use.)					
2. Verifies medical necessity for oxygen therapy					
3. Uses risk/isolation specific safe practices and personal protective equipment					
4. Introduces self, checks patient ID band, explains procedure					
5. Selects, attaches correctly colored venturi mask adapter appropriate for the ordered oxygen %					
6. Sets oxygen flowmeter rate appropriate for the oxygen % specific Ventimask adapter.					
7. Attaches mist collar to Ventimask adapter (to prevent occlusion of air entrainment ports)					
8. Analyzes VM oxygen % to verify within +/-2% of ordered oxygen %					
9. Attaches VM to patient					
10. Oxygen appliance sticker completed and attached to VM					
11. Adheres to following practice: If VM ordered with continuous aerosol component then:					
a. Aerosol unit air powered (entrainment port full open and air flowmeter set at maximum).					
b. Aerosol tubing and drainage bag properly placed (no dependent loops; bag at low point).					
c. Tubing condensate drained into drainage bag then discarded into toilet.					
d. Proximal temp for heated aerosol units within 30-34 degrees centigrade; heater warning sticker on heater cord.					
12. HR, RR, and POX changes noted and recorded.					
II. CONTINUOUS (COOL OR HEATED) AEROSOL SYSTEMS:					
1. Checks physician order for completeness					
2. Verifies medical necessity for aqueous aerosol therapy					
3. Uses risk/isolation specific safe practices and personal protective equipment					
4. Introduces self, checks patient ID band, explains procedure					
5. Sets oxygen % selector at ordered concentration					
6. Sets oxygen flowmeter at maximum					
7. Situates aerosol delivery tubing and drainage bag properly.					
8. Analyzes CA oxygen % to verify +/-2% of ordered oxygen%					
9. Attaches CA to patient via aerosol mask, face tent, trache collar, tee piece with 150cc oxygen reservoir tubing					
10. Drains tubing condensate into drainage bag and discards condensate into toilet					

Form No. 4940 Page 1 of 4 (11/93)

Appendix: Respiratory Clinical Checklist (cont.)

SCALE:

S = Satisfactory: Performs according to policy and procedure, and quality improvement standards
U = Unsatisfactory: Does not perform according to policy and procedure, and quality improvement standards
O = No opportunity to perform
NA = Not applicable

	SKILLS ASSESSMENT: TO BE COMPLETED BY THE ORIENTEE AND RETURNED TO THE PRECEPTOR		EVALUATION: TO BE COMPLETED BY THE PRECEPTOR		
	NEVER PERFORMED PROCEDURE	PROCEDURE PERFORMED	DATE	RATING	INITIALS
11. Monitors/records proximal temperature (if heated) every 2 hours; heater warning sticker on heater cord.					
12. HR, RR and POX changes noted and recorded.					
III. HAND HELD NEBULIZER (HHN) THERAPY:					
1. Checks physician order for completeness					
2. Verifies medical necessity for medicinal aerosol therapy.					
3. Places M.D. therapy evaluation sticker in progress notes every 48 hours and every 72 hours					
4. Uses risk/isolation specific safe practices and personal protective equipment.					
5. Introduces self, checks patient ID and explains procedure					
6. Assembles HHN device correctly					
7. Fills HHN with ordered meds and 1-2 mls ordered diluent					
8. Connects HHN to appropriate gas source					
9. Adjusts gas source flowmeter to correct flow of 6-8 LPM					
10. Administers HHN via mouthpiece except on intolerance requiring sealed mouthpiece or aerosol mask.					
11. Instructs patient to breath through mouth with each inhalation being slow, maximal and F/B momentary breath hold.					
12. Monitors before and after pulse, respiratory rate, BSDs.					
13. Coughs or suctions patient					
14. Solicits patient response to therapy (i.e., is patient's breathing better, same or worse).					
15. Shakes out HHN medication residual; stores in clean draw-string bag or equivalent; removes all meds from room except MDIs.					
IV. CONVERSION FROM HAND HELD NEBULIZER (HHN) TO METERED DOSE INHALER (MDI)					
1. Checks HHN order for completeness.					
2. Verifies medical necessity for medicinal aerosol therapy.					
3. Can recite MDI conversion criteria (HHN drug available in MDI, patient over 16, patient physically and mentally capable of self administer MDI).					
4. Uses risk/isolation specific safe practices and personal protective equipment.					
5. Introduces self, checks patient ID, can explain rationale for conversion.					
6. Assesses patients's ability to actuate MDI.					
7. Demonstrates proper technique to patient: a. Shakes MDI					
b. Removes cap, holds upright, simulates placement of MDIs outlet port edge on lower lip with mouth open.					
c. Explains that inhaler is fired after start of deep, slow inhalation F/B 4-10 second breath hold.					
8. Observes/coaches patient in proper technique a. Instructs patient to wait 30-60 seconds after first puff to allow airways to open so second puff goes deeper					
b. Explains/attaches aerochamber spacer to MDI for patients with coordination difficulties					
c. Instructs patient in number of ordered puffs/treatment, treatment frequency, how to access instructional MDI video (Telecare, Ch 27 at 10 am, 12 pm, 2 pm, 4 pm)					
d. Knows to enforce patient compliance at ordered frequency, reassess patient technique next day.					
9. Assesses before and after HR, RR, BSDs during first instructional session.					
10. Labels MDI with patient stamp, ordered frequency, places within patient reach.					
11. Enters physician notification of HHN to MDI conversion in order section of chart.					
V. CHEST PHYSIO THERAPY (CPT):					
1. Checks CPT order for completeness (i.e., CPT, frequency, area of emphasis, supplemental oxygen % and/or liter flow)					
2. Verifies med necessity for CPT.					

Form No. 4940 Page 2 of 4 (11/93)

Appendix: Respiratory Clinical Checklist (cont.)

SCALE:
S = Satisfactory: Performs according to policy and procedure, and quality improvement standards
U = Unsatisfactory: Does not perform according to policy and procedure, and quality improvement standards
O = No opportunity to perform
NA = Not applicable

	SKILLS ASSESSMENT: TO BE COMPLETED BY THE ORIENTEE AND RETURNED TO THE PRECEPTOR		EVALUATION: TO BE COMPLETED BY THE PRECEPTOR		
	NEVER PERFORMED PROCEDURE	PROCEDURE PERFORMED	DATE	RATING	INITIALS
V. CHEST PHYSIO THERAPY (CPT): ***(continued)***					
3. Reviews chart for: *(continued)*					
a. Postural restrictions					
b. Positional dyspnea					
c. Feeding schedules (CPT one hour before or one hour after)					
d. CXR areas of involvement.					
4. Places M.D. therapy evaluation sticker in progress notes every 48 hours and every 72 hours.					
5. Uses risk/isolation specific safe practices and personal protective equipment.					
6. Introduces self, checks patient ID and explains procedure					
7. Monitors pre-CPT, HR, RR, BSDs and POX (if available)					
8. Attaches/increases supplemental oxygen as needed to maintain POX saturation during CPT positioning					
9. Places patient in correct gravity dependent drainage positions:					
10. Manual percussion (vibrator unavailable or not tolerated):					
a. Places towel or equivalent to prevent stinging					
b. Applies 1-3 minutes of rhythmic cupping per position.					
11. Mechanical vibration (use unless ordered otherwise):					
a. Places clean cover slip over vibrator head					
b. Uses highest vibrator speed tolerated					
c. Guides (does not push down) vibrator head over areas(s) to be drained 1-3 minutes per position.					
d. Avoids spine, sternum, bony protuberances, inflamed skin, skin lesions					
12. Returns patient to pre-treatment position & oxygen status.					
13. Coughs or suctions patient					
14. Monitors post-CPT pulse RR, BSDs, POX saturation					
15. Solicits patient response to CPT (i.e., breathing better, same, worse)					
VI. INCENTIVE SPIROMETRY (SMI):					
1. Checks SMI order for completeness (i.e., SMI, or Triflo frequency)					
2. Verifies medical necessity for SMI					
3. Uses risk/isolation specific safe practices and personal protective equipment.					
4. Introduces self, checks patient ID, explains procedure					
5. Places patient in high-fowlers					
6. Coaches patient to inhale slowly and maximally, and to sustain peak inspiration for 2-3 seconds (elevating and suspending as many colored balls as possible)					
7. Repeats maneuver #6 10 times each treatment round					
8. Coughs/suctions patient (uses cough/pain pad as needed)					
9. Solicits patient response to treatment					
VII. ONE PERSON MASK/BAG RESUSCITATION (ADULT MANIKIN):					
1. Assembles bag components; can describe valve function during inspiration/expiration					
2. Performs pre-use leak check					
3. Attaches bag oxygen tubing oxygen flowmeter set near "flush" (flow indicator touches top of flowmeter tube).					
4. Attaches correct mask size					
5. Clears airway via yankhauer, suction catheter					
6. Properly inserts correct size oral airway					
7. Applies correct open airway maneuver					
8. Fits mask properly to face					
9. Maintains mask seal and open airway position while bagging					
10. Squeezes bag depth at least 400ml (on manikin indicator)					

Form No. 4940 Page 3 of 4 (11/93)

Appendix: Respiratory Clinical Checklist (cont.)

SCALE:
- **S** = Satisfactory: Performs according to policy and procedure, and quality improvement standards
- **U** = Unsatisfactory: Does not perform according to policy and procedure, and quality improvement standards
- **O** = No opportunity to perform
- **NA** = Not applicable

	SKILLS ASSESSMENT — TO BE COMPLETED BY THE ORIENTEE AND RETURNED TO THE PRECEPTOR		EVALUATION — TO BE COMPLETED BY THE PRECEPTOR		
	NEVER PERFORMED PROCEDURE	PROCEDURE PERFORMED	DATE	RATING	INITIALS
VII. ONE PERSON MASK/BAG RESUSCITATION (ADULT MANIKIN): *(continued)*					
11. Squeezes bag respiratory rate 12-20 BPM.					
12. Visually assesses chest movement (follows with auscultation if in doubt)					
13. Assesses carotid pulse after every 10 cycles of (5:1) 2 person CPR.					
VIII. SAFE USE OF TRANSPORT OXYGEN E-CYLINDERS:					
1. Unit's standby E-cylinders properly secured, contain >1000 PSIG.					
2. Knows to replace standby E-cylinders if < or = 1000 PSIG; in-use E-cylinders if < or = 500 PSIG.					
3. Verifies gas type by reading label.					
4. "Cracks"/closes cylinder valve before attaching regulator					
5. Attaches regulator correctly					
6. Stands aside (not facing) regulator pressure gauge when opening cylinder valve					
7. Correctly calculates duration of cylinder flow.					
8. Properly secures E-cylinder to transport vehicle					
9. Turns on E-cylinder flow appropriate to the patient oxygen appliance and physician order					
10. Turns off E-cylinder valve when not in use.					
11. Removes portion of label, as appropriate, to read in-use or empty.					
12. Ensures proper storage, timely replacement of empty cylinders					
IX. INTERMITTENT APPLICATION OF PULSE OXIMETRY:					
1. Checks physician order for completeness					
2. Places MD evaluation sticker in progress notes every 48 and 72 hours.					
3. Uses risk/isolation specific safe practices and personal protective equipment					
4. Introduces self, checks patient ID band, explains procedure					
5. Confirms oxygen % liter flow (to ensure POX measurement made at ordered oxygen concentration)					
6. Uses proper probe					
7. Avoids probe placement over blue tone nail polish, pierced ears; shields as necessary from ambient light					
8. Can recite 4 characteristics of reliable POX reading					
9. Can recite red flag POX and HR values that require immediate MD notification					
10. Sets POX low alarm at 90% unless ordered otherwise					
11. Sets POX and HR audio alarms at mid-level intensity					
12. Documents readings, oxygen concentration, monitoring site					
13. Cleans unit appropriately					

OVERALL PERFORMANCE RATING **PATIENT FOCUSED CARE CLINICAL CHECKLIST: RESPIRATORY MODULE**

❒ SATISFACTORY ❒ UNSATISFACTORY ❒ OTHER

Comments: ____________________

SIGNATURE OF PRECEPTOR	INITIALS	DATE	SIGNATURE OF PRECEPTOR	INITIALS	DATE
SIGNATURE OF EMPLOYEE				DATE COMPLETED	
SIGNATURE OF NURSE MANAGER/CLINICAL INSTRUCTOR OR PRECEPTOR				DATE COMPLETED	

Form No. 4940 Page 4 of 4 (11/93)

Appendix: Physical and Occupational Therapy Clinical Checklist

CEDARS-SINAI MEDICAL CENTER
ORIENTATION: STANDARDS/CRITERIA

UPON COMPLETION PLACE IN EMPLOYEE'S FILE IN NURSING RECORDS

PATIENT FOCUSED CARE CLINICAL CHECKLIST
PHYSICAL AND OCCUPATIONAL THERAPY

INSTRUCTIONS:

1. SKILLS ASSESSMENT - Employee to check appropriate column, & submit to the preceptor within (2) weeks of orientation.
2. EVALUATION - The preceptor completes the evaluation column utilizing the rating scale after observing the employee demonstrate and/or describe the procedure.
3. Upon completion of this checklist, place in employee's file in Nursing Records.

NAME OF EMPLOYEE	TITLE	UNIT	SHIFT	DATE STARTED

SCALE:

S = Satisfactory: Performs according to policy and procedure, and quality improvement standards
U = Unsatisfactory: Does not perform according to policy and procedure, and quality improvement standards
O = No opportunity to perform
NA = Not applicable

	SKILLS ASSESSMENT — TO BE COMPLETED BY THE ORIENTEE AND RETURNED TO THE PRECEPTOR		EVALUATION — TO BE COMPLETED BY THE PRECEPTOR		
	NEVER PERFORMED PROCEDURE	**PROCEDURE PERFORMED**	**DATE**	**RATING**	**INITIALS**
I. PHYSICAL THERAPY TRAINING MODULE					
A. ROLLING: STANDARD: Assists patients with rolling technique utilizing good body mechanics, verbalizes all precautions, gives patients clear instructions and observes safety precautions throughout procedure.					
1. Has pillow at hand					
2. Locks the bed					
3. Utilizes pillow between knee as appropriate					
4. Stands on side, patient is rolling towards					
5. Encourages patient to assist, use arms to push/pull on bed rails, as appropriate					
6. Assists patient at pelvis, shoulders					
7. Places pillow to leave patient positioned properly.					
B. BRIDGING: STANDARD: Assists patients with bridging technique utilizing good body mechanics, verbalizes all precautions, gives patients clear instructions and observes safety precautions throughout procedure.					
1. Observes precautions throughout procedure					
2. Assesses safety to continue/or obtain help					
3. Utilizes one or two legged technique appropriately					
4. Locks bed					
5. Assists patient at pelvis					
C. SCOOTS UP IN BED: STANDARD: Assists patients with scooting technique utilizing good body mechanics, verbalizes all precautions, gives patients clear instructions and oobserves safety precautions throughout procedure.					
1. Assesses safety to proceed or obtain assistance					
2. Places bed in flat position					
3. Assesses appropriateness of trapeze					
4. Position trapeze appropriately if used					
5. Uses appropriate position to assist patient					
6. Encourages patient to use legs and arms to assist, as appropriate					
D. SUPINE TO SIT: STANDARD: Assists patients with supine to sit technique utilizing good body mechanics, verbalizes all precautions, gives patients clear instructions and observes safety precautions throughout procedure.					
1. Assesses safety to proceed of obtain assistance					
2. Gives patient appropriate support/assistance & instruction					
3. Uses appropriate technique					
4. Uses appropriate equipment correctly					
5. Has patient sit on edge of bed with feet contacting the floor					
6. Assesses safety to continue					

Form No. 4921 Page 1 of 5 Rev. 11/93

Appendix: Physical and Occupational Therapy Clinical Checklist (cont.)

SCALE:

S = Satisfactory: Performs according to policy and procedure, and quality improvement standards

U = Unsatisfactory: Does not perform according to policy and procedure, and quality improvement standards

O = No opportunity to perform

NA = Not applicable

	SKILLS ASSESSMENT — TO BE COMPLETED BY THE ORIENTEE AND RETURNED TO THE PRECEPTOR		EVALUATION — TO BE COMPLETED BY THE PRECEPTOR		
	NEVER PERFORMED PROCEDURE	PROCEDURE PERFORMED	DATE	RATING	INITIALS
E. SIT TO STAND: STANDARD: Assists patients with sit to stand technique utilizing good body mechanics, verbalizes all precautions, gives patients clear instructions and observes safety precautions throughout procedure.					
1. Prepares equipment:					
Locks chair/bed					
Adjusts walking devices					
Removes obstacles					
Has walking device within reach					
2. Has patient scoot to edge					
3. Positions feet appropriately					
4. Assesses need for assistance or safety to continue					
5. Applies transfer belt					
6. Encourages patient to use bed/chair/rail to push with arms, as appropriate					
7. Blocks patients good leg					
8. Guards from appropriate location					
F. STAND-PIVOT TRANSFERS BED-CHAIR: STANDARD: Assists patients with stand-pivot transfer bed to chair technique utilizing good body mechanics, verbalizes all precautions, gives patients clear instructions and observes safety precautions throughout procedure.					
1. Prepares chair and bed					
Chair placed at appropriate angle/distance to bed					
Chair and bed are locked					
2. Uses transfer belt appropriately					
3. Encourages patient to push to stand					
4. Blocks knee of uninvolved leg					
5. Assesses safety to continue					
6. Pivots with patient					
7. Observes weight bearing limits					
8. Encourages patient to reach back to sit					
9. Lowers patient without "plop"					
G. AMBULATION: STANDARD: Assists patients with ambulation technique utilizing good body mechanics, verbalizes all precautions, gives patients clear instructions and observes safety precautions throughout procedure.					
1. Uses appropriate equipment per chart					
2. Identifies appropriate height					
3. Verbalizes all precautions: WB status/motion limits equipment (e.g. knee immobilizers)					
Knows assistance level					
Knows distance tolerance					
4. Prepares destination					
5. Assesses safety to continue before ambulation					
6. Applies gait belt appropriately					
7. Gives clear directions					
8. Uses appropriate technique to stand					
9. Guards from appropriate location					
10. Corrects incorrect sequence or weight bearing					
11. Stays within limits of previous therapy session					
12. Assesses safety to continue after beginning ambulation					
H. POST-OP HIP SURGERY EXERCISES: STANDARD: Assists patient with post-op hip surgery. Articulates precautions, maintains proper body mechanics, informs patients of what is happening and reinforces and assists patients as necessary with the following techniques:					
1. A quad set of 3 reps					

Form No. 4921 Page 2 of 5 Rev. 11/93

Appendix: Physical and Occupational Therapy Clinical Checklist (cont.)

SCALE:
S = Satisfactory: Performs according to policy and procedure, and quality improvement standards
U = Unsatisfactory: Does not perform according to policy and procedure, and quality improvement standards
O = No opportunity to perform
NA = Not applicable

	SKILLS ASSESSMENT — TO BE COMPLETED BY THE ORIENTEE AND RETURNED TO THE PRECEPTOR		EVALUATION — TO BE COMPLETED BY THE PRECEPTOR		
	NEVER PERFORMED PROCEDURE	PROCEDURE PERFORMED	DATE	RATING	INITIALS
H. POST-OP HIP SURGERY EXERCISES: ***(continued)***					
2. Gult set of 3 reps					
3. A/A hip flexion of 3 reps					
4. A/A abduction of 3 reps					
5. A/A knee flexion and extension of 3 reps					
6. SAQ of 3 reps					
I. PROM OF THE UNINVOLOVED LE: STANDARD: Assists patients with post-op hip surgery. Articulates precautions, maintains proper body mechanics, informs patients of what is happening and reinforces and assists patients as necessary with the following techniques:					
1. Shoulder flexion					
2. Shoulder abduction					
3. Elbow flexion and extension					
4. Finger flexion and extension					
K. ACTIVE RESISTIVE ROM OF THE UE & LE: STANDARD: Assists patients with active resistive ROM of the UE & LE technique. Articulates precautions, maintains proper body mechanics, informs patients of what is happening and reinforces and assists patients as necessary with the following techniques:					
1. Performs active resistive ROM:					
Shoulder flexion/extension					
Elbow flexion/extension					
Wrist flexion/extension					
Hip flexion/extension					
Hip abduction/adduction					
Hip internal/external rotation					
Knee flexion/extension					
Ankle dorsi/plantar flexion					
L. ACE WRAPPING: STANDARD: Demonstrates and/or verbalizes the proper technique and/or procedure on patients with BK and/or AK amputation:					
1. Demonstrates proper ace wrapping technique of the BK stump					
2. Demonstrates proper ace wrapping technique of the AK stump					
3. Demonstrates proper ace wrapping technique of stump shrinker					
TRANSFER AMPUTEE:					
1. Demonstrates supine-sit transfers					
2. Demonstrates bed-chair transfers via:					
Stand pivot					
With walker					
POSITIONING:					
1. Demonstrates proper positioning of a BKA in bed					
2. Demonstrates proper positioning of an AKA in bed					
3. Verbalizes three positions a BKA should avoid in bed					
4. Verbalizes two positions an AKA should avoid in bed					
5. Verbalizes the purpose of proning					
6. Demonstrates the proper positioning of a BKA in a chair					
STUMP CARE:					
1. Demonstrates teaching a patient how to examine their stump					
2. Demonstrates teaching a patient desensitization techniques					
3. Demonstrates a dressing change utilizing clean technique and universal precautions					

Form No. 4921 Page 3 of 5 Rev. 11/93

Appendix: Physical and Occupational Therapy Clinical Checklist (cont.)

SCALE:
S = Satisfactory: Performs according to policy and procedure, and quality improvement standards
U = Unsatisfactory: Does not perform according to policy and procedure, and quality improvement standards
O = No opportunity to perform
NA = Not applicable

	SKILLS ASSESSMENT		EVALUATION		
	TO BE COMPLETED BY THE ORIENTEE AND RETURNED TO THE PRECEPTOR		TO BE COMPLETED BY THE PRECEPTOR		
	NEVER PERFORMED PROCEDURE	PROCEDURE PERFORMED	DATE	RATING	INITIALS
II. OCCUPATIONAL THERAPY ***(* = critical behaviors must meet standard 100%)***					
A. DRESSING TECHNIQUE WITH ADAPTIVE EQUIPMENT: STANDARD: Demonstrates knowledge and application of the following techniques with patients requiring occupational therapy:					
*1. Identifies 4-5 pieces of adaptive equipment commonly used in dressing and demonstrates how equipment is used					
2. Demonstrates knowledge and application of dressing techniques for:					
Hemiplegia-upper body					
Hemiplegia-lower body					
Cardiac patients					
Amputees					
* Hip precautions					
Back precautions					
*3. Identifies patient positioning issues related to each of the above					
B. GROOMING TECHNIQUES: STANDARD: Demonstrates knowledge and application of techniques for:					
*1. Toilet/commode transfers					
2. Light hygiene					
3. Hair care					
4. Shaving					
5. Nail care					
6. Object arrangement					
7. Hemi neglect					
8. Sequencing of activities					
9. Use of adaptive equipment					
10. Demonstrates positioning of hemiparetic extremity during grooming/hygiene					
11. Demonstrates incorporation of hemiparetic extremity in grooming activities					
12. Identifies two patient reactions to grooming which requires termination of treatment					
13. Identifies how visual or preceptual problems may interfere with above activities					
14. Identifies one commonly used piece of adaptive equipment					
C. SHOWERING/BATHING: STANDARD: Demonstrates knowledge and application of the following techniques:					
*1. Tub/shower transfers					
*2. Use of adaptive equipment					
3. Body scheme problems					
4. Hemi neglect					
5. Sensory deficits					
*6. Identifies precautions to be used during bathing					
7. Identifies how body schema and preceptual problems interfere with the above activities					
*8. Demonstrates good use of body mechanics and safety awareness during tub/shower transfers					
D. COGNITION:					
1. Identifies three common behaviors in patients with a right hemiplegia					
2. Identifies three common behaviors in patients with a left hemiplegia					
*3. Identifies common behaviors that require intervention from a therapist					
4. Gives examples of appropriate therapeutic intervention in cases of:					
Perservation					
Agitation					
Poor attention					

Form No. 4921 Page 4 of 5 Rev. 11/93

Appendix: Physical and Occupational Therapy Clinical Checklist (cont.)

SCALE:
S = Satisfactory: Performs according to policy and procedure, and quality improvement standards
U = Unsatisfactory: Does not perform according to policy and procedure, and quality improvement standards
O = No opportunity to perform
NA = Not applicable

	SKILLS ASSESSMENT — TO BE COMPLETED BY THE ORIENTEE AND RETURNED TO THE PRECEPTOR		EVALUATION — TO BE COMPLETED BY THE PRECEPTOR		
	NEVER PERFORMED PROCEDURE	PROCEDURE PERFORMED	DATE	RATING	INITIALS
D. COGNITION: ***(continued)***					
4. Gives examples of appropriate therapeutic intervention in cases of: *(continued)*					
Disorientation					
Uncooperative behavior					
E. PERCEPTUAL/MOTOR:					
1. Identifies three different types of observable, visual perceptual deficits related to funtional performance					
2. Identifies three strategies for helping a patient to compensate for deficits					
3. Identifies three cueing methods for specific deficits					

OVERALL PERFORMANCE RATING **PATIENT FOCUSED CARE CLINICAL CHECKLIST: PT/OT MODULE**

☐ SATISFACTORY ☐ UNSATISFACTORY ☐ OTHER

Comments: ______________________________

SIGNATURE OF PRECEPTOR	INITIALS	DATE	SIGNATURE OF PRECEPTOR	INITIALS	DATE
SIGNATURE OF EMPLOYEE					DATE COMPLETED
SIGNATURE OF NURSE MANAGER/CLINICAL INSTRUCTOR OR PRECEPTOR					DATE COMPLETED

Form No. 4921 Page 5 of 5 Rev. 11/93

Appendix: Cross-Preparation Evaluation for Unlicensed Personnel

CEDARS-SINAI MEDICAL CENTER.

Cross Preparation Summative Program Evaluation
Nursing Research & Development

Program Title: ***PFC Education Program***
Date PFC Education initiated: __________
Date PFC Education completed: ________
Unit: ________

Preceptor: please circle your appropriate title
Nurse Manager/Clinical Nurse
Physical Therapist
Occupational Therapist
Orthopedic Technician
Dietary Technician/Supervisor
Environmental Services Technician/Supervisor

Preceptor: Please rate the performance of unlicensed patient care services personnel (SPs/CPs) in the following areas; by checking the appropriate box.

Employee: If this form is being used for the completion of a self evaluation, please rate your performance in the following areas by checking the appropriate box and please include your name and title below:

________________________ ____________
Name **Title**

A. CLINICAL CARE SKILLS: ORTHOPEDICS	Self evaluation: *Excellent*	*Good*	*Fair*	*Poor*	*No opportunity / NA*	Nurse Manager/Preceptor Competency Assessment: *Competent*	*Not Competent*
1. Follows policy and procedure, proper technique, safety and infection control precautions in the assemblage, break down and cleaning of orthopedic equipment.							
2. Follows policy and procedure proper technique, and safety precautions when assisting the nurse, patient and/or ortho technician with the following:							
a. application and care of immobility devices.							
b. application and care of traction equipment.							
c. application and care of CPM.							
3. Reports pertinent observations, patient responses to the registered nurse.							

Distribution: White=Nursing Records; Yellow=Nursing Research & Development; Pink=Manager; Gold=employee

Appendix: Cross-Preparation Evaluation for Unlicensed Personnel (cont.)

B. PHYSICAL THERAPY/OCCUPATIONAL THERAPY SKILLS/RESPONSIBILITIES	Self evaluation: Excel-lent	Good	Fair	Poor	No oppor-tunity / NA	Nurse Manager/Preceptor Competency Assessment: Competent	Not Competent
1. Checks the patient's I.D. band and asks patient to state his name at the bedside prior to the procedure.							
2. Explains the procedure to the patient, gives clear directions.							
3. Verbalizes appropriate precautions when assisting the patient with:							
a. THR							
b. TKR							
c. hip fracture							
d. post spine surgery							
4. Reports pertinent observations, patient responses to the registered nurse.							
5. Documents tasks and patient's response on the appropriate documentation forms.							
6. Properly assists the patient, using appropriate adaptive equipment:							
7. Follows correct technique, safety precautions and/or utilizes appropriate equipment when assisting patients with the following functions:							
a. bed to chair transfer							
b. positioning in bed							
c. bed mobility							
d. supine to sit							
e. sit to stand							
f. ambulation							
8. Follows correct technique and safety precautions when assisting patients with the following exercises:							
a. passive ROM of the involved and uninvolved LE							
b. active ROM UE & LE							
c. active resistive ROM UE & LE							
9. Follows the correct technique and safety precautions when performing and/or assisting the patient with the following:							
a. ace wrapping technique of BK & AK stumps							
b. application of stump shrinker							
c. amputee transfers							
d. positioning of BKA & AKA in bed/chair							
e. stump care							

Distribution: White=Nursing Records; Yellow=Nursing Research & Development; Pink=Manager; Gold=employee

Appendix: Cross-Preparation Evaluation for Unlicensed Personnel (cont.)

C. FOOD AND NUTRITION RESPONSIBILITIES	Self evaluation: *Excel-lent*	*Good*	*Fair*	*Poor*	*No oppor-tunity / NA*	Nurse Manager/Preceptor Competency Assessment: *Competent*	*Not Competent*
1. Demonstrates correct handwashing technique.							
2. Demonstrates proper use and disposal of gloves/hairnet, during preparation and distribution of water							
3. Adheres to policy and procedure regarding distribution and disposal of food items according to colored coded labels and pull dates.							
4. Follows policy and procedure regarding the storage and handling of food items.							
5. Follows correct technique/procedure and safety precautions when performing the following tasks.							
a. preparation of water containers and water distribution							
b. fluid restrictions							
c. holding trays							
d. snack, juice preparation and distribution							
e. menus, menu codes and dietary restrictions							
6. Clears bedside table and prepares patient for meals							
7. Assists patients with meal trays and/or feeds patients as appropriate							
8. Follows correct procedure and contacts appropriate staff to resolve dietary related questions and/or problems.							

Distribution: White=Nursing Records; Yellow=Nursing Research & Development; Pink=Manager; Gold=employee

Appendix: Cross-Preparation Evaluation for Unlicensed Personnel (cont.)

D. ENVIRONMENTAL SERVICES RESPONSIBILITIES	Self evaluation: *Excellent*	*Good*	*Fair*	*Poor*	*No opportunity / NA*	Nurse Manager/Preceptor Competency Assessment: *Competent*	*Not Competent*
1. Follows correct handwashing technique							
2. Organizes and stocks the environmental services cart properly							
3. Organizes and cleans the environmental control center properly.							
4. Follows the seven step cleaning method and adheres to universal precautions when performing the following functions:							
a. cleaning occupied rooms							
b. cleaning occupied, but patient not in room							
c. discharge/transfer cleaning							
d. high dusting							
e. sanitizing/spot cleaning							
f. restroom cleaning							
g. removing trash and sharps							
h. floor dusting/vacuuming & edging							
i. floor sanitizing							
j. inspecting							
5. Logs stains and spills in the shampoo log book							
6. Utilizes the "S" stroke when mopping and changes the mop and cleaning cloth appropriately							
7. Follows appropriate terminal cleaning procedure							
8. Locates and refers to MSDS appropriately							
9. Follows policy and procedure, correct technique and safety precautions when handling chemical dilutions.							
10. Follows correct technique and utilizes safety precautions when cleaning isolation rooms.							
11. *Adheres to specilized cleaning requirements when cleaning eqipment and other non-standardized items, e.g. (Isoleetes, basinets, warmers, etc.)							
12. Follow admission and discharge check out procedure							

*Specialty specific criteria - indicate not applicable, if this task is not a job requirement on your assigned unit.

Distribution: White=Nursing Records; Yellow=Nursing Research & Development; Pink=Manager; Gold=employee

Appendix: Cross-Preparation Evaluation for Unlicensed Personnel (cont.)

E. TRANSPORTATION RESPONSIBILITIES	Self evaluation: *Excellent*	*Good*	*Fair*	*Poor*	*No opportunity / NA*	Nurse Manager/Preceptor Competency Assessment: *Competent*	*Not Competent*
1. Adheres to proper body mechanics and patient safety guidelines when performing the following duties:							
a. engaging and locking wheelchairs and gurneys							
b. transporting and transferring patients via wheelchairs and gurneys							
c. accessing elevators and doorways utilizing wheelchairs and gurneys.							

I acknowledge my ability to safely perform these cross prepared procedures.

______________________ ________ ________

Signature of cross prepared staff member Title Date

______________________ ________

Unit Manager's signature Date

Comments:

____

____

____

Distribution: White=Nursing Records; Yellow=Nursing Research & Development; Pink=Manager; Gold=employee

Appendix: Cross-Preparation Evaluation for Licensed Personnel

CEDARS-SINAI MEDICAL CENTER.

Cross Preparation
Summative Program Evaluation
Nursing Research & Development

Program Title: ***PFC Education Program***

Date PFC Education initiated:_____________

Date PFC Education completed:___________

Unit:______________________________

Preceptor: Please circle your appropriate title:

Nurse Manager/Clinical Nurse
Physical Therapist
Respiratory Therapists/RCP
Occupational Therapists
Orthopedic Technician
Path/Lab Med Staff

Preceptor: Please rate the performance of licensed patient care services personnel, (RN, LVN II's) in the following areas, by checking the appropriate box.

Employee: If this form is being used for the completion of a self evaluation, please rate your performance in the following areas;

______________________________ *Name* ______________ *Title*

by checking the appropriate box and

A: *CLINICAL CARE SKILLS: ORTHOPEDICS*	Self Evaluation					Nurse Manager/Preceptor Competency Assessment	
	Excellent	*Good*	*Fair*	*Poor*	*No Opportunity / N/A*	*Competent*	*Not Competent*
1. Follows policy & procedures, safety precautions, and proper technique, in the assemblage and care of patients with the following orthopedic equipment.							
a. casts							
b. immobility devices							
c. traction equipment							
d. suspension devices							
2. Follows policy & procedures, safety precautions and proper techniques, and nursing responsibilities while performing the following orthopedic functions.							
a. application and care of casts							
b. application and care of immobility devices							
c. application and care of traction equipment							
d. application and care of CPM							
3. Initiates and documents appropriate orthopedic assessments, interventions and outcomes e.g. (neuro checks, pain assessment, body alignment checks)							

Distribution: White = Nursing Records Yellow = Nursing Research & Development Pink = Nurse Manager Gold = Employee

Appendix: Cross-Preparation Evaluation for Licensed Personnel (cont.)

PHYSICAL THERAPY/OCCUPATIONAL THERAPY SKILLS	Self Evaluation					Nurse Manager/Preceptor Competency Assessment	
	Excellent	*Good*	*Fair*	*Poor*	*No Opportunity / N/A*	*Competent*	*Not Competent*
1. Verifies completeness of PT/OT orders.							
2. Checks the patient's I.D. band and asks patient to state his name at the bedside prior to procedure.							
3. Explains the procedure and gives clear directions, corrects incorrect sequence and/or weight bearing.							
4. Verbalizes appropriate precautions when assisting the patient with:							
a. THR							
b. TKR							
c. hip fracture							
d. post spine surgery							
5. Documents tasks and patient's response on the appropriate documentation forms.							
6. Properly assists and instructs patients using appropriate adaptive equipment.							
7. Follows correct technique, safety precautions and/or utilizes appropriate equipment when assisting patients with the following functions:							
a. bed to chair transfer							
b. positioning in bed							
c. bed mobility							
d. supine to sit							
e. sit to stand							
f. ambulation							
8. Follows correct technique and safety precautions when assisting patients with the following exercises:							
a. passive ROM of the involved and uninvolved LE							
b. active ROM UE & LE							
c. active resistive ROM UE & LE							
9. Follows the correct technique and safety precautions when performing and/or assisting the patient with the following:							
a. ace wrapping technique of BK & AK stumps							
b. application of stump shrinker							
c. amputee transfers							
d. positioning of BKA and AKA in bed/chair							
e. stump care							

Distribution: White = Nursing Records Yellow = Nursing Research & Development Pink = Nurse Manager Gold = Employee

Appendix: Cross-Preparation Evaluation for Licensed Personnel (cont.)

C: *RESPIRATORY THERAPY SKILLS*	Self Evaluation					Nurse Manager/Preceptor Competency Assessment	
	Excellent	*Good*	*Fair*	*Poor*	*No Opportunity / N/A*	*Competent*	*Not Competent*
1. Verifies that respiratory therapy order is complete, current and meets medical necessity guidelines.							
2. Adheres to personal and patient safety precautions and follows respiratory therapy policies and procedures.							
3. Follows risk/isolation specifics safe practices and uses personal protective equipment.							
4. Check the patient's I.D. band and asks patient to state his name at the bedside prior to procedure.							
5. Explains and/or demonstrates the procedure; and instructs/ coaches patient during the procedure.							
6. Proper selection and assemblage of respiratory equipment.							
7. Monitors, assesses and documents nursing interventions and patient outcomes.							
8. Solicits patient's response to respiratory therapy treatments.							
9. Follows policy and procedure, safety precautions, proper technique and utilizes appropriate equipment when performing or assisting with the following respiratory treatments:							
a: oxygen venti mask therapy							
b. venti mask with continuous aerosol therapy							
c. continuous coal or heated aerosol therapy							
d. HHN therapy							
e. conversion from HHN to MDI therapy							
f. CPT - 1) manual percussions							
2) use of mechanical vibrator							
g. incentive spirometer							
h. mask/bag resuscitation							
i. use of E-cylinder							
j. intermittent application of pulse oximetry							
10. Properly maintains/cleans relevant respiratory equipment.							

Note: Preceptor/Appraiser - Please utilize the attached respiratory therapy treatment guidelines during the evaluation/ competency assessment.

Distribution: White = Nursing Records Yellow = Nursing Research & Development Pink = Nurse Manager Gold = Employee

Appendix: Cross-Preparation Evaluation for Licensed Personnel (cont.)

: *PHLEBOTOMY SKILLS*	Self Evaluation					Nurse Manager/Preceptor Competency Assessment	
	Excellent	*Good*	*Fair*	*Poor*	*No Opportunity / N/A*	*Competent*	*Not Competent*
. Verifies patient's I.D. arm band against requisition and labels.							
. Follows universal precautions and aseptic technique.							
. Proper site selection and preparation.							
. Selects correct collection tubes for test and fills tubes in the proper order.							
. Labels specimens properly.							
. Proper needle and equipment disposal.							
. Avoids traumatizing patient during the procedure (hematoma, bruises, etc.).							

I acknowledge my ability to safely perform these cross prepared procedures

____________________ Employee's Signature   __________ Title   __________ Date

____________________ Unit Manager's Signature   __________ Date

Comments: ____

Distribution: White = Nursing Records   Yellow = Nursing Research & Development   Pink = Nurse Manager   Gold = Employee

Appendix: Patient-Focused Care Educational Program Faculty

Topic	Instructor
Patient-Focused Care and Team Building	Designated Surgical Division Management Staff Nancy Nuechterlein Madeleine Bruning, RN Marilyn Shirk, RN, CNS
Organizational Skills	Eda Crosby Steve Keleman Peggy Painton
Delegation and Assignment Making/Working as a Team	Designated Surgical Division Management staff Nena Villania, RN
Specialty (Surgery) Educational Module	Barbara Fields, RN Mary Eng, RN Fe Mangila, RN
Respiratory Care Educational Module	Brian Richards, RCP Carol Thaler, RCP
Occupational Therapy Educational Module	Mary Evenson, OT Sue Bowles, OT June Petty, OT Pam Roberts, OT Karen Ozaki, OT Sara Tachmeyer, OT
Physical Therapy Educational Module	Lorraine Kimura, PT Susan Vereb, PT Helen Tsuda, PT Mima Siegal, PT Michelle Prettyman, PT Diane Salgado, PT Zahra Ghasemi, PT Carol Dobashi, PT Terry Martin, PT Carl Pitts, PT Catherine Murphy, PT
Transportation Educational Module	Dan Mendias Chris Harris Sergio Tiffer
Food & Nutrition Module	David Gomes Blesilda Masatani
Environmental Services Module	Charles Rumbut Brian Williams Shirley Houston

Appendix: Patient-Focused Care Educational Program Faculty (cont.)

Topic	Instructor
Medical Social Work	Sharon Steele, MSW
Volunteer Educational Module	Mary Meola, RN Nena Villania, RN Debra Tomaschik, RN Barbara Colner
Electrocardiology Module	Magda Bunoy, RN Ivan Velasquez
Phlebotomy Module	Rick Plasse, PhD, MT Terry Jennings, MT Monica Thomas, MT
Information System Order Entry	Chris McLaurin
Documentation Module	Terry Chamorro, RN
Expectations of Team Members	Nursing Executive Council: Linda Burnes Bolton, RN Madeleine Bruning, RN Randy Cook, RN Mary Flores, RN Barbara Karagosian, RN Robin Epstein-Ludewig Maureen Nagelhout, RN Gerry Popolow, RN Jane Ramseyer, RN Les Sampson, RN

Chapter 14

Human Resource Issues in Patient-Focused Care

Jeanne Flores, BA
Robin Epstein Ludewig, BS
Nancy Nuechterlein, MA
Cynthia Balin, RN, MSN, CNAA
Pamela Garrity, RN, MS
Marilyn Shirk, RN, MN
Madeleine D. Bruning, RN, MA
Maria Fe M. Mangila, RN, MSN, CCRN

This chapter details the human resources philosophy, challenges, and implementation strategies adopted for patient-focused care (PFC) at Cedars-Sinai Medical Center. From a human resources perspective, the design and implementation of PFC presented challenges on two main fronts. These included fundamental human resources issues (i.e., compensation, recruitment, layoff, and reassignment) as well as the issues of securing the support and "buy-in" of staff with varying, and potentially competing, perspectives and interests (e.g., managers, staff, the union, and others). In order to meet these challenges, the following three areas were addressed:

1. the development of a human resources philosophy and approach for PFC;
2. the impact of this philosophy on human resource issues in the design and implemen-

Jeanne Flores, BA—Director, Employee Relations, Human Resources, Cedars-Sinai Medical Center.

Robin Epstein Ludewig, BS—Director, Nurse Recruitment and Retention, Patient Care Services, Cedars-Sinai Medical Center.

Nancy Nuechterlein, MA—Director, Employee Assistance Program, Human Resources, Cedars-Sinai Medical Center.

Cynthia Balin, RN, MSN, CNAA—Coordinator, Patient Care Services, Cedars-Sinai Medical Center.

Pamela Garrity, RN, MS—Unit Manager, 5NW, Patient Care Services, Cedars-Sinai Medical Center.

Marilyn Shirk, RN, MN—Mental Health Clinical Nurse Specialist, Patient Care Services, Cedars-Sinai Medical Center.

Madeleine D. Bruning, RN, MA—Director, Nursing Resources (former), Director, Pediatrics (former), Patient Care Services, Cedars-Sinai Medical Center.

Maria Fe M. Mangila, RN, MSN, CCRN—Clinical Nurse Specialist, Surgical Nursing, Patient Care Services, Cedars-Sinai Medical Center.

tation of PFC, including compensation, recruitment, staffing, and other issues; and
3. strategies for staff involvement, support, and team building in the implementation of PFC models.

Each of these three areas is addressed in detail in this chapter.

Human Resources Philosophy

Patient-focused care requires a paradigm shift on the part of staff throughout the institution. Individuals need to rethink their roles, their relationships with their coworkers, and the manner in which work is completed. Since the design and implementation of PFC is accomplished not in an isolated laboratory but in an active health care environment, this paradigm shift must occur in a way that is least disruptive to the staff to ensure that the quality of patient care is protected and its high priority status retained. These considerations dictate that not only managers, but all staff need to feel that their perspectives and interests are being considered and represented in the design and implementation of PFC. In addition, the bargaining unit (union) that represents many of the employees must support the changes to minimize disruptions during design and implementation. At Cedars-Sinai, the following measures were taken to support positive employee relations:

- employees were included on the design teams;
- progress in design and implementation was communicated to all employees on an ongoing basis; and
- a human resources philosophy statement was written and published.

Human Resources Philosophy Statement

The "Human Resources Philosophy: Statement of Intent in Relation to Patient-Focused Care" provided a set of principles to guide managers in decisionmaking. It also provided a statement of intent concerning what employees could expect from the implementation of PFC (see **Table 14.1**). The "Human Resources Philosophy" was intended to confirm the value of the staff, provide them with a statement of intent to involve them in the design of the new structure, and address their concerns regarding job security through a commitment to:

- provide ample notice of the impact of PFC on their jobs,
- provide education for new and/or changed jobs,
- make information about job alternatives available, and
- make staffing reductions through attrition rather than layoff whenever possible.

This set of principles drove the design and implementation of the compensation plan and the plan for moving staff into their new roles. The following sections describe the human resources strategies that were developed based upon this philosophy.

Table 14.1: Human Resource Philosophy
Statement of Intent in Relation to Operations Restructuring

1.	Actively involve employees who are doing the work in design of the new structure
2.	Be responsive to the needs and desires of individuals, taking into account their unique talents and abilities
3.	Provide adequate notice to anyone whose job is impacted by restructuring to give them time to make choices regarding career decisions
4.	Provide opportunity for extensive (e.g., 3-6 months) training where necessary to support employees in performing new tasks and roles
5.	Make every effort to ensure continued job security and avoid layoffs as a result of restructuring
6.	Assist displaced employees in being transferred or reassigned to positions for which they are qualified (including providing first preference to internal candidates where openings exist)
7.	Support all employees in finding satisfying work of which they are capable.

Human Resources Strategies

Relations with Bargaining Unit (Union)

Overall, about 25% of the workforce at Cedars-Sinai is represented by a bargaining unit. In the areas affected by PFC, union members included the LVNs; medical-surgical technicians, critical care technicians, and nursing service technicians (nonlicensed personnel); logistics technicians and nursing communications technicians (unit clerical staff); and the service workers. The strategy for relations with the bargaining unit (union) was to:

- Communicate the intent and progress of the PFC project to the leadership,
- Include members and shop stewards (but not the leadership paid by the union) in the design teams, and
- Accommodate member and leadership concerns where appropriate within the project objectives and philosophy and the bargaining agreement; where concerns could not be accommodated, the reasons were explained.

The following sections describe the most significant bargaining unit concerns and the ways in which they were addressed.

Job Security. The union requested preference be given to internal candidates in filling new positions for PFC. It also requested that employees transferring to these new positions as part of the "pilot" unit be permitted to return to their former positions in the event of pilot or program failure (rather than be laid off). Both of these requests, which were in accord with the "Human Resources Philosophy," were accommodated.

Criteria and Process for Selection. The union also requested, and received, the opportunity to review the criteria and process for selection. It was emphasized that selection would be heavily dependent upon the quality of the employee's prior work performance including customer relations and interpersonal skills, the quality of their work product, and records of attendance. In keeping with the collective bargaining agreement, the most qualified candidates would be selected.

Education. The union was assured of Cedars-Sinai's commitment to adequate and extensive education of employees for the new positions.

Compensation. The union requested that, when promoted to new positions, employees be compensated at the higher rate during the education period. Cedars-Sinai accommodated this request. They further requested that the rates for the classifications be higher than had been determined This request was not accommodated. Cedars-Sinai maintained the practice of setting pay scales reflecting market rates for those job tasks that represented the preponderance of duties, rather than setting pay scales according to the most highly compensated duty in a job description.

Addressing Manager Concerns

The concerns and perspectives of managers were addressed by the multidisciplinary Human Resources Task Force. (See Chapter 3 for details of the project organizational structure.) This task force existed throughout the implementation period and was staffed by both a fixed membership (i.e., patient care services administrators and human resources staff) and a rotating membership of managers who were included as their units were preparing for and entering the implementation phase. Issues addressed by this task force ranged from compensation and selection criteria to uniforms. It proved to be an important forum to ensure awareness of human resource issues as they emerged. The task force was also essential in ensuring a consistent approach that served both business and employee needs and concerns.

Compensation Strategies

The strategy for establishing classifications and pay grades changed early in the design phase. Although the project began with an intent to create all new classifications and titles, project staff soon realized that this process would be both disruptive and unnecessary. Instead, it was decided to retain existing job titles and incumbents where the positions were substantially unchanged, while incorporating new and/or revised duties as appropriate. The primary classifications affected by this decision were RNs and LVN IIs. The result was that the existing RN and LVN II job descriptions remained essentially the same with an addendum added to reflect the new duties (e.g., respiratory, physical therapy, EKG, etc.) that would be performed on that unit. This strategy also permitted a consistent approach that allowed for variation based upon unit needs.

In keeping with this approach, job pay grades for these positions remained unchanged when PFC was implemented. Where multiple jobs were collapsed into a new single job (job consolidation), the pay scales were set at the market rate for the job that reflected the preponderance of duties. The pay scales for the new clinical and support partner positions were set in this way. The pay scales for these new consolidated jobs were designed with sufficient width (a 30% spread) to accommodate most current employees transferring into them. The pay rate for transferring employees was adjusted according to the following principles:

1. If coming from a job with a lower pay scale, the employee received a 5% promotional increase;
2. If coming from a job with the same pay scale, there was no adjustment; and
3. If coming from a job with a higher pay scale, the following rules applied:
   - if the employee's pay was within the new scale, no adjustment was made,
   - if the employee's rate was at or within 5% of the maximum of the new scale, no adjustment was made,
   - if the employee's rate was more than 5% over the maximum of the new scale, the employee's rate was reduced to 5% over the new maximum.

Using this approach, only one or two employees out of the hundreds transferring to new positions had a reduction in pay. Where equity adjustments were required (such as in the case of LVNs) those adjustments were made at the time of annual wage plan implementation.

Recruitment Strategies

Recruitment for PFC jobs was designed to assure clinical competence and customer service skills while minimizing disruption to the units and the staff. Based upon these objectives, the strategies described in the following sections were developed.

Retaining Incumbents on Home Units. Incumbents were retained on their home units for those positions with no change in title (i.e., RNs and LVN IIs). This strategy was key in meeting the commitment to employees under the "Human Resources Philosophy" detailed in **Table 14.1.** Although some of these employees needed to improve some aspects of their performance (frequently customer service skills), it was decided to provide them with the opportunity to do so through education with appropriate monitoring and follow up.

Retaining Nurse Managers. Nursing managers were retained on their home units in the unit manager positions. This strategy was another key to maintaining stability through the transition. The managers were assured of a position and could assist the other staff members in making a more effective transition. In addition, they knew their staffs well and could make sound decisions on the selection of new staff. The nursing managers also could help retained staff understand the changes each needed to make and support them through those changes.

Giving Preference to Employees Whose Classifications Were Eliminated. Employees in classifications that were being eliminated (e.g., medical-surgical technicians) were given preference for new jobs on their home unit. If they could not be accommodated on their home unit, they were given preference for available jobs on other units. As a result, medical-surgical technicians were given jobs as clinical partners. While a few could not successfully complete the education, most were successful and retained their jobs. This approach helped minimize disruption on the unit and employee concerns about job security.

Assistance in Completing PFC Education. While all employees were required to successfully complete the PFC education program, assistance was provided to help them. This assistance included individualized tutoring, reading and language classes, etc. Many employees were concerned about the education and the necessity of passing written exams. Nurse managers were sensitive to these issues and went to great lengths to help employees succeed. While not all did succeed, those who did not understood that they had been treated fairly. There was not one formal challenge to any decision not to pass any employee, including employees who were laid off as a result of failure to pass (and several of these were employees with fifteen years or more of service).

Position Elimination/Layoffs

Over three hundred employees were in classifications that were eliminated with the implementation of patient-focused care with no comparable PFC position in which they could easily be placed. These included transporters, environmental service technicians (housekeepers), orthopedics technicians, cardiac monitor observers, nursing service technicians, EKG technicians, and LVN Is. The potential for disruption was high and project staff wanted to take a careful approach. Human resources' approach was based upon two commitments advance notice and assistance in finding alternative positions.

Advance Notice. As much advance notice as possible (often months) was given to employees whose job classifications were being eliminated, including discussions of their options in applying for new positions. While some employees remained in denial until formal notice of job elimination/layoff was given, most began early to explore alternatives and prepare themselves for change.

Assistance in Finding Alternative Positions. Employees were assisted in finding alternative positions within the organization to the extent feasible. They were encouraged and supported by managers and received education (many employees required assistance with verbal and written language skills) early enough to substantially improve their chances to quality for new positions.

Layoffs. In cases where no other positions could be found, employees were laid off. Layoffs were postponed until PFC was fully implemented, and it was clear that no other suitable positions could be found. In addition, the layoff severance package included not only severance pay and extended insurance benefits, but outplacement assistance to help find work with another organization.

Implementation

Implementing PFC from a human resources perspective included hiring new employees and putting all of the strategies described above into action. In addition, it included developing and implementing strategies to both build effective teams and ensure that team members understood and supported PFC. This implementation section begins by describing the recruitment process and then provides details on specific staff involvement and team building strategies used to ensure successful education and involvement of all PFC team members.

Recruitment Process

Once the PFC models were created and specific skills identified for the redesign of each individual unit, Cedars-Sinai was ready to begin the recruitment process. Recruitment responsibilities were divided between the employee relations department and nurse recruitment and retention. Clinical partners and LVN IIs were recruited by the Nurse Recruitment and Retention Department, and support partners were recruited by the Human Resources Department. The institution did not historically have an extensive applicant pool for the clinical partner role or the intravenous certified licensed vocational nurse (LVN II). There was, however, a significant applicant pool for the support partner role both internally and throughout the community, and recruitment advertising was not required. Instead, Human Resources employed strategies such as posting the job internally and notifying various community agencies that retrain and place individuals with the necessary skills.

Recruitment for LVN IIs and clinical partners started with advertising in trade journals and newspapers such as the *Los Angeles Times*, *Nurseweek*, and *Attention Nurses*. Cedars-Sinai also notification of various community agencies and schools including the Metropolitan Skills Center (a division of the Los Angeles Unified School District), the Jewish Vocational Services, and Los Angeles Trade Technical Community College. Concurrent with the launch of the marketing program, project staff began to educate the nursing staff who would conduct the initial screening of all the applicants and would be responsible for referring qualified candidates to the hiring managers. The teams included unit managers and clinical nurse specialists from the divisions that were slated for the first "go-live" dates.

A special screening tool was developed to assist the interviewers in assessing the clinical and customer service skills of all applicants. Using this tool, it quickly became apparent that it would be necessary to interview a significant number of applicants for each hire. Throughout the course of the recruitment period, many applicants (both internal and external) applied who did not meet minimum qualifications. **Table 14.2** shows the number of applications and interviews necessary to hire the needed number of clinical partners and LVN IIs.

Table 14.2: Hiring Process for Clinical Partners and Licensed Vocational Nurse IIs

	Number of Applicants	Number of Interviews	Number of Hires
Clinical Partners	484	303	54
LVN IIs	430	295	77

Once applicants were identified, verbal and written reference and criminal background checks were conducted. This was done prior to scheduling a pre-employment physical examination and a start date. Specific training needs were identified for each candidate based upon their work experience and educational background. Prior to beginning the PFC training program, many of the new hires were required to complete Cedars-Sinai's LVN II course, including the IV certification portion, or the clinical partner course. New hires with experience could challenge the competency exams prior to beginning employment. (The complete education program is described in Chapter 13.)

Team Building

Team building is an ongoing process. The importance of involving staff at all stages of the design and implementation of PFC has already been emphasized in the discussion on project organization (Chapter 3) and the descriptions of the unit-specific care model development processes (Chapters 4-9). The following sections describe in detail some of the strategies employed by Cedars-Sinai to strengthen the new PFC teams being assembled for each unit. The first section focuses on the importance of team building in the health care setting and some of the issues discussed during the team building portion of the PFC educational program. This overview is followed by a description of a small group exercise (storyboarding) that was also a part of the program. Additional sections then detail a number of different strategies to encourage staff participation in different phases of the PFC design and implementation process.

Teams in a Health Care Setting. People—their behaviors, attitudes, and relationships —determine the efficiency and spirit with which the team's mission is accomplished. Anyone who works in an interdependent role knows that "[i]t all depends on who you are working with." The shift goes better or worse to a large extent because people are "in sync" or "out of sync" with one another's expectations and needs. The challenge of building teams in a health care setting means influencing the likelihood that people will treat each other in mutually agreeable ways as each goes about making a contribution to patient care. Teambuilding begins with examining the values and expectations that go into working relationships. Team members can explore these issues with one another by watching each other's behavior and talking about their concerns. Too frequently, however, people learn about their own values and expectations by focusing on what irritates or disappoints them. Any group of caregivers is likely to say things such as:

- "I just don't want to be here when I have to work with that person... She never has anything good to say...complain, complain, complain...it's exhausting!"
- "I can never find him...where could he possibly be hiding?...Somebody should do something about that guy...we are left to do all his work." or
- "I hate the way she demands rather than asks. She talks to me like I was some dog. I'm human too. I deserve respect even if I don't have a big title."

As part of the team building portion of the PFC education program, staff were asked to describe what makes the day (or shift) go better. This question stumped many staff members. They knew what ruined the day and described their "pet peeves." Most of the responses reflected strong work values, including taking responsibility, being accountable, giving and receiving help as needed, being visible and available, treating others fairly, showing respect, being courteous, being constructive and direct in confronting interpersonal issues, and making all co-workers feel as a member of the "group." All of these concepts and preferences need to be made even more explicit by team members, however, to ensure everyone knows what is meant by "acting professional."

This need for explicit definitions is especially important in a culturally diverse work group. Respect, for example, may mean something different to one person than to another. If one team member addresses another informally in an effort to be warm and collegial and the other prefers a more formal approach that acknowledges his or her status as an elder, the consequences are obvious. It is difficult for team members to know what effect they are having on one another, and the importance of communication was stressed. Information sharing is key in the business of helping people, but interpersonal information is not always easy to share. Team members want others to just "know what they mean." Some team members may even assume that others enjoy offending them by doing something they assume the other party knows irritates them. Use of a foreign language is one example of this type of misunderstanding. When individuals share a language, they naturally use it when in contact with one another. In spite of a hospital policy requesting that English be spoken in the work area, many staff still speak their primary language with one another. The consequences vary. Those who are reticent about confronting their peers and asking them to speak English may experience mounting resentment because they feel left out. More often, the same language group is oblivious to others' noncomprehension because they are more focused on what they are saying to one another. One individual suggested that not to speak in the shared language is to be hypocritical. Reminders seem the only effective intervention for this particular communication barrier in a multicultural work group.

There is also a tremendous need to encourage and reward direct communication about such matters as how one team member's behavior affects another. Personal and collective responsibility for the sense of team is exhibited in the ability and willingness to work at "reading" each other. Team members are more likely to succeed if they

- clarify what the message received was perceived to be;
- ask for what one needs in order to do one's best; and
- negotiate the conflicts that naturally occur.

The storyboarding exercise described in the following section was one of the interventions used during the PFC education program to begin the team building process.

Creating a Team Vision Through Storyboarding. Participants came to the education program with varying degrees of understanding of PFC (from the employee for whom, literally, the first day of education was the first day on the job to the individual who had been with the organization for several years, knew all of the team members, and had a good understanding of the concepts and structure of patient-focused care. All the reactions, which one would expect during a restructuring process involving much change over a short period of time, were present. Mixed with the enthusiasm, commitment, optimism, eagerness, and excitement was a healthy dose of cynicism, doubt, anxiety, fear, apathy, resentment, a "wait and see" attitude, and stolid acceptance. Also woven into the mix were different ethnic and cultural responses to change. Participants had a very real sense of the enormity of the undertaking.

Aware of these issues, project educators viewed team building as a key component of the PFC education program. The introductory group discussion on teamwork was reinforced by a small group exercise designed in part as a means of relieving tension, as well as providing an opportunity to practice some of the team building concepts that had been introduced. The employees were asked to group themselves into sets of ten to twelve, approximating the teams within which they would be working. If their unit managers were present, they were encouraged to join a relevant group.

Each participant was given a two page "Participant's Guide" to walk them through the exercise. Part I of the exercise was designed to allow team members to learn something about one another. The instructions were as follows:

A. Before you "dive into" this exercise, please take some time to learn a little bit about one another your strengths, backgrounds, and points of view about patient-focused care. You will then be able to use that knowledge to design the storyboard that you will be asked as a team to construct.

B. You will select a timekeeper (criteria: functioning watch, reasonably assertive personality).

C. Allow each person on your team two minutes to introduce themselves and give their point of view on the discussion questions.

D. The timekeeper should signal when two minutes have passed.

The discussion questions were the following:

1. Give your name, position/title, and a brief description of your role on the patient-focused care team.
2. What irritates me most as a team member is when people.............

3. When a conflict, disagreement, or difference of opinion comes up among team members, I ....
4. In being a team member, I think my strengths will be............
5. I think where I may need to improve in order to be an effective team member is ....

Everyone was then instructed to proceed to Part II. Each team was given the following materials:

- 20″ x 24″ blank posterboard
- several sets of scissors
- several glue sticks
- several marking pens
- twelve magazines (a wide variety with a good combination of pictures and headline text, e.g., *Time*, *Newsweek*, *Sports Illustrated*, *Allure*, *Cosmopolitan*, *People*, *Life*, etc.)

The teams were told: "Each of you has your own vision of what patient-focused care looks like and what it means to be a member of the team. Over the next twenty minutes, your team will create a storyboard of this vision by cutting out pictures and print, or making your own captions or drawings, that help develop a collective image of this new way of doing business and where you and your teammates fit into the picture." Each team was then instructed to pick a spokesperson who would interpret the storyboard after it was completed for the group-at-large when everyone reassembled.

The storyboarding exercise produced several results. Most team members seemed to genuinely enjoy the activity and great deal of positive energy was produced. Group processes that were evident included the following: who took the lead, who deferred, who participated fully, who held back or sat on the periphery, who needed to be encouraged to participate, how the spokesperson was chosen (usually by pointing to someone and saying "you do it"), and how groups gave themselves permission to be different with creative, reflective, funny, sarcastic, and other postures on the storyboard

During the "Show and Tell" segment, which comprised Part III of the exercise, the whole group reconvened. The spokespersons came to the front of the room with their storyboards, and they were given two minutes each to present and interpret them. The camaraderie that had developed during the creation of the storyboards was evident. The individual team members would clap and encourage their spokesperson. They displayed a collective pride and a healthy competitive spirit about their storyboards. The boards themselves revealed their feelings about patient-focused care on many levels. Some team boards were quite negative, expressing a collectively cautious approach and fairly cynical point of view. Others were more optimistic and forward-looking in their design. A third perspective balanced the negatives and positives by carefully dividing their boards in half, or using the front to express their views of the pros and the back their views of the cons.

By the end of the process, from the 300 or more stories created, the project team had a fairly complete picture of how Cedars-Sinai employees felt about this restructured way of caring for patients. The results for those charged with leading this effort to a successful conclusion included a heightened appreciation and understanding of the following:

- the variation among the teams and their approaches to patient-focused care;
- becoming a team is an evolutionary process that requires active involvement and constant attention;
- different units came to the process with varying levels of understanding and commitment;
- teams needed to be encouraged to share information among one another and get to know one another before a seamless approach to caregiving could be achieved.
- getting to know one another and share values, concerns, pet peeves, hopes, and concerns was an important part of moving toward acceptance;
- allowing participants to express negative feelings and fears in a safe manner was a valuable way of releasing tension and expressing what other felt but not said aloud;
- teambuilding is an ongoing effort, and this was only the beginning.

Strategies for Staff "Buy-in"

As the observations about team building above indicate, staff buy-in is critical to the change process. Without the participation and cooperation of the staff, no change will have a chance at success and the planning, money, effort, and time spent on the change will be wasted. This section describes a number of additional methods that may be used to gain staff buy-in. These include early staff involvement, education, celebration of events, and, most importantly, communication. Most individuals do not enjoy change, but if involved in the change process they can develop a vested interest in the success of the change. The unit manager is pivotal in all of these involvement strategies, as acting as a gatekeeper for events, scheduler for education, organizer of celebrations, and communicator of both management expectations and staff concerns. It is the unit manager who must, on a daily basis, "sell" the change idea to the staff.

Early staff involvement. Early staff involvement in development of institution-wide role changes, as well as the staffing model for the unit, begins the buy-in process. Identifying the informal leaders on the unit and involving them in the development and change process makes the transition smoother. At Cedars-Sinai, staff representatives from various job classifications were involved in building the task lists that were used to create the new roles and role changes. This involvement gave staff members a sense of control over the process. Once the models were developed, practicing assignment making according to the new unit staffing model prior to implementation also helped the staff anticipate how the changes would affect them.

Communication. Communication about the coming change also must start early and be frequent and copious. During the Cedars-Sinai PFC planning phase, the proposed changes were discussed at each staff meeting, with reports about the individual unit's progress and the units that had already made the shift to patient-focused care. Formal meetings at the unit level to discuss the issues and plan for the change were also important. By far the most effective method of decreasing staff anxiety about the proposed changes, however, was informal discussion, usually on the unit, between the unit manager and one or two staff members to review individual concerns and clarify or dispel rumors.

Work Sampling. Work sampling also took place on each nursing unit to establish baseline information on the amount of time spent by staff members in different types of tasks (e.g., patient care, transportation, documentation, etc.) for both model development and evaluation purposes. (See Chapter 15 for more details.) The work sampling process offered another opportunity for communication about the change, this time by someone other than the unit manager. (Work sampling was done by project staff and by nurse managers, clinical nurse specialists, and selected staff members from other units.) It was essential, however, to ensure that all were giving the same message and clarification of the purpose of work sampling was important. At the beginning, it was viewed by some staff members as spying on them to report what they were doing wrong to the unit manager. When it was explained that the unit manager would only see aggregate data and not individual performance information, this fact, coupled with the explanation that the data would be a means of evaluating how successfully PFC met it goals of decreasing documentation time and increasing the time spent at the bedside, anxiety did decrease. When only the aggregate data were made available and no individual repercussions resulted, faith in the system also increased.

Preceptors and Super Trainers. Identification of preceptors and super trainers on each unit also increased staff involvement and commitment to the process, since they were now a part of it. Preceptors and super trainers were identified on all shifts to ensure that resources would be available at all times. These roles were designed to help new staff integrate into the unit as well as to assist in role transition to the new tasks and completion of the task list checkoffs. Some of the new tasks were not performed frequently enough on each unit to ensure that the staff could all complete the checklists in a timely fashion. To assist with these competencies, cross unit checkoffs on units where the tasks were performed very frequently (e.g., EKGs on the cardiac step-down unit), rounding with other job classifications (e.g., respiratory therapists), and/or the creation of patient simulations were instituted. All of these assisted in increasing staff comfort with the new tasks and the development of a new team that went beyond the traditional "nursing" team.

Incorporating New Staff. Incorporation of the new personnel classifications and new roles presented a challenge. On each unit there was an influx of new staff at the same time that previous staff members were adjusting to their new roles. Communication was again a major intervention. Team building and learning to trust each other in the new roles were also important. Tests of the team and management's ability to perform as expected in the new staff model occurred frequently. Following guidelines established prior to implementation assisted with this transition, as well as quick action with either re-education or termination from the position when a staff member could not perform a task or was not making the role transition successfully.

Celebrations. Celebration of events was important in creating team spirit. Pot lucks for new staff as they joined the unit helped them feel welcome as part of the team. Celebration of the unit going "live" with a ribbon cutting ceremony including the presence of upper management, pictures to commemorate the occasion, and, of course, food made the transition a festive occasion. It also served to separate the old from the new.

Maintaining the New. Post-implementation communication and reinforcement of the new roles and personnel are essential. Maintaining the new is difficult and much effort is needed to ensure that staff do not slip back into the old, comfortable ways. The unit manager's role includes monitoring and reinforcing the new roles, incorporating new personnel into the team, and fine tuning the staffing model for the unit. Communication both in formal and informal meetings with staff is essential for the smooth and orderly transition to PFC.

Pace of Implementation. At Cedars-Sinai as the roll out speed increased, the PFC classes became larger and larger. Multiple units were going "live" on the same day to meet implementation deadlines. Advantages included a shortened period during which the institution was running two care delivery systems. The time period for staff to anticipate the change was also shortened, and everyone felt like they were in the same boat. Disadvantages included the large class sizes, and the strain placed on the available resources such as teaching personnel, classrooms, and coverage of the units to allow staff to attend class. This meant that more reinforcement, clarification, follow up, coordination, and communication fell to the unit manager and PFC implementation team.

Lessons Learned

In reviewing the process, project leaders became aware of the factors that were critical to the success of the project and what might have been done to make implementation smoother. These factors covered a wide range of issues including the following:

- Cedars-Sinai's decision not to require employees to reapply for positions which were substantially unchanged (e.g., RN, LVN II) was essential. While employees still had some fear of change, at least they were not afraid of job loss. This allowed them to concentrate on the education, and it minimized the disruptions to patient care.
- In some areas the impact of the changes may have been underestimated, even on individuals whose classifications remained the same. Team building interventions and on-site seminars in coping with change held later in the process were very helpful, but they could have been implemented earlier.
- Managers responsible for hiring sometimes were confused by the fact that some employees did not have to formally apply for jobs while others did. This led to premature commitments or mixed messages to some candidates. It was impor-

tant to carefully communicate the status of each category to the hiring managers.

- While the institution's recruitment and hiring approaches were straight forward, the large number of applicants and tight timeline presented a challenge in meet ing PFC deadlines. It was not anticipated that a review of such a large volume of applicants and new graduates was necessary to meet the hiring needs. These issues also had a large impact on the education program and timeline.
- Written communication skills needed to be carefully assessed in the recruitment process. It was also important for hiring managers to understand the importance of this skill in order to avoid giving mixed messages to applicants (i.e., some applicants had very high customer services skills, but they did not have sufficient communication skills—particularly written skills—and could not successfully complete the education or do the job).
- Employee participation in design teams was critical to acceptance of the changes. In order to gain full acceptance, it was important to go beyond simple participation to actively considering their issues. Cedars-Sinai had to hold extensive discussions and initiate repeated communication about the steps in the transition to PFC. Cedars-Sinai also had to assist employees in coping with the change once it occurred.
- It was also essential to research the labor market prior to finalizing staffing models and new job designs to ensure that expectations for multiskills jobs were realistic and available in the market.

Overall, the Cedars-Sinai's human resource philosophy and commitment to cross-preparation of existing staff and keeping them informed about the change process served the institution well. In addition, Cedars-Sinai's experience emphasizes the importance of the unit manager as the key to staff buy-in and a successful transition. The units that had the smoothest transitions had unit managers who actively supported PFC, involved key staff early, and kept the lines of communication open. These observations are also supported by the PFC evaluation findings detailed in Chapter 16. Team building and the maintenance of the interdisciplinary team provide both the greatest benefits and the greatest challenges to PFC. They must be recognized as an ongoing process that cannot end with PFC implementation.

Chapter 15

Evaluating the Effectiveness of Patient-Focused Care: Evaluation Methodology

Linda Burnes Bolton, DrPH, RN, FAAN
Carolyn E. Aydin, PhD
Harriet Udin Aronow, PhD

This chapter gives a brief outline of the rationale and methodology for the evaluation of patient focused-care restructuring at Cedars-Sinai Medical Center.

Evaluating Innovations in Health Care Delivery

Evaluation, "an integral part of program planning, enables ... health care providers to make informed decisions regarding the efficacy of health care. Evaluation should not be considered an end in itself, but rather, an ongoing process by which the strengths and weaknesses of a program are identified, resulting in informed systematic changes."[1] This description of the process of evaluation is especially appropriate for innovations in the delivery of health services.

With the emergence of health services research methods, new models of patient care, like other new medical technology, can be subjected to rigorous evaluation and held accountable for their intended results. Unlike other technological innovations that are amenable to controlled experimental trials, organizational change efforts are complex and imbedded in multiple management processes. Yet the search for quality in health services demands that programs be evaluated systematically, held accountable, and changed to improve outcomes. The evaluative framework for the quality of health care, which was first articulated by Avedis Donabedian, preserves the complexity of organizational

LINDA BURNES BOLTON, DRPH, RN, FAAN—Director, Nursing Research and Development, Director, Surgical Nursing, Cedars-Sinai Medical Center and Research Institute; Assistant Clinical Professor, University of California-Los Angeles, School of Nursing; and Associate Professor, California State University, Los Angeles.

CAROLYN E. AYDIN, PHD—Assistant Administrator for Nursing Research, Cedars-Sinai Medical Center and Research Institute; Assistant Clinical Professor, University of California-Los Angeles.

HARRIET UDIN ARONOW, PHD—Research Associate, Nursing Research and Development, Cedars-Sinai Medical Center and Research Institute; Assistant Researcher, University of California-Los Angeles, Department of Medicine.

change and permits the placement of the evaluation in the context of total quality management efforts.[2] Health care, in this framework, is a system with measurable structures, processes, and outcomes.

Summative vs Formative Evaluations

It is useful, at this point, to make the distinction between summative and formative evaluation. In summative evaluation, one designs a study with a fixed design, fixed intervention, and fixed start and end time. Data are collected until the end time, analyzed, and a conclusion is drawn about the effect of the intervention. The traditional clinical trial is a form of summative evaluation. The advantages of summative evaluation are that the owners of the intervention receive a final conclusion in a fixed time schedule and that the outcomes measured are likely to be linked to the intervention and not some extraneous, unmeasured phenomena. The disadvantages are that the intervention receives only one chance of success. If it is judged a failure, the intervention is unlikely to get a second chance, and intervention experiments, outside a laboratory setting, are more likely to be "out of control" trials.

Formative evaluation, also called program evaluation, is an ongoing iterative process in which repeated measurements of expected outcomes are built into a process of periodic review, judgment, and adaptation of the intervention. The advantages of formative evaluation are that they are flexible and accommodating to complex organizational settings. The disadvantages are that the process is ongoing (i.e., must be maintained over long periods of time), and the intervention is typically less controlled during a period of observation. Elements that may have been well articulated initially may have changed in small ways in response to periodic feedback in the evaluation cycle.

Improving Organizational Performance (IOP)

Organizational efforts to improve the model of hospital-based health services are typically supported by a formative evaluation framework. The measurement of cost and effectiveness of health care organizational redesign projects is made difficult because each small aspect of care delivery change is embedded in a complex organizational context. Several authors argue that costs and outcomes of hospital care innovations cannot be fully estimated without considering the total organizational context of the delivery of care.[3,4,5,6,7] It is essential to evaluate the impact of change efforts directed at improving efficiency, sustaining quality and lowering costs by utilizing both formative and summative evaluation methods.

The information generated from the evaluation of PFC serves dual purposes to facilitate judgments on the success of restructuring (summative) and to guide decisions on future adaptations of the care-delivery model (formative).

PFC Evaluation Plan

The goal of patient-focused care (PFC), is to redesign hospital care to be more consumer responsive, fiscally prudent, and guided by feedback on the quality of patient outcomes.[8,9] The organizing principles of PFC include ***managed demand***—grouping patients with similar needs in stable numbers; ***redesigned work***—deploying staff to care units and cross-preparing where possible; and ***empowered employees***—developing unit-centered care teams, care models, and accountability. These goals and key features of the PFC redesign provide the link between the planning for restructuring, measuring its successful implementation, and the outcomes of the change effort. Consistent with complex interventions that result in organizational change and affect the quality of health care, the evaluation of PFC was designed to measure both the technical quality and interpersonal quality of health services.

Orthopedic Surgery - Pilot PFC Unit

After an eight-month planning process, in October 1993, the pilot orthopedic surgery unit at Cedars-Sinai implemented a PFC model (see Chapter 4). During the planning phase a smaller multidisciplinary task force was convened to develop an evaluation plan. This plan expanded on the elements developed under the "Strengthening Hospital Nursing" grant and use of unlicensed assistive personnel on nursing units (see Chapter 2). Working with the goal and key features of the PFC model redesign, the evaluation task force set down basic categories of quality service and outcomes of care that either would have positive intended or potentially negative unintended effects associated with the new PFC model of care delivery. Within each category, the task force operationalized the effects of PFC restructuring into measurable variables. The task force set its own goal to both inform the PFC management at specific time points post-implementation (e.g., at 3-, 6-, and 12-months) whether PFC met its objectives and to fit the PFC restructuring into an ongoing process to improve organizational performance.

Guiding Principles

The evaluation of PFC was guided by a set of principles established by the task force. They are the following:

Multidisciplinary Leadership. The evaluation was accountable to a multidicipilinary task force that included representation from clinical management, quality management, financial management, information systems, nursing, and health services research. This task force, in turn, reported to the management task force for PFC (Steering Committee).

High Standards of Data Validity and Reliability. The process and outcome measures for PFC objectives were selected on the basis of their known validity and reliability. Staff and management needed to be assured that the data upon which PFC was to be judged actually reflected the new care model and that the observations over time could be linked to real changes in the care model, and not random variation or other systematic change processes. This went hand-in hand with the next principle.

Minimize New Data Collection. The attempt was made to rely as much as possible on known and existing hospital generated data sources. These data were familiar to the staff and had preexisting data collection and reporting mechanisms (with the associated hardware, software and human resources). The overall effect would be to minimize the cost of new data collection and to work within existing sources. Where data had been "suspect" the task force worked with the sources to improve the quality of the data, so that users would be confident in their validity and would be more likely to believe results for PFC and for continuing quality evaluation efforts.

Promote Ongoing IOP Effort. The task force set as its goal to fully integrate the evaluation of this one particular organizational experiment (albeit a major event in a natural sequence of organizational adaptations) into the ongoing efforts to *Improve Organizational Performance.*

PFC Purpose Operationalized

Consistent with the principles of the PFC model and its outcomes objectives, the evaluation plan included five general categories of quality:

Competency. In every instance where there were cross-prepared or newly educated tasks, staff were evaluated after education and on the care unit for the competency of their performance.

Clinical Quality. Each service area selected patient-focused, clinical quality measures that reflected the specific patient population aggregated in that area. Specific time and care process-sensitive indicators were chosen for each aggregated patient population. For example, surgical areas typically chose to monitor survival site infection rates and medicine areas selected incidence of dermal ulcers.

Service. Service, the direct manifestation of care delivery in a PFC model, was a major focus of outcome evaluation. Service encompassed measures of the how the model appeared on the unit, such as the proportion of staff work time spent with value-added (patient care) tasks vs. documentation or transportation, and in patient-focused perceptual issues, such as call light response and the cleanliness of the environment.

Customer Satisfaction. Customers of the new care model were defined to include all those affected by the way in which restructured care was delivered—patients, physicians, and employees. A comprehensive evaluation of PFC must monitor their reaction to PFC and provide this feedback to the PFC management team because, without customer satisfaction, there would be little hope of sustaining the model or delineating the model's ability to sustain quality.

Financial Impact. Changes in staff mix, patient re-aggregation, and efficiencies associated with deployed central services were expected to reduce the overall cost to deliver care. Although not included in original PFC efforts, in today's health care market this outcome has emerged as a particularly important measure of PFC success.

PFC Evaluation Measures

Figure 15.1 displays the set of measures that were adopted for the evaluation of the orthopedic pilot Unit PFC model and the time frame over which each measure was reported. Each subsequent service area tailored this plan to meet specific patient characteristics. However, the basic plan remained consistent throughout the Cedars-Sinai. In the following section, each performance area and its measures are discussed in turn.

Detailed Description of Evaluation Measures

The PFC model was evaluated as a complex organizational innovation for both its technical and interpersonal quality objectives. Technological quality would be achieved by demonstrating competency in staff knowledge and performance, good clinical outcomes, and efficient care delivery. Interpersonal quality would be assessed by changes in structure and processes of care; communication within teams among care providers and between care providers and patients; and customer satisfaction.

Technical Quality

I. Competency for Redesigned Jobs

Organizational Goal. To deploy previously centralized, departmentalized tasks to the nursing unit and create effective cross-prepared clinical teams.

Evaluation Process. The education required for new tasks and new staff is formidable, and the evaluation of competent performance is essential. In every instance where Cedars-Sinai cross-prepared or developed new roles, staff were evaluated for competency of performance both following education and on the care unit. For example, simple physical therapy and respiratory therapy interventions were cross-prepared to nursing staff on the orthopedic unit. Competency was assessed by a combination of self-evaluation, written examination, and demonstration of performance in labs and with patients. Competency was also assessed early in implementation, and again at one year, to monitor acquisition and sustainability.

Figure 15.1: Sample Evaluation Plan for the Patient-Focused Care Orthopedic Model and Time Frame of Data Collection

Quality Category *Evaluation Element* Measurement Method	Baseline	3-months	6-months	12-months
Competency for Redesigned Jobs	X		X	X
Skills assessment of cross-prepared staff				
Clinical Quality of Care				
Length of Stay per Diagnostic Guidelines	X		X	X
% Low Risk Hips with LOS <= 5 days				
% Low Risk Knees with LOS <= 4 days				
Functional Status	X	X		X
Functional Status in Transfers at Discharge				
Functional Status in Ambulation at Discharge				
Average Improvement in Walking Distance				
Patient Care Quality Indicators	X	X	X	X
Rate (per 100 procedures) Surgical Site Infections				
Rate (per 100 proc's) Post-operative Pneumonia				
Rate (per 1,000 pt days) Unattended Falls				
Rate (per 100 discharges) Acquired Dermal Ulcers				
Rate (per 100 discharges) DVT				
Rate (per 100 disch's) Respiratory Complications				
Rate (per 100 disch's) Unplanned Readmit <8days				
Service Outcomes	X		X	X
Responsiveness				
Call Light Response Time (average/median)				
% RN Time in Direct Patient Care & Support				
Teamwork/Coordination				
Number of Different Staff Interacting with Patient				
% RN Time in Scheduling & Coordination				
% Missed PT Treatments				
Environment/Amenities				
Litter Counted in Two Sampled Hours				
Information/Communication				
% RN Time in Documentation				
Customer Satisfaction	X		X	X
Physician Satisfaction with Nursing Staff				
Patient Satisfaction with Nursing/Service Area				
Employee Satisfaction with Role, Job, Team				
Financial Impact				
Managed Demand	X	X	X	X
Diagnostic Mix on Unit				
Average Daily Census				
Resource Consumption	X	X		X
Target Total Cost Reduction				
FTE Staff On and Off Unit				
Labor Cost per Discharge				

II.Clinical outcomes

Organizational Goal. To maintain or improve the technical quality of care while creating a new model of patient care in which (1) patients are aggregated by similarity of problems and needs and (2) staff with specialized skills and knowledge are deployed to the unit and function as a clinically coordinated team. On the pilot orthopedic unit, the net effect of these care model changes was to reduce the licensed physical therapy staff needed to care for the orthopedic surgery patients by approximately two full-time equivalents (FTEs). In addition, patients were likely to see only two different therapists during their stay, instead of a daily cycle of centralized staff. Furthermore, with all patient care staff prepared in getting patients out of bed and practicing transfers and walking, functional recovery should be as good or better than before PFC. The potential risks could be quantified as well: Would there be an increase in falls? Would the newly prepared staff be too afraid to get patients out of bed and walk them? Would patient outcomes suffer as a result?

Evaluation Process. Patient-focused, clinical quality measures were selected to reflect the specific patient population needs and risks. In orthopedics, clinical quality measures included surgical site infection, pneumonia and deep vein thrombosis (DVT) rates; functional status at admission, discharge, and post-discharge; unattended falls; acquired dermal ulcers; unplanned readmission within seven days; and length of stay for patient groups being managed on clinical pathways. Clinical outcomes, except for functional status, were reported at baseline and three-month intervals thereafter. Functional status was abstracted from physical therapy notes at baseline, three months post-implementation, and one year post-implementation. The management team was especially interested in monitoring the effects of deploying licensed physical therapists and cross-preparing unlicensed unit staff for simple practice in transfers, ambulation, and therapeutic exercise.

III. Financial Impact

Organizational Goal. The goal was to decrease the cost to provide care during a hospital admission. Three PFC principles were hypothesized to have cost-reduction potential. Reaggregating patients by special need would reduce the travel time of ancillary staff. Controlling the average daily census of patients with similar needs would stabilize the demand for staff. Permanent deployment of some of those staff on patient care units, where volume of services allowed, would reduce dispatch and travel time. And cross-preparation of unit-based staff to do simple physical activity tasks, respiratory tasks, and assist the patient with self-care needs would both reduce the need for ancillary therapy staff and even out census-related and acuity-related variations in demands for patient care.

Evaluation Process. Financial measures evaluated the following: diagnostic mix on the unit; average daily census; total operating costs per discharge; and number of FTEs (both on and off the unit) providing care to patients on the unit. Staffing was assessed at baseline, just after implementation of the new model, and one year later. The remainder of financial measures were reported in regular three-month intervals. The achievement of the total expected cost reduction was evaluated at the end of one year.

Interpersonal Quality

I. Service Outcomes

Organizational Goal. The Cedars-Sinai's goal was to maintain or improve service provided by the cross-prepared team member implementing PFC restructuring. Service outcomes directly measure the changes in processes, consistent with principles of PFC. Since Cedars-Sinai would be more patient-focused, the following should occur:

1. There should be more people (including licensed and unlicensed staff and deployed therapists) on the unit to respond to patient needs. Therefore, more time should be spent in providing care to the patients, the unit should be tidier, and call light

response time reduced.

2. With staff providing high volume services permanently deployed to the unit (e.g., physical therapy on orthopedics or room cleaning and transportation services on all units), there should be fewer different care providers interacting with the patient.
3. With staff deployed to the unit and functioning as a stable patient care team, there should develop a sense of staff ownership and commitment to the unit. This should result in a sense of pride in service and better team work.
4. Technological enablers (including computers, redesigned patient servers, and redesigned charting) associated with the new care model should result in less time spent in nonvalue-added activities, such as documentation and more time in patient care activities.

Evaluation Process. This one area, that most specific to the implementation of the PFC model, engendered the greatest amount of new data collection during the PFC implementation period. Direct observational methods were selected to evaluate the changes in the delivery of care in patient care area. Staffing patterns recorded by the nurse manager provided counts of patient care staff interacting with each patient. Simple litter counts were used to assess cleanliness. Research staff observed and measured the time between call light initiation and resolution of the patient's needs in a sample of hours on the unit. Work sampling was selected as the method to evaluate the degree to which delivery of care changed with the model.

The work sampling method has its roots in industrial engineering, but there is a recent rise in use in hospital settings as a method to support planning and evaluation of service delivery innovations.[10,11,12,13] First described by Tippett in 1935, work sampling is a less obtrusive and more efficient derivative of time-and-motion studies.[14] Work sampling involves systematically observing a group of workers and coding a probability sample of their work activities. The resulting statistics reflect the proportion of time spent by each worker in each category of activity. The precise amount of time spent in a category of activity can only be inferred by this method; and the accuracy of the estimate is directly related to the frequency and total number of observations and the number of categories of activity.[15]

The work sampling method has been especially useful in hospital settings where specific innovations have been designed to directly impact the amount of work-time spent in a particular activity (e.g., documentation time, travel time within or between units , or preparation of medications).[16,17,18] Work-sampling methods have been used widely as tools for guiding PFC development, but they have had limited use in detailed evaluations of the outcome of PFC. However, the principles of work redesign, use of licensed and unlicensed care providers, and the use of technological "enablers" make work sampling an attractive evaluation strategy.

Work-sampling at Cedars-Sinai focused on classifying work activities into those which were seen as "value-added" (i.e., patient care and patient supportive activities); and "non-valued added" (i.e., documentation and waiting time). Six broad categories were identified in preliminary method development, including: ***patient care*** – activities that consist of direct interaction or physical contact with the patient (e.g., changing dressings, administering medication, patient education); ***patient support*** – activities where direct interaction does not occur, but that directly support the provision of care (e.g., change linens, prepare medications, family teaching, preparing specimen); ***scheduling and coordination*** – activities that involve planning for patient's care, admission, discharge (e.g., entering orders, scheduling ancillary services, conferring with team members); *transportation* – activities that are directly concerned with transfer of patients, supplies, meals, self, etc. (e.g., moving patients, delivering meals, looking for supplies); ***documentation*** – activities that require paperwork or computer data entry (e.g., charting medications, writing patient care notes); ***ready and waiting*** – on the unit, but no meaningful activity, idle, nonwork related conversations.

Work-sampling was planned as a baseline premeasure and for repeated assessment at 6-months and 12-months post-implementation. Two 12-hour day shifts were randomly selected, and observations of activities were recorded every five minutes by trained staff. The same work sampling strategy was used for each unit in the subsequent housewide implementation.

II. Customer Satisfaction

Organizational Goal. The PFC model, while it represented organizational change, was expected to result in maintained or improved customer satisfaction. In times of momentous change in the health care delivery system, it is difficult to sort out the cause and effect relationship between a single restructuring effort and customer satisfaction. By focusing on aspects of the delivery of care that were most changed by PFC restructuring, however, the survey responses described below would provide a sense of the reaction of three diverse customers—patients, physicians, and employees of the medical center.

Evaluation Process. Patient satisfaction was assessed using a patient satisfaction survey sent to all patients after discharge. The results were available quarterly. Cedars-Sinai had used the consulting services of Press, Ganey Associates, Inc., prior to and shortly following PFC implementation. However, the institution changed vendors to NCG, Inc. With both of these vendors, institutions may receive not only their own results but also comparisons with peer hospitals. Institutions are also provided with the opportunity to benchmark their own findings against similar organizations nationwide.

Physician satisfaction was measured using a survey adapted specifically for PFC by the service standards design team (see Chapter 2) from a previous Cedars-Sinai physician survey. The new survey focused on physician perceptions of clinical and technical competence, responsiveness, coordination, and teamwork on the unit (see **Figure 15.2**). The survey also asked for ratings of other services, such as housekeeping, admitting, laboratory services, radiology, billing, and operating room services. Physicians completed the surveys prior to PFC implementation and at six months and one year post-implementation.

Figure 15.2: Physician Survey

Date________________

As part of the evaluation plan for Patient Focused Care at CSMC, we need to know how well we are <u>currently</u> meeting <u>physician needs</u>. Please take a few minutes to complete this survey and return it in the enclosed envelope. You: response is important. If you have any questions, please call Carolyn Aydin (855-3694) or Linda Burnes Bolton (855-5191), Nursing Research & Development

I. Evaluation of Nursing Services

Please <u>check only</u> the <u>three</u> units where you practice <u>most</u> frequently:

Special Care Units

[ ] Neonatology ICU 4NIA
[ ] Pediatric ICU 4PIC
[ ] Medical ICU 5CCE
[ ] Medical ICU 5CCW
[ ] Medical ICU 5MIC
[ ] Respiratory ICU 5RIC
[ ] Cardiovascular ICU 6CSI
[ ] Surgical ICU 7ICU
[ ] Surgical ICU 8ICU

Definitive Observation Units

[ ] Maternal Fetal Care Unit 3ACU
[ ] Intermediate Neonatology 4NIB
[ ] Intermediate Neonatology 4NIC
[ ] Cardiac Observation 5COU
[ ] Cardiovascular DOU 6PIU
[ ] Medical Observation 6SCU

[ ] Labor and Delivery 3LDR

Routine Care Units

[ ] Skilled Nursing SNAC
[ ] Psychiatry 2W
[ ] Psychiatry 3E
[ ] Psychiatry 3W
[ ] Obstetrics 3N
[ ] Gynecology-Oncology 3SW
[ ] Pediatrics 4N
[ ] Medicine-Hem/Onc 4SW
[ ] Medicine-Cardiology 5NW
[ ] Medicine-Pulmonary 5SE
[ ] Medicine-GI 5SW

[ ] IDC/Infectious Disease 6SE
[ ] Medicine-Nephro/Endocrn 6SW
[ ] Cardiovascular-Thoracic/Liver 6NW
[ ] Orthopedics 7NE
[ ] General Surgery 7NW
[ ] Neuro/HEENT/Trauma 8N
[ ] Rehabilitation Rehab

Please list the three units selected in the spaces indicated below.

Then rate nursing services on each unit using the following scale:

Ratings: Excellent=5 Good=4 Neutral=3 Fair=2 Poor=1 No Opinion=0

	The 1st Unit which is: ______	The 2nd Unit which is: ______	The 3rd Unit which is: ______
1. Courtesy and attentiveness toward patients..........................	[ ]	[ ]	[ ]
2. Responsiveness of nurses to physicians' orders......................	[ ]	[ ]	[ ]
3. Communication between nurses and physicians..........................	[ ]	[ ]	[ ]
4. Quality of patient care provided........	[ ]	[ ]	[ ]
5. Quality of nursing unit management......	[ ]	[ ]	[ ]
6. Nurse staffing levels on the unit.......	[ ]	[ ]	[ ]
7. Teamwork among unit staff..............	[ ]	[ ]	[ ]
8. Courtesy and responsiveness to physicians...........................	[ ]	[ ]	[ ]
9. Quality of patient education............	[ ]	[ ]	[ ]

Figure 15.2: Physician Survey (cont.)

Ratings: Excellent=5 Good=4 Neutral=3 Fair=2 Poor=1 No Opinion=0

	The 1st Unit which is: ______	The 2nd Unit which is: ______	The 3rd Unit which is: ______
10. Courtesy and responsiveness to visitors..............................	[ ]	[ ]	[ ]
11. Availablity of equipment and supplies to meet physician needs.................	[ ]	[ ]	[ ]
12. Willingness of staff to meet physician needs..........................	[ ]	[ ]	[ ]
13. Staff's authority to meet physician needs without referring the problem to someone else..........................	[ ]	[ ]	[ ]
14. Overall performance of nursing staff....	[ ]	[ ]	[ ]

II. Evaluation of Other Services

Housekeeping	Excellent	Good	Neutral	Fair	Poor	No Opinion
1. Housekeeping in public areas	(5)	(4)	(3)	(2)	(1)	(0)
2. Housekeeping in patient rooms and patient care areas	(5)	(4)	(3)	(2)	(1)	(0)
3. Overall Housekeeping Evaluation	(5)	(4)	(3)	(2)	(1)	(0)

Admitting

1. Responsiveness and courtesy of admitting personnel	(5)	(4)	(3)	(2)	(1)	(0)
2. Ease of admitting patients	(5)	(4)	(3)	(2)	(1)	(0)
3. Ease of scheduling patients	(5)	(4)	(3)	(2)	(1)	(0)
4. Overall Admitting Evaluation	(5)	(4)	(3)	(2)	(1)	(0)

Laboratory Services

1. Range of services provided	(5)	(4)	(3)	(2)	(1)	(0)
2. Timeliness of services provided	(5)	(4)	(3)	(2)	(1)	(0)
3. Courtesy and responsiveness of staff	(5)	(4)	(3)	(2)	(1)	(0)
4. Overall Laboratory Evaluation	(5)	(4)	(3)	(2)	(1)	(0)

Radiology

1. Range of services provided	(5)	(4)	(3)	(2)	(1)	(0)
2. Timeliness of services provided	(5)	(4)	(3)	(2)	(1)	(0)
3. Courtesy and responsiveness of staff	(5)	(4)	(3)	(2)	(1)	(0)
4. Overall Radiology Evaluation	(5)	(4)	(3)	(2)	(1)	(0)

Billing

1. Accuracy of bills	(5)	(4)	(3)	(2)	(1)	(0)
2. Courtesy and responsiveness of billing personnel	(5)	(4)	(3)	(2)	(1)	(0)
3. Overall Billing Evaluation	(5)	(4)	(3)	(2)	(1)	(0)

Figure 15.2: Physician Survey (cont.)

III. Evaluation of Services and Facilities that Impact on Surgical Practice

(If you do not perform surgical procedures on a regular basis, please skip to Section IV below.)

Please rate the following services and facilities that impact on surgical practice:

	Excellent	Good	Neutral	Fair	Poor	No Opinion
General						
1. Coordination of admissions with surgery scheduling	(5)	(4)	(3)	(2)	(1)	(0)
2. Scheduling procedures for operating rooms	(5)	(4)	(3)	(2)	(1)	(0)
3. Surgical facilities/equipment	(5)	(4)	(3)	(2)	(1)	(0)
4. Patient waiting time for routine elective surgery	(5)	(4)	(3)	(2)	(1)	(0)
5. Availability of operating room time	(5)	(4)	(3)	(2)	(1)	(0)
Nursing Specialty Areas						
1. Operating room nursing: quality of patient care	(5)	(4)	(3)	(2)	(1)	(0)
2. Recovery room nursing: quality of patient care	(5)	(4)	(3)	(2)	(1)	(0)
3. Intensive care unit (ICU) nursing: quality of patient care	(5)	(4)	(3)	(2)	(1)	(0)

IV. *Principal area of medical practice?* ____________________
(please specify)

How many years have you practiced medicine? ________*years*

How many years has your medical practice been associated with Cedars-Sinai Medical Center?

______ *(Please include years with former Cedars of Lebanon and Mt. Sinai Hospitals.)*

What is your current hospital medical staff affiliation at Cedars-Sinai?

____*Attending* ____*Associate* ____*Courtesy* ____*Provisional* ____*Other*

Approximately what percent of your total admissions last year (1992) went to Cedars-Sinai Medical Center?

______%

Thank you. Your cooperation is greatly appreciated. Please return the survey in the enclosed envelope to Nursing Research and Development, Room 2033.

Staff members also completed a survey probing specific issues such as job satisfaction, role clarity, and teamwork (see **Figure 15.3** for post-implementation version). This survey, developed using items from the work experience literature,[20] was first used at Cedars-Sinai to evaluate the assistive personnel program in 1991 and has been used at regular intervals since that time. The items on the survey form a number of scales, each of which has an 0.80 or higher Cronbach's alpha coefficient of reliability . These include patient care job satisfaction[21] (**Figure 15.3**: questions 1-5 in section I), general job satisfaction[22, 23] (questions 6-9), job clarity (questions 12-13), role tension[24] (4 items in section II), and teamwork[25] (7 items in section III). A short form (**Figure 15.4**) was also used for staff in centralized departments (e.g., housekeeping, food and nutrition, respiratory therapy, and so on). A number of the single items (e.g., question 10 in section I is a one-item teamwork question) were included specifically to match those items used in the short form so comparisons of the opinions of staff in different areas would be possible. Unit-based staff completed the surveys prior to PFC implementation and at six months and one year post-implementation.

PFC Evaluation and the Process of Improving Organizational Performance

The process of implementing PFC substantially rearranged the focus of improving organizational performance (IOP) at Cedars-Sinai. PFC, with its continued development of guidelines and pathways, encompassed a complete restructuring of the work-teams and processes of care. The IOP process has remained constant, with a complete shift in the management groups involved in IOP from departmental level to interdisciplinary team management groups – some with a clinical program (or service line) focus, others with a system-wide focus. The hospital-wide implementation of PFC took place during the year after the orthopedic unit went up. During this time the focus of the evaluation moved from the single pilot unit to the larger framework of Improving Organizational Performance.

Data from a variety of hospital sources were used to evaluate the implementation of PFC. Each measure was selected for a specific link to the expected desirable effects and potential undesirable effects of PFC restructuring. Many of the measures selected for the pilot orthopedic unit were generalized to the hospital-wide implementation of PFC models. Over the hospital-wide planning period, evaluation measures were consolidated into service line report cards, often incorporating multiple units with similar service needs. For example, the pilot orthopedic unit was grouped with all surgery except for cardiothoracic surgery.

The report cards were developed to include and communicate sufficient management information to monitor, evaluate, and adapt the process of care in a multidisciplinary team. Report cards look very much like the PFC evaluation plan (**Figure 15.1**) and are produced every calendar quarter. Patient-focused care, as other innovations and adaptations in the delivery of care, will become an event in a continuous process of organizational monitoring, evaluation and improvement.

Figure 15.3: Job Satisfaction for Unit-Based Staff

Patient Focused Care Job Satisfaction Survey

Unit: ________ **Date:**____________

This survey asks you to rate different aspects of your job. Your responses will provide information to help us evaluate how well Patient Focused Care meets your needs and the needs of your patients. Your responses are confidential and your opinions are important to us.

Please check the number that indicates whether you agree or disagree with each statement.

I. The following statements rate your general job satisfaction.

	Strongly Agree		Uncertain		Strongly Disagree
1. The patient care delivered on my unit is excellent.	[5]	[4]	[3]	[2]	[1]
2. I am able to provide the amount of direct patient care I desire.	[5]	[4]	[3]	[2]	[1]
3. I am satisfied with the types of activities that are included in my job.	[5]	[4]	[3]	[2]	[1]
4. I am satisfied with my role on the unit.	[5]	[4]	[3]	[2]	[1]
5. I make a significant contribution to patient care on my unit.	[5]	[4]	[3]	[2]	[1]
6. The job offers me the opportunity to use my personal initiative or judgement in carrying out my work.	[5]	[4]	[3]	[2]	[1]
7. The job gives me considerable opportunity for independence and freedom in how I do the work.	[5]	[4]	[3]	[2]	[1]
8. I am satisfied with the nature of the work I perform.	[5]	[4]	[3]	[2]	[1]
9. I am satisfied with my relations with others in the organization with whom I work--my coworkers.	[5]	[4]	[3]	[2]	[1]
10. Personnel in my area work together as a team.	[5]	[4]	[3]	[2]	[1]
11. I am kept informed about important things that are happening at CSMC.	[5]	[4]	[3]	[2]	[1]
12. I am clear of just what the scope and responsibilities of my job are.	[5]	[4]	[3]	[2]	[1]
13. I know what others who work with me expect from me.	[5]	[4]	[3]	[2]	[1]
14. There is cooperation and communication between nurses and physicians on my unit.	[5]	[4]	[3]	[2]	[1]
15. I would never go back to the old way of doing things.	[5]	[4]	[3]	[2]	[1]

-over-

Figure 15.3: Job Satisfaction for Unit-Based Staff (cont.)

	Very Satisfied		Neutral		Very Dissatisfied
All in all, how satisfied are you with your job?	[5]	[4]	[3]	[2]	[1]

II. How often do you feel bothered by:	Always		Sometimes		Never
1. Being unclear of just what the scope and responsibilities of your job are?	[5]	[4]	[3]	[2]	[1]
2. Not knowing just what others who work with you expect from you?	[5]	[4]	[3]	[2]	[1]
3. Being unable to prioritize work because of the workload?	[5]	[4]	[3]	[2]	[1]
4. Thinking that you'll not be able to satisfy the conflicting demands of various people around you?	[5]	[4]	[3]	[2]	[1]

III. To what extent:	To a very great extent		To some extent		To a very little extent
1. Does your unit plan together and coordinate efforts?	[5]	[4]	[3]	[2]	[1]
2. Does your unit make good decisions and solve problems well?	[5]	[4]	[3]	[2]	[1]
3. Do persons in your unit know what their jobs are and how to do them well?	[5]	[4]	[3]	[2]	[1]
4. Is important information shared within your unit?	[5]	[4]	[3]	[2]	[1]
5. Does your unit really want to meet its objectives successfully?	[5]	[4]	[3]	[2]	[1]
6. Is your unit able to respond to unusual work demands placed upon it?	[5]	[4]	[3]	[2]	[1]
7. Do you have confidence and trust in the persons on your unit?	[5]	[4]	[3]	[2]	[1]

What works best in Patient Focused Care?____

____

____

What things about Patient Focused Care still need to be worked out?__________________________

____

____

IV. Your current job: [1] RN [2] LVN [3] Clinical Partner [4] Support Partner [5] NCT [6] Other__________ (specify)

Unit:_____ Shift:______ Years on present unit:________ Years at CSMC:__________

PLEASE RETURN TO CAROLYN AYDIN, Ph.D., NURSING RESEARCH AND DEVELOPMENT, ROOM 2021
10/27/94 (reformatted 5/95)

Figure 15.4: Job Satisfaction for Central Staff

Patient Focused Care Job Satisfaction Survey

Dept:______________________ Floor:__________ Date:_____

This survey asks you to rate various aspects of your job. Your responses will help us evaluate how well Patient Focused Care is meeting your needs. Your responses are confidential and your opinions are important to us.

Please check the number that indictes whether you agree or disagree with each statement.

	Strongly Agree		Uncertain		Strongly Disagree
1. Personnel in my area work together as a team.	[5]	[4]	[3]	[2]	[1]
2. I am kept informed about important things that are happening at CSMC.	[5]	[4]	[3]	[2]	[1]
3. I am clear of just what the scope and responsibilities of my job are.	[5]	[4]	[3]	[2]	[1]
4. I know what others who work with me expect from me.	[5]	[4]	[3]	[2]	[1]
5. I am satisfied with the types of activities that are included in my job.	[5]	[4]	[3]	[2]	[1]
6. I am satisfied with my role.	[5]	[4]	[3]	[2]	[1]
7. I make a significant contribution to patient care.	[5]	[4]	[3]	[2]	[1]
8. The job offers me the opportunity to use my personal initiative or judgement in carrying out my work.	[5]	[4]	[3]	[2]	[1]
9. The job gives me considerable opportunity for independence and freedom in how I do the work.	[5]	[4]	[3]	[2]	[1]
10. I am satisfied with the nature of the work I perform.	[5]	[4]	[3]	[2]	[1]
11. I am satisfied with my relations with others in the organization with whom I work--my co-workers.	[5]	[4]	[3]	[2]	[1]
	Very Satisfied		Neutral		Very Dissatisfied
All in all, how satisfied are you with your job?	[5]	[4]	[3]	[2]	[1]

Job Title:______________ Years on this floor:_____ Years at CSMC:_____ Years of experience:_______

Education: (Please check highest educational level)

(1) High School Diploma (2) Certification Program (3) AA (4) Bachelors (5) Masters (6) Other

Please return to Carolyn Aydin, Ph.D., Nursing Research and Development, Room 2021

(3/8/94-reformatted 5/95)

Lessons Learned

PFC was the institution's first experience with fundamental organizational redesign. As such it has provided the context for discovery of those internal and external factors that facilitate or impede the process of improving organizational performance to meet patient care needs.[19]

Patient-focused care, a major planned organizational redesign, must be evaluated in a total quality framework; for outcomes resulting both from implementation of redesigned patient care delivery teams and the interpersonal/communication functions of those teams. Change consistent with PFC principles must be continuously monitored and reinforced. Report cards on organizational performance will assist in fostering the continued development of PFC models, because: (1) they are a concrete link between the process of care (what the team is and does) and the outcome of care (clinical outcomes and satisfaction); and (2) they reinforce the multidisciplinary team management of patient care delivery. Overall, the experience of the development of PFC evaluation at Cedars-Sinai supports the need to evaluate innovations in hospital care delivery models in their organizational context, over time and within a framework of ongoing improvement of organizational performance.

References

1 Johnson JH, N Olesinski. "Program Evaluation: Key to Success." *Journal of Nursing Administration.* 1995; 25:53-60.

2 Donabedian A. "Evaluating the Quality of Medical Care." *Milbank Memorial Fund Quarterly* 44 (Part II) 1966:166-196.

3 Arndt M, B Bigelow. " The Impact of Individual and Contextual Factors on Nursing Care and the Implementation of AHCPR Practice Guidelines." *Medical Care Review.* 51 1994:61-82.

4 Goughnour BR. "Cost Considerations of Analgesic Therapy: An Analysis of the Effects of Dosing Frequency and Route of Administration." *Postgraduate Medical Journal.* 67(suppl. 2) 1991:S87-S91

5 Kibbe DC, AD Kaluzny, CP McLaughlin. "Integrating Guidelines with Continuous Quality Improvement: Doing the Right Thing The Right Way To Achieve The Right Goals." *Journal on Quality Improvement.* 20 1994:181-91

6 Manuel P, K Alster. "Unlicensed Personnel: No cure for an Ailing Health Care System." *Nursing & Health Care.* 15 1994:18-21

7 Wakefield DS, ST Cyphert, JF Murray, T Uden-Holman, et al. "Understanding Patient-Centered Care in the Context of Total Quality Management and Continuous Quality Improvement" *Journal on Quality Improvement.* 20 1994:152-161

8 Moffitt GK, PB Daly, L Tracey, M Galloway, TC Tinstman. "Patient-Focused Care: Key Principles to Restructuring." *Hospital & Health Services Administration.* 38 1993:509-21

9 Townsend MB. Patient-Focused Care: Is It for Your Hospital?" *Nursing Management.* 24 1993:74-80

10 Correnti DM. "Work Sampling and Professional Nurses." *Journal of Nursing Administration.* 231993:11

11 Finkler SA, JR Knickman, G Hendrickson, M Lipkin, WG Thompson. A Comparison of Work-Sampling and Time-And-Motion Techniques for Studies in Health Services Research." *Health Services Research.* 28 1993:577-97

12 Quist BD. "Work Sampling Nursing Units". *Nursing Management.* 23 1992:50-51

13 Scherubel JC, AF Minnick. "Implementation of Work Sampling Methodology." *Nursing Research.* 43 1994:120-123

14 Tippit LHC. "Statistical Methods in Textile Research. Uses of the Binomial And Poisson Distributions: A Snap Reading Method of Making Time Studies of Machines and Operatives in Factory Surveys." *Journal of Textile Inst Trans.* 26 1935:51-5

15 Finkler SA, et al, 1992

16 Sittig DF. "Work-Sampling: A Statistical Approach to Evaluation of the Effect of Computers on work patterns in Healthcare." *Methods of Information in Medicine.* 32 1993:167-74

17 Minnick A, K Pischke-Winn, MB Sterk. " Introduing a Two-Way Wireless Communication System." *Nursing Management.*25 1994 25:42-47

18 Seidel AM, TW Woller, S Somani, PW Abramowitz. "Effect of Computer Software on Time Required to Prepare Parenteral Nutrient Solutions." *American Journal of Hospital Pharmacy.* 46 1991:270-5

19 Farris BJ. "Converting a Unit to Patient-Focused Care." *Health Progress.* 1993 (April):22-25

20 Cook JD, SJ Hepworth, TD Wall, and PB Warr. The Experience of Work: A Compendium and Review of 249 Measures and their Use. New York: Academic Press, Harcourt Brace Jovanovich, Publishers, 1981.

21 Adapted from Slavitt DB, PL Stamps, EB Piedmont, and AMB Haase. "Nurses' Satisfaction with their Work Situation." *Nursing Research* 27 1978: 114-120.

22 Adapted from Hackman JR. and GR Oldham. "Development of the Job Diagnostic Survey." *Journal of Applied Psychology* 60 1975: 159-170.

23 Adapted from Schriesheim C. and A Tsui. Development and Validation of a Short Satisfaction Measure for Use in Survey Feedback Interventions. Paper presented at the Academy of Management Western Region Meeting, April 1981.

24 Adapted from Brosnan J. and M Johnston. "Stressed but Satisfied: Organizational Change in Ambulatory Care. Journal of Nursing Administration November 1980: 43-46. Brosnan and Johnston adapted their version from Rizzo JR, et al. "Role Conflict and Ambiguity in Complex Organizations." *Administrative Science Quarterly* 15 1970: 150.

25 "Group Process" scale adapted from Taylor JC. and DB Bowers. Survey of Organizations: A Machine Scored Standardized Questionnaire Instrument. Institute for Social Research, University of Michigan, Ann Arbor, MI: 1972.

Chapter 16

Impact of Patient-Focused Care: Evaluation Findings

Linda Burnes Bolton, DrPH, RN, FAAN
Harriet Udin Aronow, PhD
Carolyn E. Aydin, PhD

This chapter presents results from the evaluation of the pilot orthopedics unit to date and preliminary results from the housewide implementation of patient-focused care. As presented in Chapter 15, the evaluation employed multiple measures sensitive to changes in the processes of care and the expected outcomes of PFC restructuring. The PFC model was evaluated as a complex organizational innovation for both its technical and interpersonal quality objectives. Technological quality would be achieved by demonstrating competency in staff knowledge and performance, good clinical outcomes, and efficient care delivery. Interpersonal quality would be assessed by changes in structure and processes of care; communication within teams and between caregivers and patients; and customer satisfaction.

The PFC restructuring represented a fundamental change in the way in which patient care was delivered. Corresponding to the complex intervention, the evaluation was multidimensional as well. Results from the pilot orthopedic PFC model are reported first to provide a comprehensive overview of the elements in the evaluation design. Preliminary results from the first six months of the housewide evaluation are then reported. A discussion of our conclusions and the future of the evaluation plan follows.

Methods Review

To summarize, the PFC models represent a restructuring of the delivery of hospital-based care into self-governing units designed around the specific needs of well-defined

LINDA BURNES BOLTON, DRPH, RN, FAAN—Director, Nursing Research and Development, Director, Surgical Nursing, Cedars-Sinai Medical Center and Research Institute; Assistant Clinical Professor, University of California-Los Angeles, School of Nursing; and Associate Professor, California State University, Los Angeles.

HARRIET UDIN ARONOW, PHD—Research Associate, Nursing Research and Development, Cedars-Sinai Medical Center and Research Institute; Assistant Researcher, University of California-Los Angeles, Department of Medicine.

CAROLYN E. AYDIN, PHD—Assistant Administrator for Nursing Research, Cedars-Sinai Medical Center and Research Institute; Assistant Clinical Professor, University of California-Los Angeles.

patient groups. Tasks and activities of patient care are tailored to achieve the therapeutic goals of similar patients, and as many activities as feasible are permanently deployed to the care unit. PFC care units are self-regulating and can respond to changing external demands. The goal of PFC is to ensure that the patient receives the best, most appropriate hospital care as efficiently as possible. The goal and principles of PFC contain key statements that were implemented into an evaluation plan.

Consistent with the principles of the PFC model and its outcome objectives, the evaluation plan included five general categories of measures: (1) competency of performance of newly prepared skills; (2) clinical outcomes general to all hospitalized patients and specific to the specific patient characteristics on the PFC unit; (3) characteristics of the service delivery system that directly corresponded to the PFC model changes; (4) satisfaction of the customers of the new care models including patients, physicians, and patient care staff; and (5) financial impact of the new care model both in terms of stabilizing the patient care demand by regulating census and patient mix, as well as the overall cost to treat patients on the PFC unit.

The following section presents the results of the orthopedic PFC model implementation over its first year of implementation. The broad scope of results are presented and discussed.

Orthopedic Pilot Unit

Technical Quality

I. Competency for Redesigned Jobs

By six-months post-implementation 100% of staff were competent in simple physical therapy tasks, but only 20% of staff had been checked out as competent in respiratory tasks. Respiratory interventions occurred with relative infrequency, and specific staff had assumed the responsibility for all respiratory tasks. The others had no opportunity to demonstrate performance to the educators. Yet the unit manager believed it was important for all licensed staff to be capable of delivering respiratory care. A special effort was made to bring educators to the unit to evaluate all staff. By one year 100% of staff had been assessed as competent.

Summary. Competency in newly prepared skills is clearly a key to successful PFC restructuring. Because of the high volume need for physical interventions supporting functional recovery these cross-prepared skills, aspects of the multidisciplinary team work, received expedited attention. The professional physical therapy staff were on the unit and available to coach, reinforce, and test competencies for the new skills. In contrast, competencies for the low volume respiratory tasks were established more slowly. Without deployed respiratory therapists, the logistics of coordinating appropriate patients with staff members who still needed competency testing, and the licensed respiratory therapy staff were formidable.

II. Clinical Quality

Length of Stay and Initial Evaluation. During the year of PFC implementation the median length of stay for patients referred for physical therapy (PT) on the orthopedic unit dropped by one day (i.e., from six days to five days). During the same time period, the delay between hospital admission and PT evaluation also dropped by one day. The therapists were evaluating patients one day sooner on average than before the PFC model.

Patient Functional Status. A patient's functional status was measured on a 10-point scale (1=unable ... 5=moderate assistance of one person ... 8=contact guard ... 10=independent) in three areas — bed to chair transfers, sit to stand transfers, and ambulation on even surfaces. **Figure 16.1** illustrates the median discharge ratings at baseline and the two post-implementation periods for a randomly selected sample (approximately 20%) of patients receiving physical therapy on the orthopedic unit. Patients in all three quarters were discharged at quite similar levels of independence in physical functioning. Half the patients were discharged at or above a "minimal assistance" or "contact guard" assistance level.

There was a trend (non-significant) for shorter ambulation distances at discharge (see **Figure 16.2**) over the post-implementation period. Evidence in physical therapy documentation pointed to a considerable increase in activities with home health care staff and physicians around discharge planning for continued home and outpatient therapy. Decreased walking distance might be expected with a reduction of one day in length of stay. The team response of increased discharge planning and communication was reinforced by having deployed staff on the unit and emphasis on patients' needs consistent with the PFC model.

Other Clinical Outcomes. There was a total of 1,856 patients discharged from the orthopedic unit for a total of 10,153 patient days during the year following implementation of the PFC model. Post-implementation rates of falls, infections (surgical site and post-operative pneumonia), dermal ulcers, DVTs, unexpected deaths and readmissions, etc., were compared to baseline rates using control limits (three standard deviations) calculated from the year prior to implementation. Rates, calculated for all patients and reported quarterly, were well below control limits. There was one exception; in the first quarter post-implementation the rate of surgical site infections exceeded control limits. For the remainder of the year the rate was well below one per one-hundred procedures (the baseline level).

Summary. The results of the clinical quality outcomes evaluation suggest that the PFC model was implemented without negative impact on previous hospital indicators of quality. Furthermore, there was some indication of increased efficiency and effectiveness of the patient care team interventions to promote functional recovery. This finding validates the concept of the specialized interdisciplinary care team associated with PFC. The maintenance of the care team's effectiveness lies in continued team building and the skill in team management.

Figure 16.1: Patient Functional Status Scale

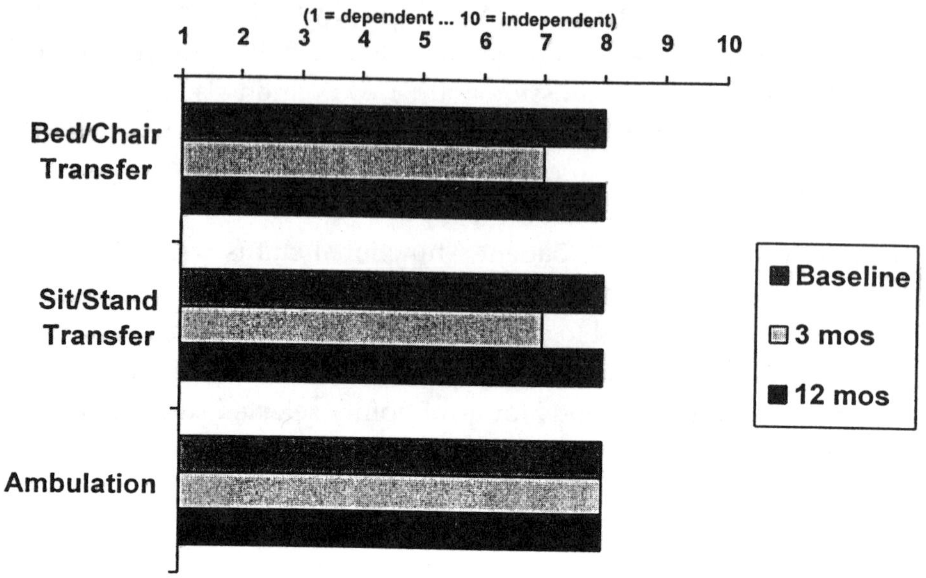

Median Functional Status Rating at Discharge for Patients Receiving Physical Therapy on the Orthopedic Unit at Baseline, Three-Months and Twelve-Months After Implementation of PFC.

(Note. Median scores are reported in the figure. Mean scores were 7.1, 7.0, and 7.1 for bed to chair transfers over the three time periods; 7.1, 7.0, and 7.1 in sit to stand transfers; and 7.0, 6.9, and 6.8 in ambulation.)

Figure 16.2: Patient Ambulation Distance at Discharge

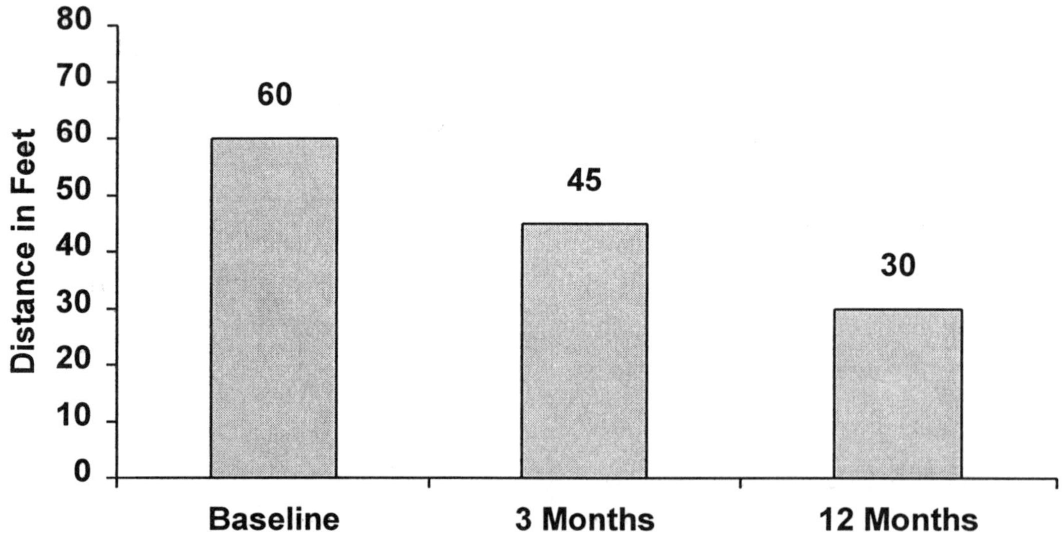

Distance Walked at Discharge for Patients Receiving Physical Therapy on the Orthopedic Unit at Baseline, Three Months, and Twelve Months After Implementation of PFC.

III. Financial Impact

Managed Demand. Findings relative to aggregation of orthopedic patients with similar needs in one unit were equivocal. Patient census rose during the first six months, then it fell back to baseline levels by one year post-implementation. This trend paralleled the total hospital census trend, and it probably reflected external market pressures more than restructuring trends. The percentage of patients on the unit that were orthopedic diagnoses did not change systematically over the year post-implementation. But within orthopedic diagnostic categories hospital-wide, the percentage of patients admitted to the orthopedic unit increased for all diagnostic groups except total hip replacements (see **Table 16.1**).

Table 16.1: Number and Percentage of Orthopedic Patients in Hospital Discharged from the Orthopedic Unit at Baseline, Three-months, and Twelve-months Post-Implementation of PFC

Orthopedic Diagnosis	Baseline		First Quarter Post-Implementation		Fourth Quarter Post-Implementation	
	N	%	N	%	N	%
Hip Fracture	26	83.9	25	86.2	76	93.8
Total Hip Replacement	50	98.0	44	93.6	43	87.8
Total Knee Replacement	23	88.5	31	88.6	25	100.0
Amputation	2	25.0	5	38.5	9	60.0
Other Orthopedic Surgery	204	77.0	185	74.9	147	81.2
Orthopedic Medicine	71	37.6	62	30.7	53	46.9
Total	**376**	**66.0**	**352**	**61.4**	**353**	**76.1**

Cost to Deliver Care. There was a total net reduction of 4.5 full-time equivalent staff (on and off-unit) delivering care to patients associated with restructuring to a PFC model. With changes in mix of licensed and unlicensed staff, there was a corresponding 9.6% reduction in unit staff costs to deliver care. The restructured PFC orthopedic model held to its target cost reduction of $300,000 from the previous year's operating costs.

Summary. These results suggest the PFC restructuring on the orthopedic unit had variable success in stabilizing demand and patient mix on the orthopedic unit. Average daily census was not consistently brought to PFC budget level, although there were some changes in diagnostic reaggregation. Changes in admissions management and response to census changes are likely to need a more hospital-wide management response. The findings in financial outcomes reinforced the need for continued work on adapting the entire organization and not individual patient care models to meet the principles of PFC, so that PFC will better meet its objectives.

Interpersonal Quality

I. Service outcomes

Work Sampling. Changes in the distribution of daily work activities by nurses on the orthopedic unit are depicted in **Figure 16.3.** Between pre-implementation and six months post-implementation, there was a noticeable increase in patient care and decrease in documentation. An unexpected increase in time spent in coordination and scheduling activities was attributed to the new multidisciplinary patient care team (including licensed physical therapists and unlicensed care partners and support partners) and the role of team leader played by the RN; increased discharge planning efforts associated with decreases in patient length of stay; and the cross-preparation of RNs to do computer order entry for their patients. By one year post-implementation, the percentage of work samples in direct patient care for RNs returned to baseline levels, while time spent in coordination and scheduling continued to increase.

Figure 16.4 displays the one-year trends of work activities by patient care staff (licensed and unlicensed) on the orthopedic pilot unit. In this graph, one can observe a modest increase in patient care activities (direct and support), the trend for increased time spent in coordination and scheduling, and sustained decrease in time spent documenting.

Summary. The statistical validity of work sampling as a method of measuring organizational change in care delivery model is currently being investigated by the authors. However, the descriptive results reported above support the value of directly examining the way work is completed during formal implementation of PFC or other restructuring of the care model.

The sustained trend for reduced time in documentation suggests the successful implementation of technological enablers and work space reengineering, and hospital-wide revisions to increase the efficiency of multidisciplinary documentation in the medical record. The modest gains recorded for the entire care team in direct patient care and support activities highlight the need to continue to revisit the principles of PFC in ongoing IOP reviews of the care model.

Figure 16.3: Work Sampling of RN Activities

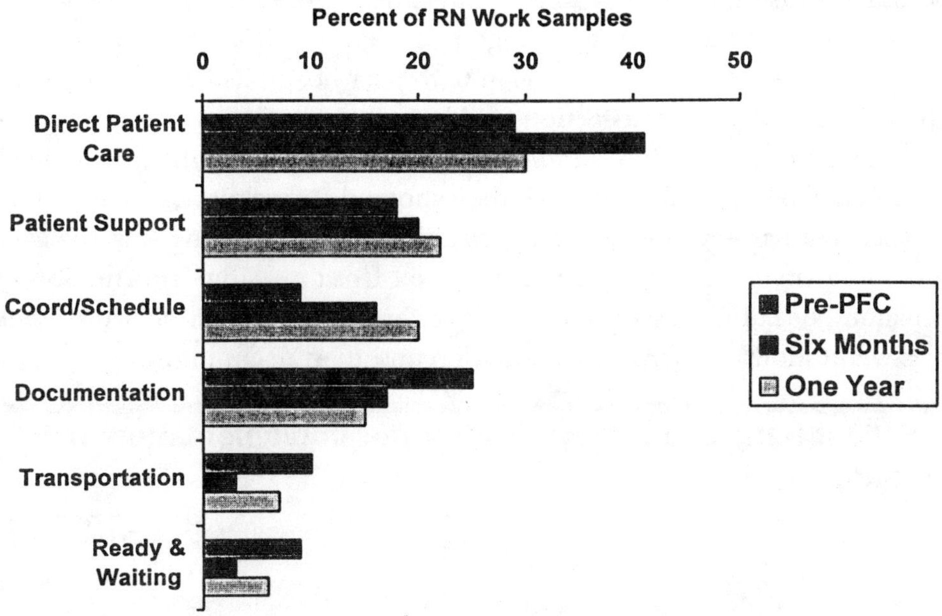

Distribution of Registered Nurses' Work Activities on the Orthopedic Unit Before and After Implementation of PFC.

Figure 16.4: Work Sampling of All Orthopedic Staff

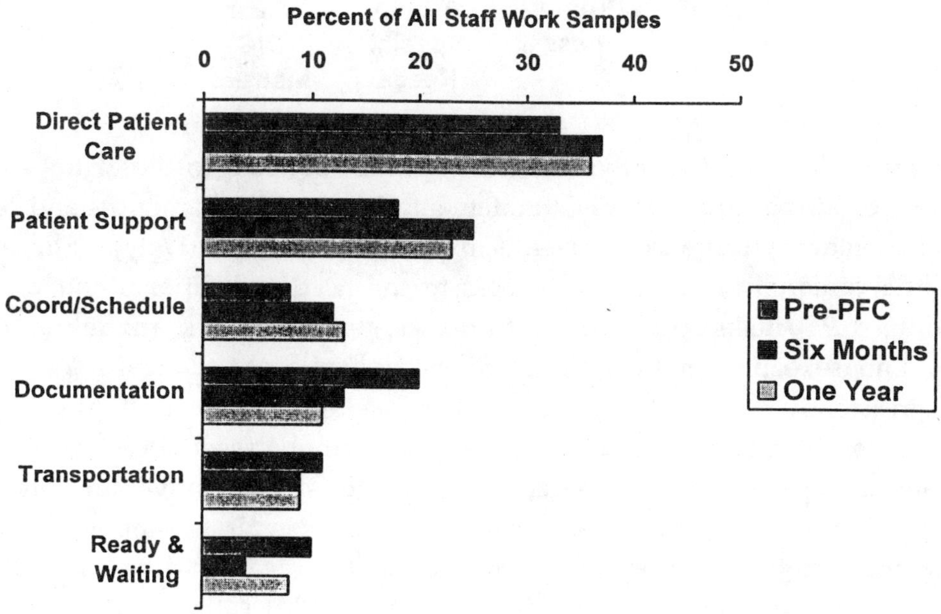

Distribution of All Nursing Staff (licensed and un-licensed) Work Activities Before and After Implementation of PFC on the Orthopedic Unit.

II. Customer satisfaction

Patient Satisfaction. Patient satisfaction was measured quarterly by the Press, Ganey Associates, Inc. surveys used by numerous hospitals throughout the United States. As noted in Chapter 15, Cedars Sinai has recently changed vendors to NCG, Inc. Institutions may receive their own results as well as a comparison with peer hospitals (600+ beds) and all hospitals using the service. Patient satisfaction with the orthopedic service (see **Figure 16.5**) increased immediately following PFC implementation, declined slightly in the following quarter but remained above pre-PFC levels. It then showed a precipitous decline in the summer of 1994. Aspects of patient satisfaction specifically related to changes in the care model (e.g., promptness in answering call, attention received from nursing, information given by nurses, daily cleaning of bathrooms) followed a similar pattern, reaching scores well above pre-PFC levels several months after implementation and then declining.

Figure 16.5: Patient Satisfaction Before and After Implementation of PFC on the Orthopedic Unit

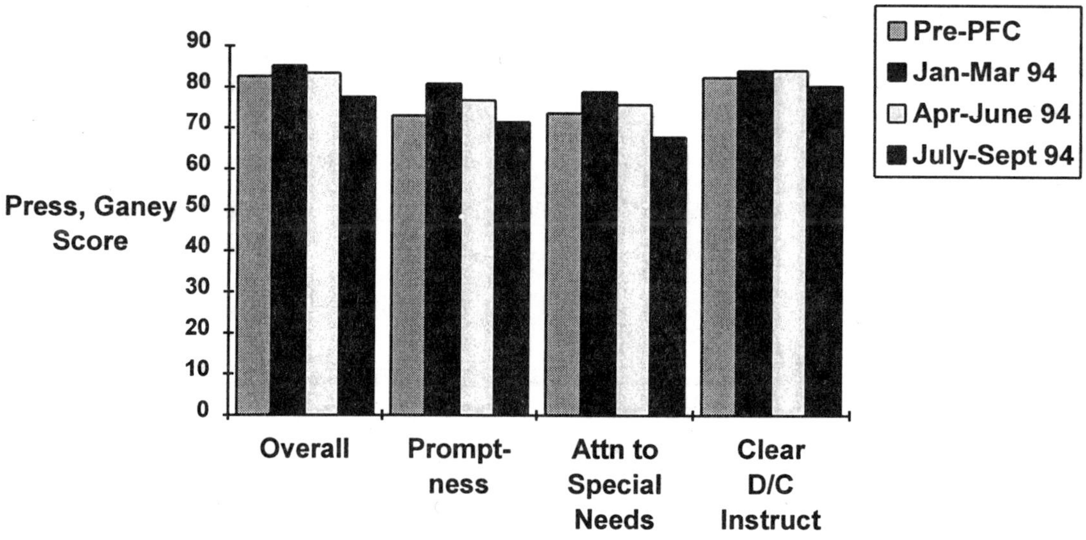

Physician Satisfaction. Fifty-two physicians, who admit patients to the orthopedic unit, received satisfaction surveys prior to PFC implementation, and at six months and one year following implementation (response rates=48%, 52%, and 38% respectively). Survey items included a 5-item scale covering responsiveness to the needs of patients and physicians (Cronbach's alpha=0.94), items on nursing performance, staff teamwork, and ratings of physical therapy and housekeeping on the unit. Findings showed slight changes in ratings at six months with consistently positive ratings at one year (see **Figure 16.6**). Both physician comments and responses to scale items indicated polarization among respondents at six months, with fewer neutral responses, some physicians overwhelmingly positive, and others very negative about changes to the unit. By one year, most of the negative comments had disappeared. These findings corroborate Lathrop's observations regarding the early PFC pilot hospitals where, while the majority of physicians were reasonably satisfied with the new procedures, there was also a minority that was very vocal and very unhappy.[1]

Staff Satisfaction. Staff on the orthopedic unit completed job satisfaction surveys prior to implementation and at six months and one year post-implementation. Findings showed slight changes at six months with a downward trend (although not statistically significant) in all items except role clarity at one year (see **Figure 16.7**). There were no systematic differences in responses between licensed and unlicensed patient care staff.

An item analysis of the adapted seven-item teamwork scale indicated increased satisfaction with the technical aspects of teamwork (i.e., solving problems well, knowing their jobs, and meeting objectives and demands).[2] However; the item analysis also indicated a decline in satisfaction with the interpersonal aspects of teamwork (i.e., planning together, sharing information, and trusting other team members). Furthermore, written comments indicated an overwhelming consciousness of both the benefits of good teamwork and the effort and difficulties involved in maintaining the team. At six-months post-implementation close to 25% of the comments concerned the new caregiver roles, including confusion about role descriptions, delegation, performing new tasks, etc. At one year these were no longer issues and teamwork became the overriding focus of both positive and negative comments. Despite any concerns, however, 66% of staff at six months post-implementation and 74% of staff at one year agreed with the survey item, "I would never go back to the old way of doing things."

Summary. The group of orthopedic surgeons, who admit patients and practice at Cedars-Sinai, were included in the planning and implementation of the orthopedic PFC model. It was not unexpected that a few were not happy with the early changes in the process of care on the unit. However, the majority were satisfied, and the level of satisfaction grew over the first year post-implementation. The consistent physician involvement and the fact that the surgeons were a fairly homogeneous and cohesive group probably contributed to the overall good level of satisfaction. Again, emphasizing the interaction effects of PFC changes in other organizational changes, a significant PFC restructuring of the operating room care model was undertaken during the same time frame (see Chapter 6). The physicians' satisfaction with the operating room rose substantially, and some of their positive attitude may have generalized to the care model on the orthopedics unit.

The decline of patient satisfaction scores on the orthopedic unit in the summer of 1994 mirrored patient satisfaction results for the entire institution in a time of rapidly decreasing lengths of stay and turmoil within the hospital, as staff from the twenty-seven remaining units went through PFC education, using per diem and floating staff to provide direct patient care. New care models were planned and implemented in rapid succession over the spring, summer, and early fall of 1994. Long-term monitoring of patient satisfaction will help separate the effects of the immediate change process from the longitudinal impacts of PFC on patient satisfaction.

Staff satisfaction results suggest a dynamic process of PFC implementation that extends months and perhaps years beyond the "ribbon cutting" ceremony opening the PFC model unit. Initial staff concerns about knowing what their role is and whether the new staff are competent are at some point set to rest. They are replaced by concerns about the distribution and delegation of work and the smooth functioning of the patient care team. It is imperative to address these continuing concerns in ongoing model development, while focusing on the patient and patient goals.

Figure 16.6: Physician Satisfaction Before and After Implementation of PFC on the Orthopedic Unit

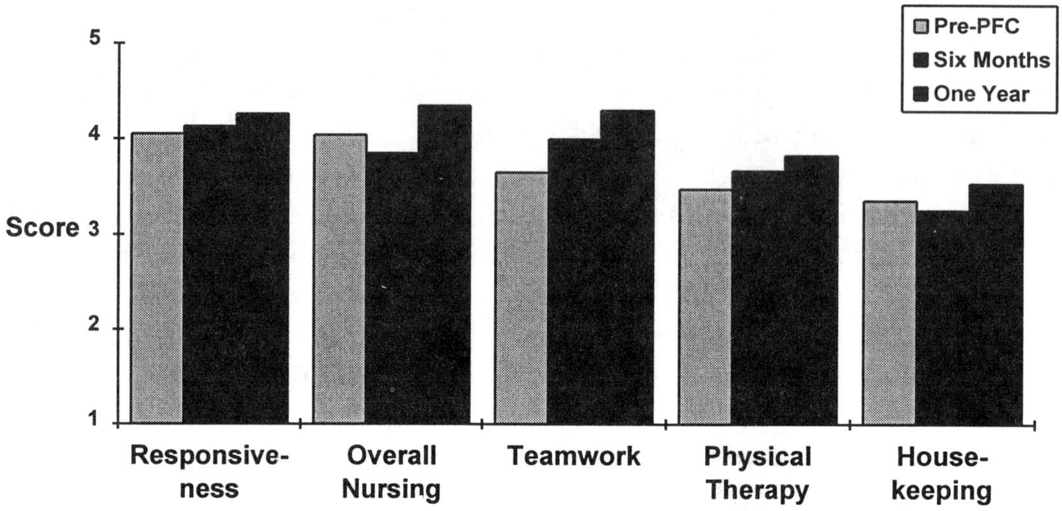

(Scale: 1=Poor, 2=Fair, 3=Neutral, 4=Good, 5=Excellent)

Figure 16.7: Staff Job Satisfaction Before and After Implementation of PFC on the Orthopedic Unit

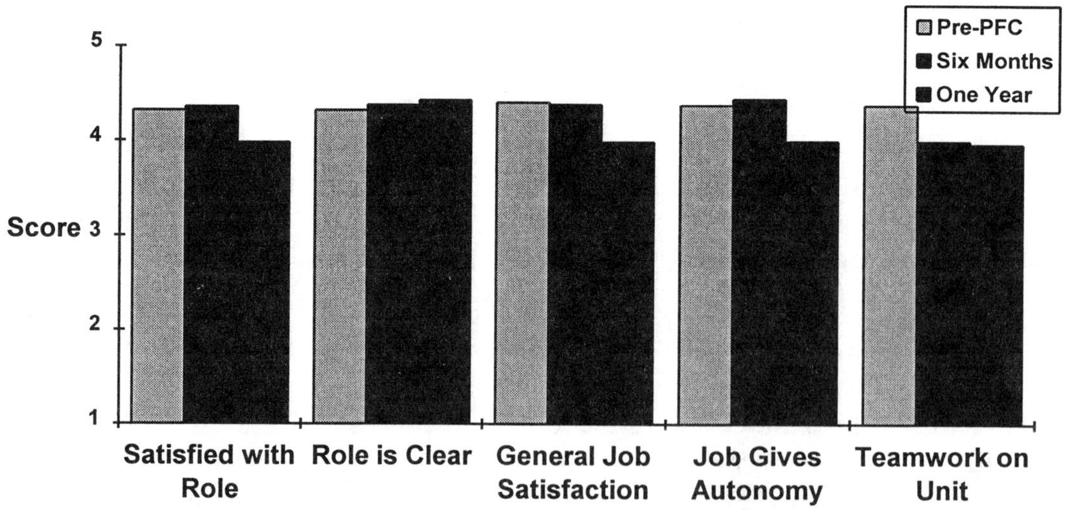

(Scale: 1=Strongly Disagree, 3=Uncertain, 5=Strongly Agree)

Preliminary Results from the Hospital-Wide Implementation

Data tracking the outcome of the hospital-wide implementation of PFC were collected in the same format as those from the orthopedic pilot unit. However, hospital-wide data is incorporated into service line report cards, so that a multidisciplinary outcome management team might review the data on a regular basis and change appropriately the care model. An example of a report card is displayed in **Figure 16.8.** Most measures have an associated target of performance, while some are monitored to establish a trend or expected variation.

Figure 16.8: Excerpt from the IOP Report Card from the General Surgical Service Area

Improving Organizational Performance: General Surgical Service Area		*1994*
Key Indicators	**Jan-Mar (PFC Baseline)**	**Apr-Jun (PFC Implementation)**
I. Competency for Redesigned Jobs		
Orientation Checklist	*na*	100%
Preceptor Evaluation of Cross-Prepared Staff	*na*	100%
II. Clinical Outcomes		•
Length of Stay per Diagnostic Guidelines		•
ALOS Mastectomy	3.9 days	•
ALOS TURP	3.7 days	
% of Low Risk Hip Pts with LOS ≤ 5 days	74%	
% of Low Risk Knee Pts with LOS < 4 days	79%	
Quality Indicators		
Rate (per 100 procedures) surgical site infections	•	
Rate (per 100 procedures) post-op pneumonia	•	
Rate (per 1,000 patient days) unattended falls	•	
Rate (per 100 discharges) acquired dermal ulcers		
Rate (per 100 discharges) readmission w/in 7 days		
•		
•		
•		

While PFC specific measures have been incorporated into the service line report card and will be collected and reported for at least one year after implementation, gradually the multidisciplinary outcomes management team will have to decide if continued data collection of measures designed to evaluate the implementation of PFC are cost-effective to maintain for the long-term development and adaptation of the models. Periodically, the management team will review all outcome measures in the report card to assess their value in measuring the quality of outcomes in each service line. Currently, with the inclusion of pathways and guidelines into the PFC models, there is a stronger focus on measurement and evaluation of length of stay, operational costs per discharge, and rates of complications within specific diagnoses managed in clinical pathways (see Chapter 23).

Two areas of particular interest for the evaluation of PFC restructuring efforts have been work sampling and customer satisfaction. The pilot orthopedic unit experience indicated that work sampling can give managers a direct look at how the PFC model has been implemented on each unit and in each service line area. Satisfaction data should provide insight into the teamwork issues hospital-wide. The data should also suggest whether the issues raised on the orthopedic unit have generalized to the hospital-wide changes and might generalize to other institutions. Because of the importance of monitoring these two particular outcomes of PFC restructuring, the results for six-month post-PFC outcomes in work sampling and in customer satisfaction were analyzed, and they are reported in preliminary form below.

Work Sampling

Beginning in April 1994 and continuing until September 1995, twenty-seven additional nursing units restructured along principles of PFC and implemented their care models. Work sampling was conducted on the restructured PFC units before implementation (during the planning phase) and at six-months post-implementation. During the interval between baseline observations and six-month follow-up, several events occurred that forced substantial structural changes in the delivery of care at Cedars-Sinai. They included an earthquake that closed the building housing post medical/surgical rehabilitation and skilled nursing units and a continued drops in patient census that resulted in moving, closing, and combining some patient care units. Despite these changes, the work sampling observations of patient care delivery continued, as did the implementation of PFC models.

Baseline Work Activities. Figure 16.9 displays the distribution of RN work activities in four key categories in seven service line areas, including ICU and post medical surgical levels of care. Most noticeable in this graph is the large variations between service area specializations and levels of care in the fundamental distribution of patient care activities. These variations have face validity considering the areas of specialization and underscore the differences inherent in both the culture and patient care demands among different types of units. For example, ICUs and pediatric care areas had the highest percentage of direct patient care samples, while psychiatry units, where much of the patient care was provided by physicians and other ancillary care providers, had the lowest. Corresponding to this care model difference, psychiatry also had substantially more of its patient care staff time spent in scheduling and coordinating. The post medical surgical service area also had a large proportion of patient care provided by ancillary therapies. However, the low involvement of RNs in scheduling and coordinating reflects the system developed by the Department of Physical Medicine and Rehabilitation to schedule all patient rehabilitation therapy treatments. The relative large proportion of time allocated to patient support activities in the medicine service line area is probably attributable to the increased use of medications and diagnostic testing on these units.

Six Months Post-Implementation. In all units, the addition of the support partner was evident in the shift of patient care team activities to include the room cleaning and patient transport activities that this new role contributed to the unit. Observed in total, the percentage of work activities by the expanded care team rose in patient support and in transportation categories. To directly compare the baseline work sampling results to the six-month results, the support partner activities were excluded from the analysis. However, to reflect the changes in the team composition and the way work was distributed in the new PFC models, the remainder of the care team (RNs, LVNs, care partners) were combined in these analyses. The results from the two largest service lines medicine and surgery are briefly presented in this section.

There were ten units in the medicine and surgery areas for which there were comparable data from the baseline to six-month periods. In four of the units increases in the percentage of time the care team provided direct patient care and patient support were observed; the two categories of work activities judged as "value-added" in the PFC planning process. The increases in the patient support category, however, were more consistent and dramatic than in the provisions of direct patient care. In the same four units, there were corresponding decreases in the percentage of time spent documenting and ready and waiting. Unlike the pilot orthopedic unit, these four units demonstrated no substantial change in the time spent coordinating and scheduling (two increased slightly and two decreased slightly).

Figure 16.9: RN Work Samples by Category of Work and Service Area Specialization (Pre-Implementation of PFC).

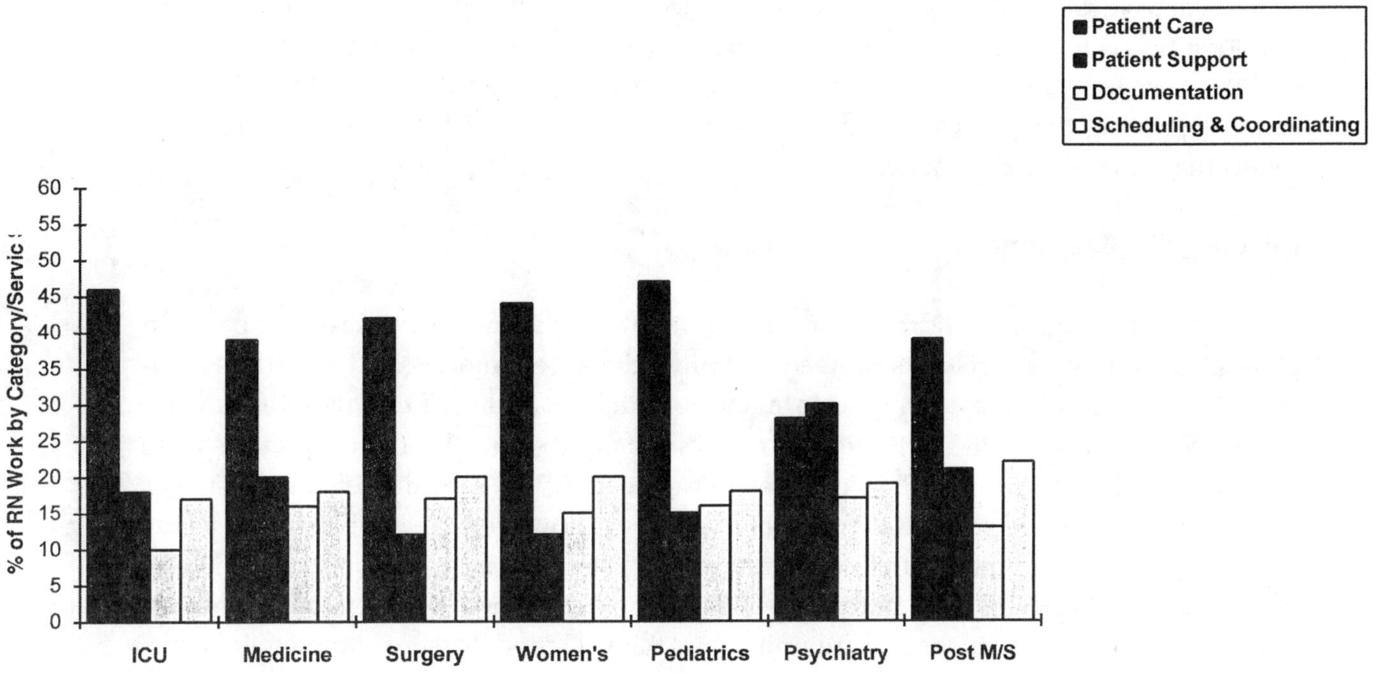

In the remaining six patient care units, work sampling results demonstrated mixed success at the six-month mark. While none had increases in direct patient care time, three units were observed with increases in indirect patient support activities. The percentage of work time spent documenting was reduced on all four units. The proportion of activities in the scheduling and coordination category on three units rose substantially.

Observing across all ten units, the proportion of work samples in documentation dropped in eight units. The drop in time spent documenting and waiting for others to perform work allowed more patient care and support time. While transportation was not a large proportion of the work day for any unit (under 10% for all units), there was a small increase in the proportion of work activities in transportation in eight of the units, including the four that demonstrated the most PFC changes.

Summary. The preliminary six-month look at the selection of medicine and surgery PFC units revealed a dynamic process of conversion. Four of the ten units appeared to be well underway into a more patient-focused model of care. Two additional units appeared to have made few changes in the distribution of work activities, although all had made changes in the licensure mix of the care team. This, in itself, suggests that these six units had made model changes consistent with the principles of PFC during the first six months after implementation. Repeated observations at one-year will indicate if movement toward a PFC model is sustained.

For four units, work sampling results at six months suggest that more work needs to be done on implementing the PFC model. In one or two of the units, patient mix changes may account for some of the observed changes. But in three units, the dramatic increase in work activities spent in coordinating and scheduling activities may indicate that more attention needs to be paid to teamwork issues and management of the daily routine. In each of these four units, direct patient care activity dropped by approximately 10% percent, suggesting that the care team staff were focusing more on indirect or care team issues than directly on the patient.

Customer Satisfaction

Physician Satisfaction. Findings from the six-month physician surveys were mixed. In general, the intensive care units showed that physicians were more satisfied with responsiveness of unit staff, the overall performance of nursing, and staff teamwork following the implementation of PFC, although samples sizes were small and the differences were not statistically significant. Physician responses to the PFC care models on the floors were generally unchanged. At the time of the survey, however, the enablers such as the desks and PCs at the quads and consolidation of patient charts, innovations generally popular with physicians, had not yet been implemented. These enablers were not part of the PFC plan for the intensive care units, thus the ICU models were completely implemented at six months, which was not the case for the patient care floors.

Staff Satisfaction. Staff satisfaction varied from unit to unit, even within the same service line. Some staffs showed increased satisfaction with their roles, jobs, and teamwork on the unit, while on other areas satisfaction decreased. **Figures 16.10** and **16.11** show findings for two units in the same service line. Clearly, some unit teams were adjusting to the PFC models better than others.

Patient Satisfaction. Because of the institution's change in vendors for patient satisfaction surveys (see Chapter 15) comparisons of pre- and post-implementation patient satisfaction data was not possible. Patient data are being tracked on an ongoing basis, however.

Figure 16.10: Staff Satisfaction on Unit A

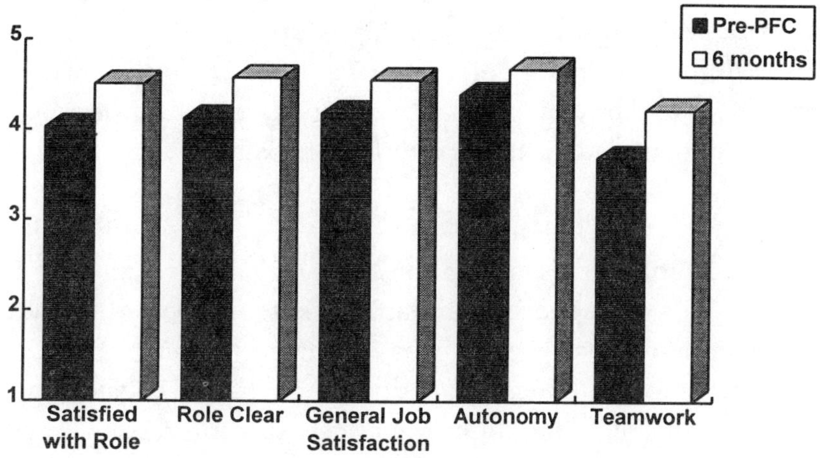

Figure 16.11: Staff Satisfaction on Unit B

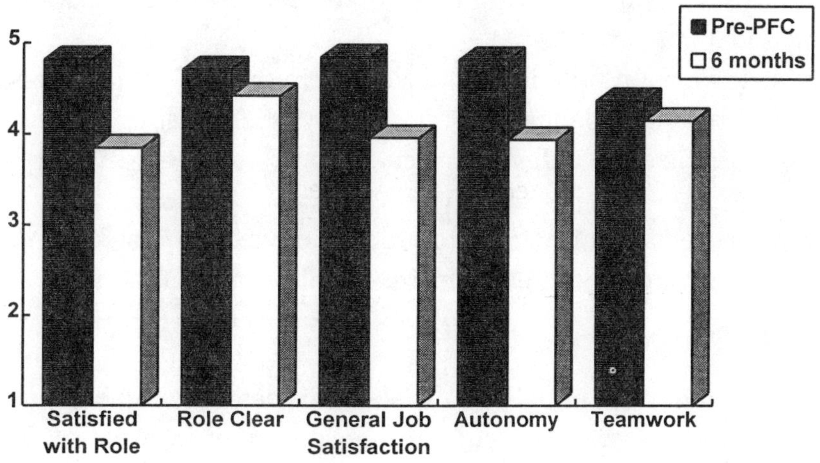

Lessons Learned

PFC was Cedars-Sinai first experience with fundamental organizational redesign. As such it has provided the context for discovery of those internal and external factors that facilitate or impede the process of improving organizational performance to meet patient care needs.[3] Perhaps foremost in the lessons learned from evaluation data, reinforced by anecdote and observation, is the need for a close and continual examination of the communication and interaction issues within newly formed, multidisciplinary care teams.

Team building and maintenance are especially important in the context of redesigned or expanded processes of care delivery. The people involved in organizational change must own the change process, both individually and collectively.[4] As team members they must receive skills and information on the "how to's" of team functioning as well as the "how to's" of core clinical tasks. Lack of adequate preparation of care teams—the people who do the work—can impair a restructuring effort.[5] Specific recommendations for additional team building efforts are detailed in **Table 16.2.** Four efforts are being pursued simultaneously at Cedars-Sinai—quality action teams; multidisciplinary outcomes management teams, patient and customer simulation exercises, and focused team building.

In addition to the need for increased team building, evaluating all staff for competent performance in new skills was a more formidable task than expected. For the subsequent house-wide implementation, the process was facilitated by integrating the clinical performance evaluations into the education sequence itself. In considering clinical outcomes, evaluation findings also highlight the effects of compressed lengths of stay on patient functional status at discharge. These outcomes underscore the importance of appropriate discharge planning and the continuum of levels of care in the community.

Table 16.2: Recommendations for Additional Team Building and Maintenance

- Include the development of well functioning self-directed service teams as an organizational goal in redesign
- Identify specific team functioning objectives in the design and planning phases
- Identify and provide adequate resources (personnel, training costs, group facilittation and organizational development support) to develop interpersonal team functioning
- Communicate, communicate, communicate; develop and sustain vertical and horizontal communication mechanisms for all team members

PFC appears to have met its expectations for staff competency, clinical quality, and efficiency of care delivery. Patient satisfaction ratings did not reflect the expected improvement. Although other major changes taking place in the hospital organizational environment (downsizing and introduction of resource management initiatives) may have had some effect on patient satisfaction, clearly patient education and patient-staff relationships are key features in any major organizational restructuring. Patient-staff relationships are even more difficult to maintain as lengths of stay in the hospital drop. Recent research has shown that the most frequent patient complaints concern areas of communication between staff and patients. The following are examples of patient concerns: patient education about what to do after discharge, explanations of the daily hospital routine, and communication about the side effects of drugs, test results, and how much pain or discomfort to expect from a test or procedure.[6] Clearly, the interpersonal aspects of the quality of care, including staff relationships to maintain the integrity of the patient care team, require increased attention.

Conclusion

Patient-focused care, a major planned organizational redesign, must be evaluated in a total quality framework, for outcomes resulting both from implementation of redesigned patient care delivery teams and the interpersonal/communication functions of those teams. Change consistent with PFC principles must be continuously monitored and reinforced. Evaluation results suggest that team function processes are more complex and require a longer period of transition and support to achieve expected care model outcomes. Report cards on organizational performance will assist in fostering team work, because they are a concrete link between the process of care (what the team is and does) and the outcome of care (clinical outcomes and satisfaction). Overall, the findings support the need to evaluate innovations in hospital care delivery models in their organizational context, over time and within a framework of ongoing improvement of organizational performance.

References

1. Lathrop JP. *Restructuring Healthcare: The Patient Focused Paradigm.* San Francisco: Jossey-Bass 1993.

2. Taylor JC, DB Bowers. *Survey of Organizations.* Institute for Social Research, University of Michigan: Ann Arbor, MI 1972.

3. Farris BJ. "Converting a Unit to Patient-Focused Care." *Health Progress.* (April) 1993: 22-25

4. Smeltzer CH, NN Fornella , H Beebe. "Work Restructuring: The Process of Decision Making. *Nursing Economics* 11(4) 1993:215-222

5. Hines PP, CH Smeltzer, M. Galletti "Work Restructuring: The Process of Redefining Roles of Patient Caregivers." *Nursing Economics* 12(6): 1994 346-350

6. Charles C, M Gauld, L Chambers, B O'Brien, RB Haynes, R Labell. "How Was Your Hospital Stay? Patients' Reports About Their Care in Canadian Hospitals. *Canadian Medical Association Journal* 150(11): 1994 1813-1831

Section III

Applying Clinical Practice Guidelines and Outcomes Research

Section III focuses on clinical guidelines, pathways, and outcomes research, beginning with a detailed introduction to evidence-based practice, drawing from and synthesizing seminal publications in the field. This introduction is followed by practical information based on Cedars-Sinai's experience in the development, implementation, and evaluation of clinical practice guidelines. Chapter 19 details Cedars-Sinai's comprehensive resource management initiative, in which multidisciplinary teams participate in a structured process to develop clinical guidelines and pathways and measure appropriate outcomes for specified patient populations throughout the institution's service lines. Chapter 20 closes the section with a description of the Quality of Well-Being Scale, which is currently being tested in a self-administered format (QWB-SA1.0). The authors present information on the scale's proven usefulness in measuring outcomes of clinical trials, and discuss its potential application in evaluating the outcomes of changes in health care delivery and practices brought about by initiatives such as patient-focused care and clinical guidelines and pathways.

Chapter 17

Introduction to Evidence-Based Practice

A. Gray Ellrodt, MD
Michaela Cho, PharmD

This chapter presents an overview of evidence-based medicine (EBM) and its application to selected patient populations. Although the chapter will emphasize the approach to groups of patients, it is essential to maintain the focus on individual patients as care is provided on an individual basis. Much of this chapter will be based upon the pioneering work of the members of The Evidence-based Medicine Working Group and their numerous publications. This group has provided an operational definition of evidence-based medicine. They note: "A new paradigm for medical practice is emerging. Evidence-based medicine de-emphasizes intuition, unsystematic clinical experience, and pathophysiologic rationale as sufficient grounds for clinical decision making and stresses the examination of evidence from clinical research. Evidence-based medicine requires new skills of the physician, including efficient literature searching and the application of formal rules of evidence evaluating the clinical literature."[1]

Evidence-based medicine could therefore be considered scientific clinical medicine. When appropriately practiced, evidence-based medicine emphasizes findings from clinical research in conjunction with the art of medicine and reasoning from pathophysiology and experience. When one attempts to practice EBM, many challenges and limitations soon appear. These include significant gaps in the clinical literature and significant controversy among reports. On the other hand, busy clinicians often do not go to the literature for routine questions and often feel ill-prepared to critically appraise the clinical literature because medical school and residency training have often failed to provide training in clinical epidemiology, a "basic science for clinical medicine." [2] Although many of the principles and tools of evidence-based medicine are from clinical epidemiology, the actual practice of EBM draws from even broader disciplines including outcomes research, total quality management (TQM), systems analysis, theories of behavioral change, and finally from the foundation of doctor-patient relationships and the art of medicine. The blending and balancing of these disciplines form the basis of self-learning resulting in optimal practice. This chapter will, therefore, draw from all of these disci-

A. Gray Ellrodt, MD—Vice Chairman for Clinical Affairs, Department of Medicine, Director, Division of Internal Medicine, Cedars-Sinai Medical Center; Professor of Medicine, University of California-Los Angeles, School of Medicine.

Michaela Cho, PharmD—Pharmacy Resident, Department of Pharmacy Services, Cedars-Sinai Medical Center.

plines in presenting an approach to evidence-based care (practice) for populations and ultimately for the individual patient.

Why Use Evidence-Based Medicine?

Although there may be multiple reasons not to use evidence-based medicine in the approach to populations of patients through clinical guidelines and pathways, there are clearly several important potential advantages. These include the following:

1) **By encoding optimal practice from the medical literature the individual practitioner or team is most likely to improve patient outcomes**: Many groups employ clinical guidelines and pathways to reduce variation. Although this is a reasonable goal, the simple reduction in variation may not necessarily improve outcomes but, rather, simply make them more homogeneous. Reducing variation around the wrong practice serves no useful purpose. Reducing variation around optimal practice derived from the medical literature through an evidence-based approach is most likely to improve clinical and economic outcomes.

2) **Empowers all members of the multidisciplinary team to shape care**: When a multidisciplinary team consisting of providers from different facets of patients' care (i.e., medicine, nursing, pharmacy, microbiology, etc.) begins to shape care through guidelines or pathways, it is often confronted by individuals who appear to have the greatest experience or expertise or who have the most inflexible ideas about "optimal care." The team may thus be intimidated by this individual (often a physician) and not be able to significantly change care from this person's preconceived notions. Using an evidence-based medicine approach, however, the team can use the clinical literature as a neutral arbiter of optimal practice and potentially avoid conflicts based upon ego rather than best science. This approach empowers all members of the health care team and places them on an equal footing in designing optimal care.

3) **Provides the maximum opportunity to change practice**: By empowering the entire team and providing a more even playing field, there is a greater opportunity to actually change rather than simply encode current practice.

4) **Avoids micromanaging those aspects of care that are unlikely to affect patient outcomes**: If the team is unable to find any literature to support a particular practice or no evidence that outcomes are improved, it may decide not to focus scarce resources on tracking or attempting to change practice around this particular element of care. An important result of comprehensive literature reviews and critical appraisals is often the recognition that the issue at hand has not been adequately studied and that protracted discussions of these issues and the embracing of firm stands is not productive.

Operational Definitions of Clinical Practice Guidelines and Clinical Pathways

There are many definitions of clinical practice guidelines and pathways. For purposes of discussion, this chapter will use the following:

Clinical Practice Guidelines *are "systematically developed statements to assist practitioner and patient decisions about appropriate health care for specific clinical circumstances."* [3]

Clinical Pathways *are tools to coordinate the daily progress of a "typical, uncomplicated" patient across many clinical departments.* [4]

Clinical guidelines can be inserted as essential elements of a pathway to inform specific decisions about patient care. For example, a pathway for the management of patients with upper gastrointestinal hemorrhage might contain a guideline recommending prompt UGI endoscopy and another using the findings of UGI endoscopy and clinical observation to risk-stratify patients and determine the optimal length of hospital stay.

Evidence-Based Practice for Populations of Patients

Although many of the principles and techniques of evidence-based medicine have been developed for and applied to individual patients, they are equally useful for populations. This is not surprising given evidence-based medicine's foundation in clinical epidemiology. The use of EBM to develop clinical guidelines and pathways has been well described. [5-9] The use of evidence-based medicine to optimize care for the individual patient has also been presented in detail. [1, 10-11] It is not surprising that many of the same principles apply for, ultimately, evidence-based care is always applied to one patient at a time in the decisionmaking process of the practitioner and patient (and/or family). **Table 17.1** outlines the steps in applying an evidence-based approach to caring for a population of patients. Potential differences in the practice of EBM between populations and individuals include the type of literature searches performed (i.e., breadth and depth) and the use of a multidisciplinary team to initially judge the relative value of the expected benefits, harms, and costs. Literature searches for populations may pull multiple articles addressing many elements of care to develop guidelines and pathways for groups of patients. For the individual patient, the practitioner may be most interested in the single "best" article to address a specific issue for the individual patient. The following sections describe the steps in applying evidenced-based care to a population.

Table 17.1: Summary of Evidence-Based Care for a Population.

STEP NUMBER	ACTIVITIES
1	Formulate a clear problem statement
2	Perform a formal literature search
3	Assess the quality of the article(s)
4	Multidisciplinary team judges the relative value of the expected benefits, harms, and costs of the critically appraised interventions
5	Develop Clinical Practice Guideline(s) for each important element of care
6	Place guidelines to form the backbone of a Clinical Pathway
7	Develop a systematic approach to process measurement and reporting
8	Develop a systematic approach to outcomes measurement and reporting
9	Implement guidelines and pathway
10	Measure and report process variation and clinical and economic outcomes
11	Use process and outcomes measures with updated literature searches and appraisals to continually improve care of population

Adapted from references [5-9]

1. Formulate a Clear Problem Statement

The first step in utilizing clinical studies is to formulate the medical issue into a clear question.[2] This entails expressing the question in the most specific terms possible. Questions pertaining to a population of patients may include the following: *What is the optimal length of stay for uncomplicated patients undergoing total hip replacement?* or *Should selected asthma patients receive corticosteroids in the emergency department?* Questions can be categorized into those relating to diagnosis, prevention, or therapy harm and prognosis. Categorizing the clinical question can not only help prioritize its significance, but also clarify the target of the literature search, allow an appropriate evaluation of the validity of relevant studies, and, ultimately, help find answers in an efficient and timely manner.

If a multidisciplinary team has been formed to address the care of patients with a certain condition, they may wish to address multiple elements of care that are, from experience or knowledge of the clinical literature, likely to have a significant impact on clinical outcomes. For example, a team developing a clinical pathway for total hip replacement may prioritize formal literature searches in the areas of DVT prophylaxis, timing and intensity of physical therapy, length of stay, and level of care. The team can then assign members to perform the searches with the assistance of a medical librarian if available.

2. Perform a Formal Literature Search

Upon formulating a clear, pertinent clinical question, a search can then be conducted for available evidence. Several routes of inquiry are available: asking a colleague or consultant, checking reference lists in textbooks, finding relevant articles in personal files, and using a bibliographic database such as MEDLINE.[12] Seeking a colleague or consultant is a viable alternative if a question arises from an event that is unlikely to be encountered again. Textbooks are only as current as their most recent references, and, usually, by the time they are published, their material may be outdated. Furthermore, there is no guarantee that the methods used to assess the referenced citations were valid.[13] Personal files in general, have become obsolete since new and faster methods of retrieving a wide range of current medical literature have become available.

The United States National Library of Medicine (NLM) produces and maintains several biomedical databases (see **Table 17.2**).[12] The Medical Subject Headings (MeSH) vocabulary, which consists of approximately 17,000 terms, is used to index citations (i.e., the title, authors, source, and abstract of an article) in these databases. When used properly, MeSH is a powerful tool for improving access to the medical literature. Because approximately ten to twenty MeSH terms are indexed to a citation, a search using the appropriate term can retrieve a citation and others indexed with the same term.

Table 17.2: Major National Library of Medicine Databases

AIDSLINE
AIDSTRIALS
HEALTH
MEDLINE
TOXLINE

Adapted from Lowe and Barnett [12]

Source: Figure was reprinted with permission from "Understanding and Using Subject Headings (MeSH) Vocabulary to Perform Literature Searches," by H.J. Lowe and G.O. Barrett in the Journal of American Medical Association 271 (14) 1994: 703-705 (Copyright 1993/1994, American Medical Association).

In addition to MeSH indexing terms, text words may also be used to search for articles. This method is useful if no appropriate MeSH terms are applicable or if a search requires modification by the combination of MeSH terms with title or abstract words. Because the text word search method relies on an uncontrolled vocabulary, it will limit a search to only those articles containing a specific word in its title or abstract. Therefore, despite any relevance to the subject, citations without a particular text word will not be retrieved. For instance, using the word "hyperlipidemia" in a text word search will exclude those citations with the narrower term "hypercholesterolemia" in its text.

Limiting techniques may be applied to further narrow the search. MeSH subheadings include eighty terms that limit the number of citations to those related to certain aspects of biomedicine. Examples of MeSH subheadings include administration and dosage, diagnosis, therapy, etc. (see **Table 17.3**).[12]

Table 17.3: Medical Subject Headings (MeSH) Topical Subheadings[a]

Administration & Dosage	Drug Therapy	Pathogenicity
Adverse Effects	Economics	Pharmacokinetics
Blood	Epidemiology	Physiology
Chemically Induced	Etiology	Prevention & Control
Complications	Immunology	Radionuclide Imaging
Diagnosis	Mortality	Transmission
		Utilization

[a]List is not all inclusive.

Adapted from Lowe & Barnett. [12]

Source: Figure was reprinted with permission from "Understanding and Using Subject Headings (MeSH) Vocabulary to Perform Literature Searches," by H.J. Lowe and G.O. Barrett in the Journal of American Medical Association 271 (14) 1994: 703-705 (Copyright 1993/1994, American Medical Association).

Citations may also be limited to those published in a particular year, English language articles, human studies, and specific publication types such as clinical trials, reviews, guidelines, and randomized controlled trials (see **Table 17.4**). Considering that most clinicians have limited time to conduct literature searches, it is generally recommended that a search begin with a valid overview, meta-analysis, or practice guideline; however, if these are not available, original studies should then be sought. If a team is developing guidelines it is reasonable to search for and utilize original studies.

Table 17.4: Medical Subject Headings (MeSH) Publication[a]

Abstract	Comment	Letter
Bibliography	Consensus Development Conference	Meeting Report
Clinical Trial	Editorial	Meta-analysis
Clinical Trial, Phase I	Guideline	Practice Guideline
Clinical Trial, Phase II	Journal Article	Randomized Controlled Trial
Clinical Trial, Phase III		Review
Clinical Trial, Phase IV		

[a] List is not all inclusive.

Adapted from Lowe & Barnett. [12]

Source: Figure was reprinted with permission from "Understanding and Using Subject Headings (MeSH) Vocabulary to Perform Literature Searches," by H.J. Lowe and G.O. Barrett in the Journal of American Medical Association 271 (14) 1994: 703-705 (Copyright 1993/1994, American Medical Association).

Generally, study designs fall into two categories: observational and interventional. Observational types include case control or retrospective studies and cohort studies. Case control or retrospective studies have the advantage of studying rare conditions or diseases. Cohort studies, which may be concurrent or nonconcurrent, have the advantage of evaluating one or more etiologic factors on multiple outcomes. Concurrent cohort studies are inherently time-consuming and expensive since they require concurrent follow-up of patients over long periods of time. On the other hand, nonconcurrent cohort studies require less time to conduct since individuals are evaluated after assignment to groups based on patient-specific parameters. By their very nature, observational studies are prone to methodological errors and biases.

Interventional studies include randomized clinical trials. When properly conducted, they may support the three criteria for contributory cause: (1) the characteristic, or the "cause," is associated with a disease, or the "effect," more often than by chance alone; (2) cause predicts the effect; (3) altering only the cause affects the probability of the effect.[16] When these criteria are met, the inference that the intervention alone affected the study outcomes is strengthened. Randomized, controlled trials provide the strongest evidence in support of treatment effects.

3. Assess the Quality of the Article

A quick screening of the title and abstract may assist in determining the general scope and relevance of the article. This process is particularly important when a large number of citations requires screening. Guides have been established for quick assessments of primary, which provide original data, and integrative studies, which summarized primary data, for the selection of those articles that are more likely to provide valid results (see **Table 17.5**).

Table 17.5: Guides for Selecting Articles Most Likely to Provide Valid Results

Primary Studies	
Therapy or Prevention	- Was the assignment of patients to treatments randomized? - Were all patients who entered the study accounted for and attributed at its conclusion?
Diagnosis	- Was there an independent, blind comparison with a reference standard? - Did the patient sample include an appropriate spectrum of patients to whom the diagnostic test will be applied in clinical practice?
Harm	- Were the comparison groups clearly identified and similar with respect to important determinants of outcome? - Were the outcomes and exposures measured similarly in the groups being compared?
Prognosis	- Was a representative patient sample identified at a well-defined point in the course of the disease? - Was follow-up sufficiently long and complete?
Integrative Studies	
Overview	- Did the review address a clearly focused question? - Were the criteria used to select articles for inclusion appropriate?
Practice Guidelines	- Were the options and outcomes clearly delineated? - Did the guideline use an explicit process to identify, select, and combine evidence?

Decision analysis	- Did the analysis model a clinically important decision? - Was valid evidence used to develop the baseline probabilities and utilities?
Economic analysis	- Were at least two clearly described alternatives compared? - Were the expected consequences of each alternative based on valid evidence?

Adapted from Oxman et al. [10]

Once an article has passed the initial screening, the validity of the study results and their usefulness in clinical practice may then be more critically assessed. Three basic questions may be posed at this point to better determine study strengths and weaknesses.[15,16]

Source: Figure was reprinted with permission from "User's Guide to the Medical Literature. I. How To Get Started," by A.D. Oxman, D.L. Sackett, and G.H. Guyatt in the Journal of American Medical Association 270 (17) 1993;2093-2095. (Copyright 1993/1994. American Medical Association).

These include the following:

(1) Are the study results valid?
(2) What were the results?
(3) Will the results help me care for my patients?

The approach to answering these questions is specific to the type of study being evaluated (see **Tables 17.6** and **17.7**).

Table 17.6: Guides to Critically Appraising Articles on Therapy or Prevention

Are the study results valid?

Was the assignment of patients to treatments randomized?
Were all patients who entered the trial accounted for and attributed at its conclusion?
Was follow-up complete?
Were patients analyzed in the groups to which they were randomized?
Were patients and study personnel "blind" to treatment?
Were the groups similar at the start of the trial?
Were the groups treated equally aside from the study intervention?

What were the results?

How large was the treatment effect?
How precise was the estimate of the treatment effect?

Will the results help me care for my patients?

Can the results be applied to clinical practice?
Were all clinically important outcomes considered?
Are the treatment benefits worth the potential harms and costs?

Adapted from Guyatt et al. [15]

Source: Figure was reprinted with permission. "User's Guide to the Medical Literature. II. How to Use an Article About Therapy or Prevention. A. Are the Results of the Study Valid?" by G.H. Guyatt, D.L. Sackett, and D.J. Cook in the Journal of American Medical Association 270(21) 1993 2598-2801. (Copyright 1993/1994, American Medical Association).

Table 17.7: Guides to Critically Appraising Articles on Diagnosis

Are the study results valid?

Was there an independent, blind comparison with a reference standard?

Did the patient sample include an appropriate spectrum of patients to whom the diagnostic test may be applied in clinical practice?

Did the results of the test influence the decision to perform the reference standard?

Were the methods for performing the test described in sufficient detail to permit replication?

What were the results?

Are the likelihood ratios for the test results or data necessary for their calculation provided?

Will the results help me care for my patients?

Will the reproducibility of the test result and its interpretation be satisfactory in my setting?

Are the results applicable to my patient population?

Will the results change management of this population?

Will patients be better off as a result of the test?

Adapted from Jaeschke et al. [17]

Source: Figure was reprinted with permission from "User's Guide to the Medical Literature.III. How to Use Article About a Diagnostic Test. A. Are the Results of the Study Valid?" by R. Jaeschke, G.H. Guyatt, and D.L. Sackett in the Journal of American Medical Association 271(5)1994; 389-391. (Copyright 1993/1994, American Medical Association).

The following is a description of the methods used to evaluate articles on therapy or prevention and diagnosis.

Critical Appraisal of Articles on Therapy or Prevention

Are the study results valid? Several steps are involved in the process of analyzing the effects of a therapeutic (i.e., reducing symptoms or curing disease) or preventive (i.e., reudicng the risk of disease or complication) intervention on study outcomes.

- **First, determine if the assignment of patients to groups was randomized.**

Nonrandomized studies provide much weaker evidence than randomized ones. The randomization process minimizes the effects of comorbidities, underlying severity of illness, and other factors on the overall study outcomes. Therefore, as long as the sample size is sufficient, random allocation of study participants insures an even distribution of patient characteristics between treatment and control groups.

A sufficient sample size is determined by several factors including the following:[16]

1. The magnitude of Type I and Type II errors that readers and investigators are willingto tolerate. Type I (or Alpha) error is the error of identifying a significant difference in outcomes between treatment and control groups when no true difference exists. The

cause is generally by chance. Investigators set a significance level which indicate how large an alpha error will be tolerated. The alpha level is usually set at 5% with the P value < 0.05. Type II (or beta) error is the failure to find a statistically significant dif ference in outcomes between treatment and control groups when a true difference exists. The cause of this error is usually chance or an insufficient sample size. Most investigators choose to accept a Type II error occurrence rate of no greater than 20%.

2. The percentage of individuals in the control group who are expected to experience adverse outcomes. If this percentage, estimated from previous studies, is large, the sample may be small but sufficient to show statistical significance if one truly exists.
3. Magnitude of the difference in outcomes between treatment and control groups. If this difference is small, a large sample size is required to demonstrate this difference.

Table 17.8 outlines the sample size required in controlled trials based on the probabilities of adverse outcomes in the treatment and control groups and the acceptable probability of a Type II error.[16] In summary, when the frequency of a particular adverse outcome (e.g., death) in the treatment and control groups is expected to be low and the difference in these outcomes is expected to be small, the sample size must be sufficiently large to limit the possibility of Type I and II errors. A power analysis calculation permits the reader to determine if a large enough sample has been studied to avoid a Type II (or Beta) error.

- **Assess if all the patients that entered the study were accounted for at its conclusion.**

When a significant number of patients are lost to follow-up, significant patient characteristics may be distributed unevenly between the treatment and control groups. Furthermore, a large number of patient exclusions may affect study outcomes, particularly if those excluded may have had a different prognosis than those included in the final analysis. Therefore, patients lost to follow-up should continue to be attributed to the group to which they were originally randomized in order to preserve the value of the randomization process and to allow an intent-to-treat analysis.

Readers may assess for themselves the effect of follow-up losses on study outcomes by performing an informal sensitivity analysis. For instance, in positive trials (i.e., studies that demonstrate statistically significant treatment benefits), the outcomes of the study can be recalculated after assuming that all patients lost from the treatment group fared poorly while all those lost from the control group did well. If the conclusions do not change, the loss to follow-up may not be excessive. If the conclusions do change, however, the follow-up loss may be significant enough to weaken the causal relation between intervention and outcomes.

Table 17.8: Sample Size Requirements Based on Probabilities of Adverse Outcomes and Type II Errors

			Probability of adverse outcome in study group			
		Type II error	1%	5%	10%	20%
Probability of adverse outcome in control group	2%	10%	3696	851	207	72
		20%	2511	652	161	56
		50%	1327	351	90	38
	10%	10%	154	619	-	285
		20%	120	473		218
		50%	69	251		117
	20%	10%	62	112	285	-
		20%	49	87	218	
		50%	29	49	217	
	40%	10%	25	33	48	117
		20%	20	26	37	90
		50%	12	16	22	49
	60%	10%	13	16	20	34
		20%	11	13	16	27
		50%	7	8	10	16

Riegelman & Hirsch. Studying a Study and Testing a Test: How to Read the Medical Literature.[16]

Source: Figure was reprinted with permission from Studying A Study and Testing A Test by R.K. Reigelman and R.P. Hirsch which was published by Little, Brown and Company. (Copyright 1989, Joseph G. Rubenson and Kenneth A. Wasch, Trustees, Riegelman Children's Trust).

- **Determine if the patients and study personnel were blinded to the interventions.**

Double-blind evaluations are optimal for minimizing treatment bias in terms of patient and provider opinion of treatment efficacy, compliance, placebo effect, measurement of treatment outcomes, and interpretation of study results. If double-blinding is not possible in the study protocol, bias may be minimized in other respects such as blinding those study personnel who assess clinical outcomes. Furthermore, patient population characteristics may be evaluated in unblinded studies. If they appear similar between the treatment and control groups, the strength of the study conclusions may be increased.

- **Evaluate the similarity of the groups at the start of the trial.**

Randomization may not always insure similar groups. Consequently, in smaller studies, there is a greater chance of finding differences in baseline characteristics between the treatment and control groups. When the magnitude of these differences is large, the effects of treatment may be exaggerated. Therefore, if substantial dissimilarities between these groups are identified, investigators should conduct an analysis that adjusts for these differences. Multivariable analysis technique, such as regression analysis, is recommended—even when no substantial differences exist between groups.[16]

- **Determine if the treatment and control groups were treated equally with the exception of the study intervention.**

Interventions other than the one under study are referred to as cointerventions. If differentially applied, they may distort study outcomes, particularly if the cointerventions are effective treatments. Therefore, in order to evaluate the impact of cointerventions, their use should be clearly described and the frequency of their occurrences documented.

What were the results? Results may be expressed in a variety of ways. **Incidence** describes the number of events (e.g., myocardial infarction, bleeding, death) that have occurred during a given interval of time divided by the number of persons at risk for that same event during that time interval. Incidence may also be described as the risk of an outcome event with treatment (Y) and without treatment (X) (see **Table 17.9**).

Table 17.9: Definition of Incidence

	Number of Events	Number of Non Events	Incidence
Treatment	A	B	Y=A/(A+B)
Control	C	D	X = C/(C+D)

Other expressions of study results include **absolute risk reduction** (ARR) which describes the difference in the number of events (i.e., incidence) between the control (X) and treatment (Y) groups (see **Table 17.10**):

$$ARR = X - Y.$$

Relative risk (RR), a comparative value, describes the risk of an event among individuals receiving treatment compared to those receiving no treatment (control):

$$RR = Y/X.$$

Relative risk reduction (RRR), the most commonly reported measure of treatment effects, describes the reduction in the number of events in patients receiving treatment compared to those receiving control. It is expressed as a percentage or a ratio (e.g., 0.25):

$$RRR = [1 - Y/X] \text{ or } [1 - RR].$$

The reported RRR is only an estimate (i.e., point estimate) of the true treatment effect. Therefore, investigators will often calculate confidence intervals (CIs) to report the accuracy (i.e., "precision") of the point estimate by describing a range within which the true effect most likely lies. Generally, a 95% CI is chosen. This means that there is a 95% probability that the true result lies within the defined range. On the other hand, there is a 5% probability that the true treatment effect lies outside the range. This aspect of CI relates to the P value (Type I error) which is usually set at < 0.05.

Table 17.10: Summary of Measures Used To Report Effects of Interventions

Absolute risk reduction (ARR)	Relative risk (RR)	Relative risk reduction (RRR)
X - Y	Y/X	[1 - Y/X] or [1 - RR]

A larger sample size provides greater numbers of outcome events which increase the probability that the true treatment effect is close to that observed in the study. This is the concept of study "power": the larger the sample size, the greater the study power. Adequacy of the sample size with respect to probability of outcomes and Type I and II errors has been discussed previously. Confidence intervals are also useful in determining whether the sample size is sufficient. For studies that conclude treatment benefits (i.e., positive trial), the lower boundary of the CI may be assessed. If this value appears to be statistically significant, the sample size is adequate. On the other hand, for studies which conclude no benefit from treatment (i.e., negative study), the upper boundary of the CI may be assessed. If this value would be significant if it were true, the study requires a larger sample size because it has failed to exclude the possibility of significant treatment effects.

If no CIs are reported, alternative methods may be used to assess the precision of the results:[18]

(1) If the *P* value is 0.05 or greater, the 95% CI must include one if relative risk is reported (see **Figure 17.1**). This means that there is the possibility of no treatment benefits. However, if the *P* value falls below 0.05, the upper boundary of the CI must fall below one and the possibility of no treatment benefits is reduced.

Figure 17.1: An Example of Relative Risk with Confidence Intervals

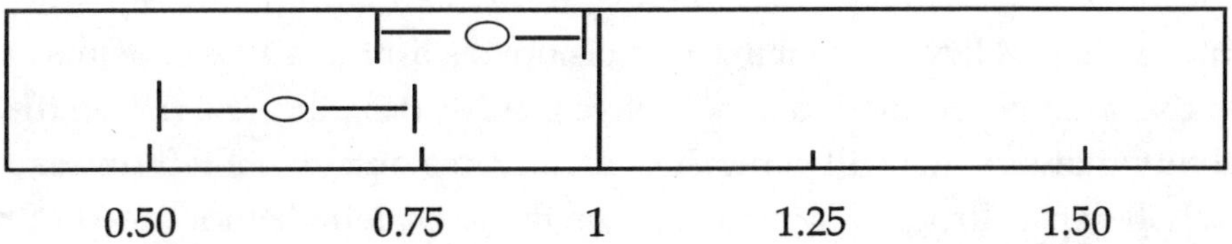

(2) If the article includes standard error (SE) values of the treatment effect, the upper and lower boundaries of the 95% CI may be calculated as the point estimate plus and minus twice the SE, respectively. The CI can then be assessed appropriately.

(3) The third, less desirable, alternative is to formally calculate the CI.

Will the results help me care for my patients? The final step is determining whether a study has clinical significance. Using the study inclusion and exclusion criteria, comparisons of a population of patients in clinical practice to those in the study may be conducted. However, this method may not only be tedious and time-consuming but may also produce variable results when different practitioners apply their own clinical skills and expertise. A more simple approach to evaluating study relevance is to ask, "Are the patients in this study so different from my patients that I could not apply the study results in my practice?"[2]

In order to determine clinical relevance of a subgroup analysis, a closer evaluation of the validity of the analysis is warranted. Guides have been published for this purpose, and the following is a summary:[19]

> The subgroup is more likely to have benefited from the intervention if the difference in the outcomes among subgroups is
> (1) large,
> (2) unlikely to have occurred by chance,
> (3) a result of an analysis defined as a hypothesis before the start of the study,
> (4) one of few subgroup analyses in the study, and
> (5) evaluated in other studies.

As more of these criteria are fulfilled, more confidence can be placed in extrapolating the results of the subgroup analysis to a population of patients in the practice setting.

All clinically important outcomes must be considered in the evaluation of study results before they are applied. "Substitute end points," which include measures such as cardiac output, blood pressure, lipid profiles, and the like, are important in assessing clinical outcomes, but, from the patients' perspective, significant benefits of treatment include measures such as reduction in the frequency of shortness of breath, number of hospitalizations, risk of myocardial infarction, improved survival and health-related quality of life. Therefore, it is imperative to consider all clinically important outcomes even when only one favorable effect of treatment is reported.

If a study is applicable to clinical practice and its outcomes have been determined to be important, the next step is to weigh the benefits of treatment against the potential harms and costs. Before treatment is initiated, patient risk of adverse events, if no treatment is rendered, must be considered even if the RRR associated with the therapeutic intervention appears impressive. A key element in the decision to start therapy is consideration of a concept called the "number needed to treat" (NNT). NNT describes the notion that the greater the probability that patients will experience an adverse outcome if left untreated, the more likely they will benefit from treatment and the fewer patients would need to be treated to prevent one adverse event. Mathematically, NNT is the inverse of the absolute risk reduction (ARR):

$$NNT = 1/(X\text{-}Y).$$

Several properties of NNT enhance its clinical usefulness:[2] (1) NNT quantifies decisions to treat select patients; (2) it expresses costs related to treatment including the costs of the regimen, monitoring, side effects, and toxicity; and (3) it may be useful for comparing different treatments for different disorders. Consequently, the number of adverse events per life saved or the number of lives saved per adverse event may provide useful insight into the benefits and risks associated with a therapeutic or preventive intervention.

Grades of Evidence

After all the pertinent articles on therapeutic or preventive interventions have been carefully evaluated, recommendations can then be formulated based on the evidence presented in the studies. Evidence varies from opinion to systematic, reproducible scientific research; therefore, evidence varies in its ability to produce predicted outcomes. Because a recommendation based on multiple randomized controlled trials is more likely to result in the predicted outcome than one based on personal experience, recommendations may be weighed or stratified (i.e., graded) based on study design and validity (see **Table 17.11**). There are several approaches to grading the quality of evidence supporting a particular recommendation. The approach in **Table 17.11** is used for the grading of evidence by the Cedars-Sinai Center for Applied Health Services Research and is used in Cedars-Sinai's resource management project. It is based upon the work of Cook, et al.[14]

A **Grade A** recommendation is based on a randomized, prospective, controlled study with low false-positive and low false-negative errors. A low false-positive error indicates a trial that demonstrates a statistically significant benefit from an intervention. An example is the randomized trial in which captopril given to patients with depressed left ventricular ejection fraction (LVEF) after an acute myocardial infarction (MI) produced statistically significant reductions in both total and cardiovascular mortality and morbidity including the frequency of severe congestive heart failure (CHF) and recurrent MI.[20] A low false-negative error indicates a trial that demonstrates no therapeutic benefits from the intervention and was large enough to exclude the possibility of a clinically important benefit. Therefore, in the absence of Type II error calculations (power analysis), studies without treatment benefits cannot be Grade A quality. The ISIS-3 trial was a large study (with adequate power) that demonstrated no clinically significant difference in the efficacy of streptokinase, tissue plasminogen activator (t-PA), and anisoylated plasminogen-streptokinase activator complex (APSAC) after an acute myocardial infarction.[21]

A **Grade B** recommendation is based on a randomized, prospective, controlled trial with high false-positive and/or high false-negative errors. A high false-positive error indicates a trial that demonstrates a positive trend but does not show a statistically significant benefit. For instance, early trials of aspirin following myocardial infarction showed positive, but statistically nonsignificant, trends demonstrating favorable effects of aspirin on survival. A high false-negative error indicates a study that shows no therapeutic benefits from an intervention, although the sample size is too small to rule out the possibility of a clinically significant benefit.

A **Grade C** recommendation is based on a nonrandomized, prospective, controlled trial which compares contemporaneous or current and former patients. This category also includes noncontrolled case series with ten or more patients. A **Grade D** recommendation is based on a retrospective analysis. A **Grade E** recommendation is supported by information based on indirect evidence, personal experience or expert opinion, and case reports with fewer than ten patients. Indirect evidence constitutes those findings derived from studies that found evidence of treatment benefits that were not the primary end points of the study. An example is a study that supports the use of trimethoprim-sulfamethoxazole (TMP-SMX) as prophylaxis for toxoplasmosis in patients with the acquired immune deficiency syndrome (AIDS).[22] This study primarily evaluated the use of TMP-SMX as prophylaxis for Pneumocystis carinii pneumonia (PCP) in patients with AIDS. The incidence of PCP was reduced in those patients who received this agent; furthermore, the incidence of toxoplasmosis was also found to be reduced in the same patient population. Indirectly, the benefit of TMP-SMX as primary prophylaxis for toxoplasmosis in patients with AIDS was demonstrated.

At least one meta-analysis supports a **Grade M** recommendation, while at least one cost-effectiveness or decision-analysis study supports a **Grade Q** recommendation. Cost- and decision-analysis studies evaluate all relevant courses of action and their consequences, in terms of outcomes and costs, in order to identify a single course of action that is in the best interest of the patient. Finally, a **Grade S** recommendation is supported by at least one study that summarizes and pools data from other articles.

A well-designed retrospective study may provide more information than a poorly designed prospective trial; therefore, both the study design as well as the validity of the outcomes must be considered when grading the evidence.

Table 17.11: Grades of Recommendations Are Supported by Evidence

Grade	Supported by
A	Randomized, prospective, controlled trial with low false-positive and low false- negative errors
B	Randomized, prospective, controlled trial with high false-positive and/or high false-negative errors
C	Non-randomized, prospective, controlled trial comparing contemporaneous patients or current and former patients Non-controlled case series with ten or more patients
D	Retrospective analysis
E	Indirect evidence, personal experience, or expert opinion Case reports with fewer than ten patients
M	At least one meta-analysis
Q	At least one cost-effectiveness or decision-analysis study
S	At least one study that summarizes and pools data from other articles

Adapted from ACCP - Cook DJ et al. [14] and Cedars-Sinai Medical Center: Center for Applied Services Research - unpublished.

Critical Appraisal of Articles on Diagnostic Tests

Are the study results valid?

- **First, determine if the diagnostic test was compared with a reference standard.**

Accuracy of a diagnostic test is determined by comparing it to an accepted reference test or a "gold" standard. This reference standard refers to a definitive diagnosis attained by biopsy, surgery, autopsy, or the like.[2] The concept of blindness means that those study personnel who conduct or interpret the test results should not know whether the patient does or does not have the target disorder. Furthermore, those applying the reference standard should not know the results of the diagnostic test. This is to avoid or at least minimize "diagnostic suspicion" bias. The results of the test and reference standard should also be assessed independently; therefore, study interpreters should be blinded to the results of one test when evaluating the results of the other.

- **Evaluate the patient sample.**

The study population should resemble those patients most likely to be encountered in clinical practice. This insures that the diagnostic test may potentially be applicable to a population of patients in question. For instance, the results of a study examining the usefulness of ferritin levels in diagnosing iron-deficiency anemia in patients over the age of sixty-five years would potentially be relevant and useful in determining the likelihood of iron-deficiency in the elderly population.[23]

- **Determine if the test result influenced the decision to perform the reference standard.**

"Verification bias" or "work-up bias" describes the influence of the diagnostic test results on the decision to use the reference standard.[17] Frequent use of the reference standard to confirm the results of the diagnostic test reduces the value of the test and further limits the usefulness of the study results.

- **Assess the methods of performing the test.**

Methods for applying the diagnostic test should be described in sufficient detail such that issues regarding patient preparation, such as special requirements for fluids, diet, or physical activity; avoidance of concomitant drugs; handling of specimens for analysis; and other precautions are clearly outlined. Techniques for conducting the test as well as methods for analyzing and interpreting the results should also be described

What were the results? If the results of the study appear to have been measured through a valid process as described above, the next step is to appraise the actual results of the study.

- **Evaluate the likelihood ratios for the test results.**

The **pretest** probability of a target disorder is determined by patient presentation of signs and symptoms and their overall clinical status. Application of a diagnostic test may modify this probability and yield a **post-test** probability of the target disorder. A measure of the accuracy with which a diagnostic test can identify the target disorder is quantified in terms of the likelihood ratio or the specificity/sensitivity of the diagnostic test.

The likelihood ratio (LR) indicates how much the test result will alter (i.e., increase or decrease) the pretest probability of a target disorder. An LR of 1 means the post-test probability is unchanged from the pretest probability. LR greater than 1 indicates an increase from the pretest to the post-test probability of the presence of the target disorder, while an LR less than 1 indicates a decrease in the post-test probability. **Table 17.12** summarizes a rough guide for interpreting LRs.[24] The further the LR value is from 1, the greater the likelihood of the presence or absence of the target disorder.

Table 17.12: Interpreting Likelihood Ratios

LR	Change from pretest to post-test probability
>10 or <0.1	Large and conclusive
5-10 or 0.1-0.2	Moderate
2-5 or 0.2-0.5	Small, sometimes important
1-2 or 0.5-1	Small, rarely important

Adapted from Jaeschke et al. [24]

Source: Figure was reprinted with permission from "User's Guide to the Medical Literature III. How to Use an Article About a Diagnostic Test. B. What Are the Results and Will They Help Me in Caring for My Patients?" by R. Jaeschke, G.H. Guyatt, and D.L. Sackett in the Journal of American Medical Association 271(9) 1994: 703-707. (Copyright 1993/1994, American Medical Association).

The LR may be used to mathematically calculate the post-test probability from the pretest probability. This calculation involves (1) converting pretest probability to pretest odds, (2) multiplying the result by the LR to obtain the post-test odds, and (3) converting the post-test odds to a post-test probability (see **Table 17.13**).

Table 17.13: Using Likelihood Ratio To Convert Pretest Probability to Post-test Probability

	Step	Equation	Comment
1	Convert pretest probability (A) to pretest odds (X)	X = A/(1-A)	Ratio of probability of having the target disorder to the probability of not having the target disorder
2	Convert pretest odds (X) to post-test odds (Y)	Y = X(LR)	-
3	Convert post-test odds (Y) to post-test probability (B)	B = Y/(Y+1)	-

-Adapted from Jaeschke et al.[24]

Source: Figure was reprinted with permission from "User's Guide to the Medical Literature III. How to Use an Article About a Diagnostic Test. B. What Are the Results and Will They Help Me in Caring for My Patients?" by R. Jaeschke, G.H. Guyatt, and D.L. Sackett in the Journal of American Medical Association 271(9) 1994: 703-707.. (Copyright 1993/1994, American Medical Association).

An easier method involves using a nomogram of Bayes theorem which has already performed all the conversions.[25] By lining a ruler across the pretest probability and LR axises, the post-test probability lies at the point where the ruler crosses the post-test probability axis.

Sensitivity and specificity may also be used to measure the accuracy of the diagnostic test. Sensitivity represents the proportion of people **with** the target disorder of those with a positive test result. Specificity is the proportion of individuals **without** the target disorder of those with a negative test result (see **Table 17.14**).[24] Because this method of calculating the post-test probability of a target disorder relies on only two criteria of either the presence or absence of disease, it may miss other important clinical information since it does not account for varying criteria such as low, intermediate, and high probabilities of disease. Therefore, due of its efficiency and simplicity, the LR, which may be calculated from sensitivity and specificity (see **Table 17.14**), is generally the preferred method for measuring the accuracy of a diagnostic test.

Table 17.14: A Comparison of the Results of a Diagnostic Test and a Reference Standard and Definitions of Sensitivity and Specificity

		Reference Standard	
		Disease present	Disease absent
Test	Disease present	True positive (a)	Falsepositive(b)
Result	Disease absent	False negative (c)	True negative (d)

Sensitivity = a/(a+c)

Specificity = d/(b+d)

LR for positive test result = a/(a+c)/[b/(b+d)] or sensitivity/(1-specificity)

LR for negative test result = c/(a+c)/[d/(b+d)] or (1-sensitivity)/specificity

Adapted from Jaeschke et al. [24]

Source: Figure was Reprinted with permission from "User's Guide to the Medical Literature III. How to Use an Article About a Diagnostic Test. B. What Are the Results and Will They Help Me in Caring for My Patients?" by R. Jaeschke, G.H. Guyatt, and D.L. Sackett in the Journal of American Medical Association 271(9) 1994: 703-707.. (Copyright 1993/1994, American Medical Association).

Will the results help me care for my patients?

- **Determine the clinical relevance of the test.**

The test should be able to consistently identify those patients with and without the target disorder. In addition, interpreters should consistently be able to determine the value of the test results.

An evaluation of disease severity and comorbidities in the study patients must also be conducted in order to determine the relevance of the study in the practice setting. As with therapeutic and preventive interventions, a question of whether any reason exists to discourage the applicability of the results to clinical practice should be posed.

Test and treatment thresholds are based on individual practitioner's clinical judgment of the risks associated with therapy and disease, if left untreated. These thresholds, therefore, affect patient management decisions. A test threshold is the probability **below** which a practitioner would dismiss a diagnosis and discontinue further tests. A treatment threshold is the probability **above** which a clinician would confirm a diagnosis, stop further diagnostic tests, and initiate treatment.[24]

As discussed previously, test results with LRs near 1 are not very useful; therefore, the further the LR lies from 1, the greater the likelihood that the test result will move the probability of disease across a test or treatment threshold and determine further actions. On the other hand, if the post-test probability of a target disorder does not move beyond either threshold but, rather, lies within their boundaries, subsequent diagnostic testing is warranted.[2]

The value of all available diagnostic tests should be closely evaluated before any one is applied. That is, if a closely related test is applied subsequent to a diagnostic test, the new information would most likely provide little or no information.

Ultimately, the usefulness of a diagnostic test depends on its ability to improve patient management and outcomes. As with articles on therapy or prevention, both clinical judgment and analytical skills are essential when evaluating studies on diagnosis.

4. Multidisciplinary Team Judges the Relative Value of the Expected Benefits, Harms, and Costs of the Critically Appraised Interventions

The principle goal of the critical appraisal exercise is to inform the discussion of the multidisciplinary team as it develops or adapts clinical practice guidelines. The goal of the first three steps can be thought of as faithful translation of efficacy information into effectiveness. **Efficacy** can be defined as the impact of a specific intervention on patient outcomes under **ideal circumstances**. For example, the findings from a large carefully conducted drug study in which the investigators have carefully selected patients through rigorous application of inclusion and exclusion criteria, used the drug according to strict protocols, and used extensive resources to assure patient adherence with study recommendations defines **efficacy**. **Effectiveness** is the impact of an intervention when applied to patients in the "real world" of day-to-day clinical practice. For example, the same drug described above is now released following FDA approval based upon efficacy information and used in practice. The busy practitioner does not have the time to carefully review all the inclusion and exclusion criteria for drug administration and faces the real possibility that the patient may not be perfectly compliant nor adherent to rigorous follow-up. It is easy to understand how efficacy and effectiveness may be quite different. By explicitly encoding the findings from clinical trials including inclusion and exclusion criteria and potentially improving practitioner and patient compliance, guidelines and pathways are excellent tools to more faithfully translate efficacy into effectiveness.

At this point in the practice of evidence-based medicine, the multidisciplinary team assembled to develop the clinical guidelines and pathways must judge the information that has been summarized. The team must weigh the expected benefits to the patient population against the anticipated harms and costs. Ultimately, of course, caregivers in conjunction with patients and their families, will decide the appropriate course. The multidisciplinary team has, however, a significant responsibility to help inform this decisionmaking process. If the team is composed of individuals including nurses, physicians, mental health experts, pharmacists and even patients, the group will have a broader base for judgment and ultimately its recommendations will probably be more acceptable to patients and health care providers.

5. Develop Clinical Practice Guidelines for Each Important Element of Care

The faithful translation of the results of the formal literature searches, critical appraisal exercises, and judgment of value by the team is the key to development of potentially effective guidelines. Guidelines were previously defined as "systematically developed statements to assist practitioner and patient decisions about appropriate health care for specific clinical circumstances.[3] The team should also keep in mind the important principle that if guidelines are to fulfill the "practical need to translate knowledge into decisions, they must use unambiguous language, define terms precisely, and use easy to follow modes of presentation." [3] The team should remember that practitioners of various levels of sophistication will probably be using the presented guidelines and therefore they must be explicit and be presented in a way which will facilitate consistent application to patients. Additional observations on the practical applications of guidelines are contained in Chapter 18 in this book. It is the quality of evidence combined with faithful translation and clear expression which form the foundation of excellent guidelines.

6. Place Guidelines To Form the Backbone of a Clinical Pathway

The multidisciplinary team may now decide to combine the guidelines that have been developed or adapted from the clinical literature into a comprehensive clinical pathway. If there is only one important guideline, then the team may simply build the detail to drive the guideline (for example necessary diagnostic tests to determine optimal length of stay). For many conditions, however, multiple guidelines are required to optimize care. For example, in the development of a pathway to improve outcomes for patients admitted to the hospital for upper gastrointestinal bleeding, a formal literature review revealed that prompt UGI endoscopy was helpful in determining the risk status of such patients. Without endoscopy, determination of risk of rebleeding, need for surgery, or death could not be accurately determined. [26]

It is also important to consider the possible interactions that various guidelines may have on each other within a pathway. There may be strong evidence for each step in the care of a given population but the combination may not be proven or may even lead to worsened outcomes. Further discussion of these issues can be found in Chapter 19 on resource management.

7. Develop a Systematic Approach to Process Measurement and Reporting

Perhaps the most important principle in process measurement is parsimony. Measure and report only those elements which are likely to have an important impact on clinical outcomes. The team should address the following questions: [7]

- What is to be measured?
- Where is the needed information available?
- Who will collect this information?
- What is the appropriate sample of patients?
- How large is the anticipated sample?
- Who will summarize the information?
- How will the summarized information be utilized for process improvement?

A far more detailed discussion of this area is contained in Chapter 19.

8. Develop a Systematic Approach to Outcomes Measurement and Reporting

The same principles of measurement and reporting apply to economic and clinical outcomes measurement. These include the caution to be parsimonious (since outcomes measurement is expensive) and to be systematic. The broad categories of outcomes measures to be considered include the following:

- Clinical quality,
- Patient satisfaction,
- Provider satisfaction, and
- Cost.

Through process measurement it is possible to determine compliance with essential guideline recommendations. Compliance with evidence-based guidelines should improve clinical and economic outcomes, but only by measuring essential outcomes are the providers able to demonstrate improved care. The linking of process improvement to outcomes measurement provides the opportunity to optimize care. Additional discussion of outcomes measurement is contained in Chapter 18.

9. Implement the Guideline or Pathway

Now that the team has developed evidence-based guidelines and pathways and has a system of process and outcomes measurement in place it must face the challenge of implementation. It has been stated that "guidelines do not implement themselves."[3] This is an important concept that may be too often overlooked. In addition to an approval process, which should have a degree of formality, the team should consider the use of technology, including computer assisted decisionmaking, and various strategies that have been shown in the literature to change physician behavior. Using multiple strategies should be strongly considered.[8, 27] See Chapter 18 for a more detailed discussion of implementation.

10. Measure and Report Process Variation and Outcomes

Measurement, statistical analysis, summarization and reporting of both process and outcomes measures provide the basis for improvement. Although improved compliance with evidence-based recommendations is likely to improve outcomes, there is no guarantee. Some of the possible explanations for a failure to improve care despite apparent decreased variation and increased adherence to guidelines include:

- Improper implementation wherein patients are misclassified by the individuals applying the guideline. For example, patients with a contraindication to B-blockers post AMI receive them inappropriately or patients, who present with low-risk chest pain are improperly risk stratified and sent home prematurely or not promptly enough.[28]
- Guidelines have not faithfully translated high quality clinical evidence and, therefore, patients are receiving suboptimal care.

- A guideline is based upon weak evidence and the resulting practice is not best practice.
- Controversy arose because of conflicting evidence and the "wrong" practice was encoded.
- Changes, which were not covered by the path, were made for the pathway population and adversely impacted clinical outcomes. For example, modification in rehabilitation services in hospital or post-hospitalization significantly worsened functional outcomes.

For these, and other potential reasons, outcomes as well as processes must be measured. Furthermore, measuring only clinical outcomes with no knowledge of process is equally limiting when the team considers improvement. The cause of poor (or even excellent) economic or clinical outcomes will be unclear and difficult to improve.

11. Use Process and Outcomes Measures With Updated Literature Searches And Appraisals To Continually Improve Care

The team now has the ongoing responsibility to continually improve the clinical and economic outcomes of care for patients impacted by the guideline or pathway. There should ideally be a formalized approach to review the summaries of process and outcomes measures coupled with a strategy to obtain updated literature searches. A more detailed description of continuous improvement can be found in Chapter 18.

How To Learn More About Evidence-Based Medicine

There are several excellent ways to learn more about evidence-based medicine. These include the following:

- Attend a formal course. The Evidence-based Working Group puts on a course each year. The course not only teaches EBM, but trains attendees to be effective teachers of this discipline.
- Read the series of articles in *The Journal of the American Medical Association* (JAMA) entitled "Users' Guides to the Medical Literature." [1,10,15,17,18,24,29,30,31,32]
- Read the five part series "Evidence-based Care" in the *Canadian Medical Association Journal* [5-9] written by the Evidence-based Care Resource Group.
- Subscribe to ACP Journal Club, a bimonthly publication of the American College of Physicians. This is not only an excellent source of brief summaries of scientifically rigorous articles, but also contains an ongoing editorial series addressing important aspects of evidence-based care.
- Read David Sackett's textbook "Clinical Epidemiolgy: A Basic Science for Clinical Medicine."[2]
- Read the JAMA series "The Rational Clinical Examination," which uses the principles and techniques of evidence-based medicine to address various elements of the clinical history and physical examination. The first article provides an excellent overview and sets the tone for the series. [33]

- At an organizational level, the hospital can identify a few interested and enthusiastic individuals with the appropriate background and encourage them to attend courses and read the references cited. These individuals can then teach others within the institution thus further disseminating the necessary skills, tools, and attitudes.

Summary

The practice of evidence-based medicine for a population of patients can be accomplished through a rigorous approach to clinical practice guidelines and pathways. This chapter has attempted to provide an overview of evidence-based medicine and present an eleven-step approach to its practice for populations of patients. Evidence-based care includes a clear problem definition, effective literature searching, critical appraisal, and judgment of the relative value of expected benefits, harms, and costs by a multidisciplinary team. This team can then develop clinical practice guidelines and pathways coupled with a system of process and outcome measure identification, summary, and reporting to drive continuous improvement.

Although this rigorous approach may seem burdensome, it is likely to result in improved outcomes for patients. Evidence-based practice combines the best elements of the science of medicine with the art of medicine. Excellent clinical literature cannot replace experience or reasoning from pathophysiology, but it can complement them tremendously. The chapter has also attempted to provide a list of resources that may be used by interested practitioners to further refine their evidence-based practice and teaching skills. It is suggested that interested individuals or teams start conservatively and pick an important and focused project. Remember the importance of a multidisciplinary team and the ultimate need to focus on the patient and family for whom we are attempting to improve care.

References

1. Evidence-based Medicine Working Group. " Evidence-Based Medicine: A New Approach To Teaching The Practice Of Medicine." *Journal of the American Medical Association* 268(17): 1992; 2420-2425.

2. Sackett DL, RB Haynes, GH Guyatt, P Tugwell. "Clinical Epidemiology: A Basic Science for Clinical Medicine." 2nd ed. Boston, Mass: Little Brown & Co; 1991.

3. Field MJ , KN Lohr eds. Clinical Practice Guidelines: Directions for New Program (Summary) Washington, DC National Academy Press: 1990

4. Deignan M, Resource Management-Cedars-Sinai Medical Center. personal communication.

5. Evidence-based Resource Group. "Evidence-Based Care: 1. Setting Priorities: How Important Is This Problem?" *Canadian Medical Association Journal* 150 (8) 1994; 1249-1254.

6. Evidence-based Resource Group. "Evidence-Based Care: 2. Setting Guidelines: How Should We Manage This Problem?" *Canadian Medical Association Journal* 150 (9) 1994; 1417-1423.

7. Evidence-based Resource Group. "Evidence-Based Care: 3. Measuring Performance: How Are We Managing This Problem?" 150 (10) 1994; 1575-1579.

8. Evidence-based Resource Group. "Evidence-Based Care: 4. Improving Performance: How Can We Improve The Way We Manage This Problem?" *Canadian Medical Association Journal* 150 (11) 1994; 1793-1796.

9. Evidence-based Resource Group. "Evidence-Based Care: 5. Lifelong Learning: How Can We Learn To Be More Effective?" *Canadian Medical Association Journal* 150 (12) 1994; 1971-1973.

10. Oxman AD, DL Sackett, GH Guyatt. "Users' Guides To The Medical Literature: How To Get Started" *Journal of the American Medical Association* 270(17) 1993; 2093-2095.

11. Guyatt GH, RZ Jaeschke, DJ Cook. "Applying The Findings Of Clinical Trials To Individual Patients." (editorial) ACP Journal Club Mar-Apr 122 1995: A12-13.

12. Lowe HJ, GO Barnett. "Understanding And Using The Medical Subject Headings (Mesh) Vocabulary To Perform Literature Searches." *Journal of the American Medical Association* 271(14) 1994; 1103-1108.

13. Antman EM, et al. "A Comparison Of Results Of Meta-Analyses Of Randomized Control Trials And Recommendations Of Clinical Experts: Treatments For Myocardial Infarction." *Journal of the American Medical Association* 268(2) 1992; 240-248.

14. Cook DJ, GH Guyatt, A Laupacis, DL Sackett. "Rules Of Evidence And Clinical Recommendations On The Use Of Antithrombotic Agents." *Chest* 102(4) 1992; 305S-311S.

15. Guyatt GH, DL Sackett, DJ Cook. "Users' Guides To The Medical Literature: II. How To Use An Article About Therapy Or Prevention. A. Are The Results Of The Study Valid?" *Journal of the American Medical Association* 270(21) 1993; 2598-2601.

16. Riegelman RK, RP Hirsch. "Studying a Study and Testing a Test: How to Read the Medical Literature." 2nd ed. Boston, Mass: Little Brown & Co Inc; 1989.

17. Jaeschke R, GH Guyatt, DL Sackett. "Users' Guides To The Medical Literature: How To Use An Article About A Diagnostic Test. Are The Results Of The Study Valid? "*Journal of the American Medical Association* 271(5) 1994; 389-391.

18. Guyatt GH, DL Sackett, DJ Cook. "Users' Guides To The Medical Literature: II. How To Use An Article About Therapy Or Prevention. B. What Were The Results And Will They Help Me In Caring For My Patients?" *Journal of the American Medical Association* 271(1) 1994; 59-63.

19. Oxman AD, GH Guyatt . A Consumer's Guide to Subgroup Analysis. *Annals of Internal Medicine.* 116: 1992; 78-84.

20. Pfeffer MA et al. "Effect Of Captopril On Mortality & Morbidity In Patients With Left Ventricular Dysfunction After Myocardial Infarction: Results Of The Survival & Ventricular Enlargement (SAVE) Trial." *New England Journal of Medicine* 327 1992; 669-677.

21. ISIS-3 (Third International Study of Infarct Survival) Collaborative Group. "A Randomized Comparison Of Streptokinase vs Tissue Plasminogen Activator vs Anistreplase And Of Aspirin Plus Heparin vs Aspirin Alone Among 41,299 Cases of Suspected Acute Myocardial Infarction." *Lancet* 339(8796) 1992; 753-770.

22. Podzamczer D. "Thrice-Weekly Cotrimoxazole Is Better Than Weekly Dapsone-Pyrimethamine For The Primary Prevention Of Pneumocystis Carinii Pneumonia In HIV-Infected Patients." *AIDS* 7(4) 1993; 501-506.

23. Guyatt GH, et al. "Diagnosis Of Iron-Deficiency Anemia In The Elderly." *The American Journal of Medicine* 88 1990; 205-209.

24. Jaeschke R, GH Guyatt, DL Sackett. "Users' Guides To The Medical Literature: III. How To Use An Article About A Diagnostic Test. B. What Are The Results And Will They Help Me In Caring For My Patients?" *Journal of the American Medical Association* 271(9) 1994; 703-707.

25. Fagan TJ. "Nomogram for Bayes's Theorem." *New England Journal of Medicine* 293(5) 1975; 257.

26. Hay J, et al. "Upper Gastrointestinal Hemorrhage Clinical Guideline: Determining The Optimal Hospital Length Of Stay." (submitted).

27. Greco PJ, JM Eisenberg. "Changing Physicians' Practices." *New England Journal of Medicine* 329(17) 1993; 1271-1274.

28. Ellrodt AG, et al. "Measuring And Improving Physician Compliance With Clinical Practice Guidelines: A Controlled Interventional Trial." *Annals of Internal Medicine* 122(4) 1995; 277-282.

29. Levine M, et al. "Users' Guides To The Medical Literature: IV. How To Use An Article About Harm." *Journal of the American Medical Association* 271(20) 1994: 1615-1619.

30. Laupacis A, et al. "Users' Guides To The Medical Literature: V. How To Use An Article About Prognosis." *Journal of the American Medical Association* 272(3) 1994; 234-237.

31. Oxman AD, DJ Cook, GH Guyatt. "Users' Guides To The Medical Literature: III. How To Use An Overview." *Journal of the American Medical Association* 272(17) 1994; 1367-1371.

32. Richardson WS, AS Detsky. "Users' Guides To The Medical Literature: VII. How To Use A Clinical Decision Analysis. A. Are The Results Of The Study Valid?" *Journal of the American Medical Association* 273(16) 1995; 1292-1295.

33. Sackett DL. " Primer On The Precision And Accuracy Of The Clinical Examination." *Journal of the American Medical Association* 267(19) 1992; 2638-2644.

Chapter 18

Development, Implementation, and Evaluation of Practice Guidelines: Practical Applications

Scott Weingarten, MD, MPH

Health care is undergoing dramatic changes, not from federal legislation, but from shifting market forces. The most significant effects of these changes concern the immediate need to provide efficient and high quality medical care. Moreover, it is no longer sufficient to claim to have excellent quality care. Payers and purchasers of health care are requiring objective data to document quality. As a result of these changes, health care providers are reexamining the care that they provide to patients and thinking creatively about strategies that lead to better quality and less costly medical care.

As the health care delivery system undergoes this diagnostic check-up, unexplained variations in medical care have surfaced at every turn. Health care providers are all doing things differently. There are widespread variations in hospital admission rates, hospital lengths of stay, and the frequency with which certain diagnostic tests are ordered. The variations in care often cannot be explained by differences in patient severity of illness or in patient outcomes. These variations have profound implications for both the cost and quality of health care.

There is a need to reduce health care costs for health care organizations to remain competitive in today's changing health care environment. Many areas throughout the country have been affected by managed care, reductions in health care pricing, downsizing, and mergers. In analyzing strategies for reducing costs, experts have concluded that clinical decisions are responsible for between 80% and 90% of health care spending. Therefore, in order to make significant inroads in health care costs, the clinical care provided to patients must be examined and efforts must be made to optimize clinical decisionmaking. In order to accomplish these important goals, clinical care must be changed to reflect more efficient ways of caring for patients as determined by scientific study. Medical care should be changed to reflect innovations in care that promote efficiency, and those aspects of care that have been shown through scientific investigation to lead to the best patient care should be translated into clinical practice.

SCOTT WEINGARTEN, MD, MPH—Director, Health Services Research Cedars-Sinai Health System and Research Institute; Assistant Professor of Medicine, University of California-Los Angeles, School of Medicine.

As health care costs are being controlled, attention has shifted to measuring and improving quality of care. If health care providers always provided optimal quality medical care, there would be no need to participate in quality improvement programs, to develop and implement practice guidelines, or to measure physician performance through the use of "report cards." However, this is not the case. Many studies have documented that clinicians have not complied with guidelines that could lead to better patient care. Whether it is performing mammograms on women in the appropriate age range, immunizing the elderly against influenza, diagnosing depression, or providing deep venous thrombosis prophylaxis in patients undergoing total hip replacement, almost all research has disclosed opportunities to improve patient care.

Many studies have documented long delays in translating research findings into clinical practice. Despite research that has shown that new technologies and treatments can improve care and save lives, significant time often elapses between the discovery of these findings and their translation into clinical practice on a widespread basis. Studies have also demonstrated that technologies may continue to be used even after they have been demonstrated to be ineffective or harmful. Strategies that facilitate the prompt translation of new and important research findings into clinical practice can potentially improve health care and patient outcomes. Practice guidelines can serve as one of these strategies.

Despite the important advances in technology that have transpired over the last several decades, there are often gaps in learning when and when not to use these newer technologies. It has been shown that new technologies are often employed in situations when they have not been found to be safe or effective. At times, there is a mismatch between the promise of new technologies and the demonstration that these technologies improve care. For example, the resolution of radiologic imaging studies has improved significantly. However, have these improvements led to the discovery of more clinically significant findings that improve patient outcomes? Or rather, have these technologies led to the discovery of incidental findings that do not improve patient outcomes? The answer to this question may depend on the population of patients being imaged. If high resolution imaging studies are performed on patients with an extremely low probability of having a disease, the number of incidental findings may exceed the number of clinically significant findings. Therefore, improvements in technology do not guarantee improvements in patient care.

Recent developments in the evolution of practice guidelines and clinical pathways parallel the timeline for the introduction of many new technologies and drugs. The first step in the introduction of a new drug or technology is development and approval. The transition of health care into an industry that is subject to competition and market forces has generated enthusiasm and excitement over the development and implementation of practice guidelines. Over the last several years, health care organizations throughout the country have made significant strides in developing guidelines and clinical pathways, and many organizations believe that these strides have led to better quality and less costly medical care.

The next phase in the introduction of a new technology or drug can be uncritical acceptance and enthusiasm. Although studies have documented the potential of guidelines for improving practice, not all of the studies will demonstrate positive effects. Following acceptance of a new technology, limitations are often discovered. In the near future, one can anticipate many cases in which guidelines will be shown to fail to improve patient care. Significant barriers to the successful implementation of practice guidelines will be found. Examples where guidelines fail to produce sustained changes in clinical practice will surface. And, when outcomes are carefully analyzed, patient outcomes may occasionally be worsened. For example, although many early drug studies have shown the promise of certain drugs, follow-up studies sometimes show that the drugs may have unanticipated effects that may compromise patient care. It is unrealistic to believe that the thousands of guidelines and clinical pathways that have been developed will universally lead to better patient care. Similarly, one would not expect that all drugs that have been developed or are under development will improve patient care. The following sections outline fourteen basic points for developing, implementing, and evaluating the success of clinical guidelines and pathways.

Basic Steps for a Successful Clinical Guideline and Pathway Program

Use the Scientific Method

As many clinicians develop clinical guidelines, they may encode the way that they have treated patients in the past, which may or may not correspond with the optimal method of treating patients. The quickest way to develop a guideline is to simply write down the way that one has cared for patients in the past. This "quick and dirty" approach to guideline development, however, may not reflect important new research and innovations in care. An evidence-based approach can encode optimal medical practice and promote the rapid translation of innovations in patient care into medical practice. Guidelines should encode all that is currently known about the best way to care for patients based upon current scientific literature. The scientific evidence used to derive guidelines and pathways may also directly relate to their acceptability to clinicians and their ability to improve patient care.

Process Guidelines Locally

There are many excellent guidelines that have been published in the literature. The American Medical Association's *Directory of Practice Parameters,* for example, lists approximately 1,600 guidelines. However, physicians are often unaware of the existence of many of these guidelines. Furthermore, it is unrealistic to expect that guidelines taken off the shelf will automatically improve patient care. Often, guidelines are difficult to understand and to use. Physicians may lack confidence in guidelines developed elsewhere. Finally, it may be difficult to translate complex, lengthy guidelines into patient care. Guidelines may need to be "home grown" or locally processed to be adopted into clinical practice.

There also may be difficulty in transporting guidelines from one health care organization to another, and patterns of care and resources may differ in health care organizations throughout the country. For example, home health services can be easily procured in large urban areas, but it can be a significant challenge to provide home health care in isolated rural areas. Therefore, a guideline that assumes the availability of frequent home health care visits may not be applicable to settings where these resources are not readily available.

Create or Choose "Decidable" Guidelines

An important problem inherent in many practice guidelines and pathways is that they tend to be vague and lack specificity (i.e., they are not "decidable" or "executable"). Controversy often ensues when a team charged with creating or adopting guidelines attempts to make specific and explicit recommendations. To quell the controversy, the team may soften the guidelines so that there is little clinical substance, and no clinician in attendance could possibly be offended. However, vague guidelines cannot possibly change clinical practice in a meaningful manner. For example, a 1982 National Institutes of Health Consensus Development Conference issued the following guideline: "CT detection of intracranial tumors is now so well established that the suspicion of any intracranial mass lesion from history or neurological examination constitutes a strong indication for the procedure." Clearly, this guideline lacks specificity and it is unrealistic to expect that any health care provider would have his or her practice after reading this guideline.

Address the Continuum of Care

Cedars-Sinai and others have researched the clinical criteria that determine when it is safe to discharge a patient from the acute care hospital. However, the validity of these criteria depends upon the quality of medical care provided to a given patient at the time of and after discharge from the hospital. For example, it may appear safe for a patient with pneumonia to be discharged from the hospital if he or she is afebrile and meets other carefully derived clinical criteria. However, if the patient is sent home with an ineffective antibiotic, the patient's outcome may be compromised. Changing medical care without considering all aspects that contribute to the patient's outcome may fail to improve quality.

Measuring quality throughout the continuum of care is required to determine the overall effects of guidelines on patient care. If only acute hospital care is considered when evaluating a practice guideline or clinical pathway, one may miss some of the effects of a patient care intervention. For example, what happens if hip fracture patients leave the acute care hospital more expeditiously? If the patient requires more recovery time in a rehabilitation facility as a result of leaving the acute care hospital more quickly, or if the patient requires care in a nursing home rather than in their own home, overall costs may have increased rather than decreased. Furthermore, quality of care may have worsened.

Acknowledge that Guidelines Are Not for All Patients

One unresolved issue is the number of patients whose care can be improved by practice guidelines and clinical pathways. Clearly, guidelines and clinical pathways will not improve care for all patients. They work best for relatively homogeneous groups of uncomplicated patients. Guidelines often are not relevant to heterogeneous populations of patients; the complexity and clinical nuances of certain patients do not lend themselves to guidelines. For example, a guideline for mammography might improve the care of asymptomatic women who are fifty-five years of age. However, there are few clinical pathways that could improve the care of complicated patients in septic shock and who suffer from multiple organ dysfunction. The percentage of patients whose care could potentially be improved through the use of guidelines is currently not known.

Keep Guidelines "Fresh"

Another potential problem with guidelines and clinical pathways is that they will rapidly become outdated. Guideline enthusiasts often muster great enthusiasm among clinicians and administrators regarding the initial development of guidelines and pathways. However, errors may be found after the guidelines are applied to patient care. Clinicians will discover ambiguity and other limitations to the guidelines. Finally, new research will be published which will make certain guideline recommendations obsolete. An organization committed to the success of guidelines must be committed to revisiting the clinical contents of a guideline at frequent time intervals. Revisiting the guidelines based on the publication of new research findings will be critical to maintaining the relevance of guidelines to patient care, and for ensuring that guidelines remain credible with clinicians.

Achieve Physician "Buy-in"

Physician acceptance is critical to ensure that guidelines are successfully implemented. In essence, individuals creating practice guidelines believe that they have a better way of caring for patients than the way that patients have been cared for in the past. If guideline creators did not believe that there was a better way to practice medicine, then the time and effort required to create guidelines and clinical pathways would have been wasted. However, creating meaningful change in human behavior is difficult. Physicians may and should question attempts to change their clinical practice. If there is little resistance, there is a good chance that either physicians are unaware of the guideline or the guideline does not differ from what physicians had been doing in the past.

Implementation, Implementation, Implementation

A fundamental barrier that can impede guidelines and pathways is inattention to their implementation. The Institute of Medicine has said that "guidelines do not implement themselves." A number of studies have demonstrated that guidelines alone often fail to produce sustained changes in physician practice. Effective guideline dissemination strategies are required to increase the probability that guidelines are adopted into practice. Researchers have commented that a disproportionate amount of time is being spent on guideline development and relatively little time and effort has been devoted to studying methods of implementing guidelines.

Think Clinical

To engage physicians in the creation of guidelines and clinical pathways, guidelines should focus on clinical matters. For example, many physicians have limited interest in spending significant amounts of time on quality improvement projects that focus on non-clinical issues (for example, the number of lost laboratory slips). Physicians usually expect health care organizations to solve these problem without them. However, in clinical matters such as choosing the correct antibiotic for patients with pneumonia, it may be possible to interest and perhaps excite a number of physicians to participate in the effort.

Align the Incentive System

An important issue that may influence the eventual adoption or rejection of guidelines and clinical pathways concerns the incentive system. If there are disincentives to following a guideline, monetary or otherwise, these disincentives may prevent successful implementation. Therefore, the external environment may determine, in part, the success or failure of efforts to implement guidelines and pathways.

Reduce Misapplication of Guidelines

Another important concern affecting the efficacy and effectiveness of guidelines and pathways is ensuring that they are applied appropriately to the patients for whom they were intended. Guidelines and clinical pathways at times will be misapplied. For example, an evidence-based clinical pathway for patients with pneumonia will probably not improve patient care if it is incorrectly applied to patients with pulmonary embolism. In fact, it may worsen care. As is the case for any diagnostic test, guidelines and pathways will have calculable sensitivity and specificity rates when applied to patient care. Case managers may sometimes identify patients as appropriate for a guideline who were, in reality, not appropriate for the guideline. Guidelines will be misapplied in clinical practice, and organizations should take appropriate steps to monitor for and reduce the misapplication of guidelines.

Evaluate the Outcomes: Was the Guideline a Success or a Failure?

Another area that has received surprisingly little attention is the evaluation of practice guidelines. Did a specific guideline or clinical pathway improve or worsen patient care? Did the guideline enhance or worsen patient satisfaction? Did the guideline reduce or increase health care costs? The answers to these questions determine whether the guideline effort can be classified as a success or a failure. Outcome validation is particularly important when few data are available to support the validity of the guideline. In situations where there are substantial data to support the effects of the guidelines, outcome validation may become less important. For example, the benefits of mammography in reducing morbidity and mortality of breast cancer patients is well established. Because the science is sound, it can reasonably be inferred that increasing mammography rates (at the appropriate time interval) in women of the appropriate age range will improve outcomes. If resources to evaluate guidelines are constrained, using mammography rates may be a sufficiently valid surrogate outcome measure and may serve as an excellent marker for reducing breast cancer mortality.

In one example, Cedars-Sinai's Department of Resource Management (led by Marianne Deignan) examined the outcomes of a guideline project to identify a single hip implant vendor for the institution. There was a belief that using a single vendor could maintain quality medical care at a lower cost. The cost savings of this intervention could be very significant, and it was theorized that operating room time could be reduced because all health care providers would be familiar with the particular hip implant. However, the orthopedic surgeons had become accustomed to using different brands of hip implants, and many were concerned about changing hip implant vendors. The orthopedic surgeons voiced concern that quality of care could be compromised by switching to a single hip implant vendor but, in the absence of data, no physician could confirm or deny the validity of this concern. Without outcomes data, proponents of the change could argue that patient care would be improved, and opponents of this policy could argue that the change would compromise patient care. There was no way to discern which opinion was correct.

In order to measure the quality of care in this instance, Cedars-Sinai needed to define and measure patient outcomes relevant to total hip replacement surgery. For practical purposes, outcomes were measured within a one-year time period, including clinical outcomes, hospital readmission, patient satisfaction, patient physical functioning, pain, and the amount of time patients needed to return-to-work. Importantly, several of the outcome measures, including pain, physical functioning, and satisfaction, could only be measured by directly asking patients about their experiences and their health.

The information on these patient outcomes is being reported back to the orthopedic surgeons after a one year time period. A preliminary analysis of the health status data (patient physical functioning and pain) showed that patient care had not been compromised; in fact, care remained excellent. Outcomes information is still being collected and these data will continue to support or refute the wisdom of the decision to change to a single hip implant vendor.

Length of Stay Is Not Sufficient as an Outcome Variable

Many studies have chosen length of stay as an outcome variable for the evaluation of clinical pathways. However, length of stay may be inadequate when used as the only outcome variable. Lengths of stay are declining throughout the United States as a result of many factors. Guidelines and clinical pathways may be only one of those factors. It is often unclear whether a guideline or pathway is responsible for reductions in length of stay or whether reductions in lengths of stay can be attributed to secular trends that were occurring independently of the guidelines or pathways.

Quality Versus Quantity

Finally, the quality of guidelines that are developed or adapted may be more important than the number of guidelines processed. For many organizations, there may be a tendency to rapidly develop as many guidelines and pathways as possible. However, one may ask whether the guidelines have improved or worsened patient care, and how that was determined. It is better to have a single guideline that has improved patient care than to have many guidelines that have had unknown effects on patient care. Therefore, the quality of guidelines and pathways may be more important than the quantity. The following case study illustrates the steps required in developing, implementing, and evaluating successful guidelines that show demonstrable improvements in patient care.

Case Example

This case study describes a guideline developed by Cedars-Sinai that demonstrated the potential to safely reduce length of stay for low-risk patients hospitalized with chest pain based on a retrospective analysis of patient medical records.[1] The study demonstrated that by using certain clinical characteristics, clinicians could identify patients who could be discharged from the hospital relatively safely. The study was scientifically rigorous and based on clinical evidence. The guidelines were "decidable," meaning that the clinical criteria were sufficiently detailed and explicit to alter patient care. Since not all chest pain patients would be appropriate for the guideline, clinical criteria were developed to allow clinicians to decide which patients were appropriate and which patients were inappropriate for the guideline. After reviewing the data, the guideline was supported by several physician opinion leaders in cardiology. The findings were also discussed and approved at the appropriate medical staff committee meetings. The institution also acknowledged that changes in patient care might cause the guideline to be outdated and agreed to revise it at periodic intervals following implementation.

The guideline for patients with chest pain was implemented by case managers seven days-a-week on a real-time basis. Patients were identified on a daily basis and information about the contents of the guideline were communicated to the physicians treating the patient. Evaluation of the guideline demonstrated a significant reduction in length of stay for low-risk chest pain patients, resulting in a total cost savings of $1,397 per low-risk patient.[1] Importantly, these reductions in lengths of stay and health care costs were related to the guideline rather than to unrelated secular trends, since when implementation of the guideline was discontinued, lengths of stay and health care costs increased. The reduction in health care costs was accomplished while maintaining excellent quality of care. There was no increase in the hospital readmission rate. Patient quality-of-life and patient satisfaction remained excellent. Furthermore, there was no increase in diagnostic testing in patients following discharge from the acute care hospital, and, therefore, there was no evidence to suggest that health care costs had been shifted to the outpatient setting.[1]

Conclusion

In conclusion, guidelines have undergone an evolutionary cycle similar to many new technologies and drugs. At the current time, there seems to be widespread acceptance of guidelines and clinical pathways, and enthusiasm abounds for their potential to improve patient care. This enthusiasm may be justified. There have been a number of examples of how guidelines have improved quality of care. There are also examples that have demonstrated that guidelines have not resulted in sustained changes in care, and it is likely that there will be reports in the future of guidelines worsening patient care. As the field of guidelines and clinical pathways matures, the role of guidelines will be defined. Guidelines and clinical pathways will be viewed as an important tool, one of many that can be used to improve patient care, enhance patient satisfaction, and safely reduce health care costs.

Reference

1. Weingarten SR, Reidinger MS, Connor L, et al. "Practice Guidelines and Reminders To Reduce Duration of Hospital Stay for Patients with Chest Pain: An Interventional Trial." *Annals of Internal Medicine* 1994;120: 257-263.

Chapter 19

Resource Management

Marianne Deignan, MBA
A. Gray Ellrodt, MD

In April 1994, the Cedars-Sinai Health System recommitted itself to its mission of providing the highest quality clinical care coupled with education, research, and community service. At the same time, the institution committed to achieving significant cost reductions by the end of the fiscal year through several strategic initiatives. Resource management, a comprehensive clinical process redesign program, was one of these initiatives. The leaders of this project were challenged with significantly reducing clinical costs while maintaining or improving the quality of care. In addition, the institution committed to rigorously measuring these cost reductions and quantifying the changes in clinical processes of care and outcomes. This chapter reviews the development, roll-out, implementation, and early results of the clinical resource management project.

Relationship to Patient-Focused Care

Since the resource management project was gearing up just as Cedars-Sinai was completing the roll out of patient-focused care (PFC) across the medical center, resource management capitalized on the existing momentum and organizational structure of the PFC initiative. The patient-focused care restructuring effort sought to improve institutional efficiency by decreasing the cost per unit of service and streamlining those services that were appropriate to deliver. The Resource Management Project focused on the appropriateness and effectiveness of the clinical services delivered at the institution, including level of care, diagnostic testing strategies, and therapeutic interventions. It also sought to decrease costs by improving quality of care and reducing the delivery of unnecessary services. In addition, as the institution became a vertically integrated health system, both initiatives focused not only on the hospital, but took a broader view of the system's resources and their optimal utilization. **Figure 19.1** illustrates the sequence of these strategic initiatives.

MARIANNE DEIGNAN, MBA—Director, Resource Management, Cedars-Sinai Medical Center.

A. GRAY ELLRODT, MD—Vice Chairman for Clinical Affairs, Department of Medicine, Director, Division of Internal Medicine, Cedars-Sinai Medical Center; Professor of Medicine, University of California-Los Angeles, School of Medicine.

Figure 19.1: PFC/Resource Management Strategic Initiatives

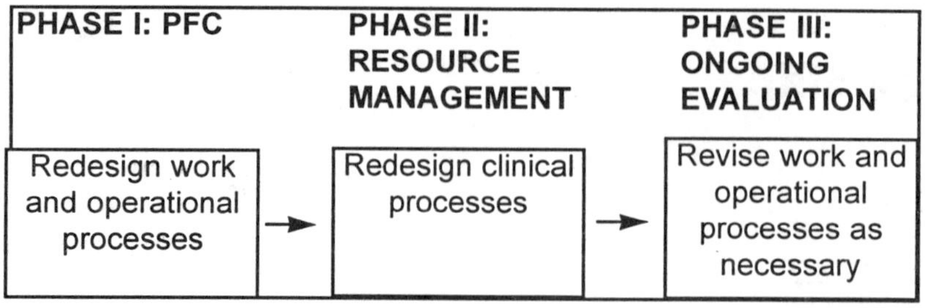

The specific cost reduction relationship between patient-focused care and resource management is demonstrated in **Figure 19.2.** The patient-focused care project at Cedars-Sinai accomplished many objectives. In attempting to streamline care and significantly reduce the number and variety of health care practitioners caring for the patient, it provided the infrastructure from which to ask several new and important questions. One of these was to challenge the project teams to differentiate between efficiency and effectiveness. **Efficiency** can be defined as accomplishing a given task with the fewest resources. **Efficacy** is the outcome of providing a service in the ideal setting (i.e., a clinical trial), while **effectiveness** can be defined as the outcome of providing the **appropriate high quality services** to the patient in a timely manner in the real world of medicine. Patient-focused care improved efficiency and sought to improve the quality of care, but did not address the issue of appropriateness of the ordered services. It did not, for example, explicitly address the optimal length of stay at the appropriate level of care and the optimal diagnostic strategy or treatment regimen for a group of patients with similar clinical conditions Resource management sought to translate efficacy into effectiveness. Furthermore, in order to meet the institution's cost and quality objectives, effectiveness and appropriateness needed to be addressed in an organized manner.

Figure 19.2: How Do RM and PFC Compare With the COST Perspective?

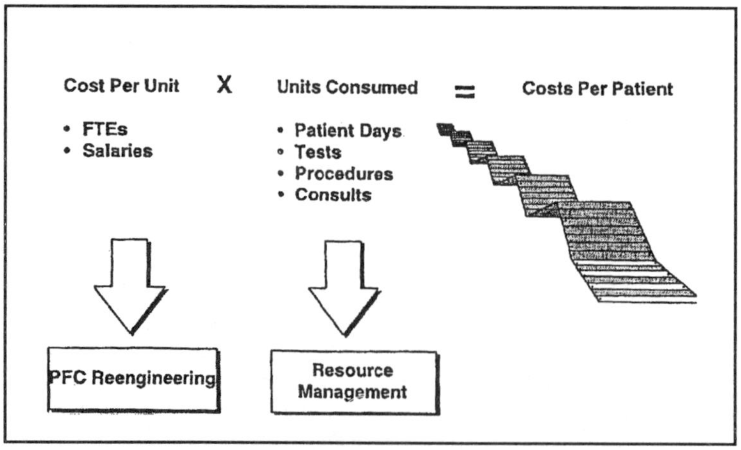

Project Strategies

In the early planning stages of the resource management project, several general and more specific strategies were identified and ultimately agreed upon. These included the following:

- Redesign clinical processes to reduce utilization of tests, procedures, consults, and days in the acute care setting for specific, targeted high volume, high cost patient populations.
- Develop clinical guidelines and clinical pathways in conjunction with key stake holders for these targeted populations.
- Develop specific implementation strategies for these populations using the literature addressing changing physician behavior.
- Select populations in which significant quality of care issues have been identified and develop clinical guidelines and pathways to address these issues.
- Develop a case management system to help support specific aspects of guideline and pathway implementation, but also to focus on "high-risk" patient populations which are (based upon the scientific literature) likely to be high cost or at significant risk for hospital and post-discharge complications.
- Develop systems to measure, analyze, and report process variation to drive ongoing quality improvement.
- Develop systems to measure, analyze, and report economic, clinical, and patient centered outcomes for use in ongoing quality improvement.

Project Structure

Figure 19.3 summarizes the organizational structure of the resource management project, which was similar to that of patient-focused care. The steering committee was chaired by the vice president for patient care services and the senior vice president for medical affairs. Significant changes included the participation of more members of the full-time and voluntary medical staff, and the organization of task forces around patient populations defined by clinical department. PFC was more centrally organized with eight major and twenty decentralized committees. In the resource management project, guideline and pathway development was more decentralized, with as many as forty teams developing guidelines and pathways as part of six task forces.

Figure 19.3

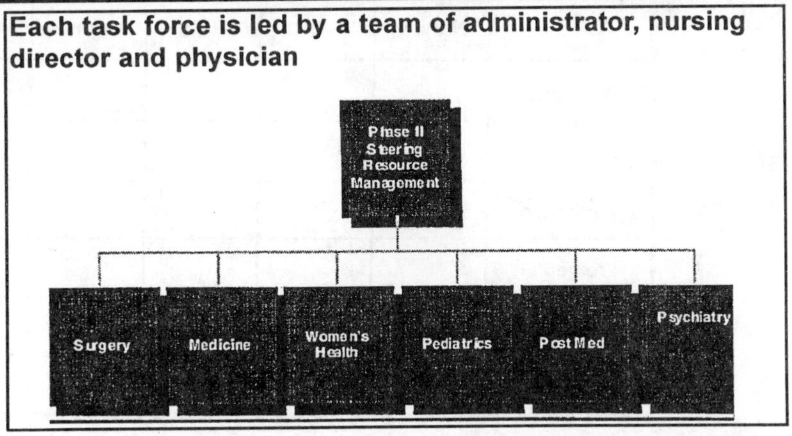

In the initial phases of the resource management project, the health care consulting firm APM (San Francisco) provided manpower and assisted in project definition and preparation of project presentations. Also integral to the project were the Clinical Pathways Committee and the existing medical staff committees. The Clinical Pathways Committee assured that all guidelines and pathways were explicit and evidence-based, had appropriate medical staff approval, and identified key process and outcome measures to be collected. The medical staff committees approved the clinical content on behalf of the large Cedars-Sinai medical staff.

Guiding Principles

The fundamental principles of the Cedars-Sinai resource management project include the following:

- Be patient-focused
- Redesign clinical processes that are linked to desired outcomes
- Use the 80/20 rule to focus on significant opportunities for improvement
- Improve quality; it leads to efficiency
- Improve efficiency; it leads to quality
- Be clear on recommendations and the underlying evidence or be silent
- Strive for best practice
- Expect deviations from best practice based on clinical judgment

Cost and Quality Issues Across Departments

The resource management steering committee agreed to the matrix management and measurement approach shown in **Figure 19.4**. This approach stressed the importance of collaboration between clinical departments (e.g., surgery, medicine) and ancillary departments (e.g., imaging, laboratory), and it formalized the shared responsibility for meeting economic and quality goals. Thus both the rows and columns had specific cost reduction targets which could only realistically be met by focused collaboration. The hospital's cost accounting and tracking system enabled groups to analyze targets and track economic outcomes in cost dollars rather than patient charges.

Figure 19.4: Set Joint Goals To Encourage the "Rows" and the "Columns" To Work Together

	Nursing	OR	Lab	Pharmacy	Etc.	TOTAL
Medicine						
Surgery						
Pediatrics						
Women's						
Etc.						
TOTAL						

Clinical Guidelines and Pathways

Why Focus on Clinical Guidelines and Pathways?

The resource management steering committee decided to focus on clinical guidelines and pathways for multiple reasons. These included the significant potential of guidelines and pathways to:

- Link tightly the processes and outcomes of care,
- Promote development of better measures of quality of care,
- Increase the predictability of demand for patient services,
- Clarify the expectations and responsibilities of care team members,
- Facilitate communication between members of the care team and patients/families,
- Decrease documentation time, and
- Promote a process for monitoring quality of care, including a systematic approach to both process and outcomes measurement.

What Are Clinical Pathways?

The project operationally defined a clinical pathway as: *A tool to coordinate the day-by-day progress of a typical uncomplicated patient across many clinical departments.*

What Are Clinical Guidelines?

The project used the definition developed by the Institute of Medicine defining clinical practice guidelines as: *"Systematically developed statements to assist practitioner and patient decision about appropriate health care for specific clinical circumstances."* [1]

How Do Clinical Pathways and Guidelines Fit Together?

Since the operational definition of a clinical guideline emphasizes the decisionmaking process involved in a specific clinical situation, multiple guidelines must be linked together to form a comprehensive plan of care over time and across departments. Therefore, the pathways typically contain multiple guidelines addressing many cost and quality issues. Each potential guideline must show promise to positively impact cost and/or quality and have a demonstrated impact on economic or clinical outcomes.

Figure 19.5: How Clinical Pathways and Guidelines Fit Together

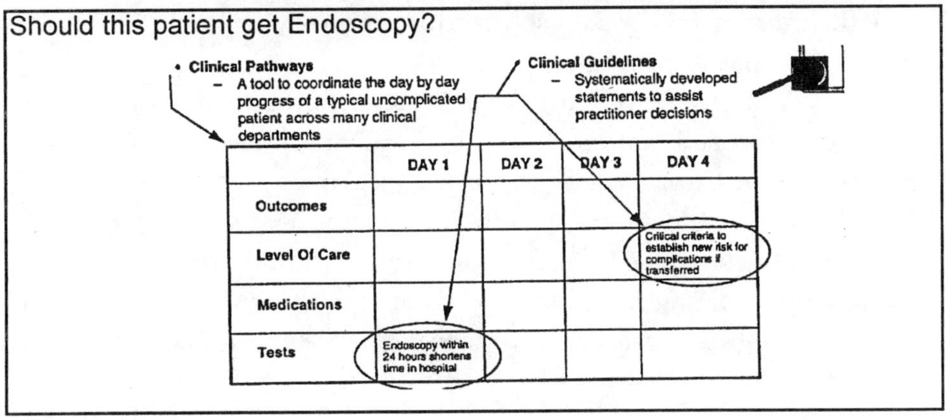

The potential guidelines are then placed in a matrix which forms the backbone of the clinical pathway. This backbone (or preliminary pathway) is shown in **Figure 19.5.**

Why Use Evidence-Based Medicine (EBM)?

The decision to use an evidence-based medicine approach in the development of clinical guidelines and pathways was not taken lightly. The leaders of the resource management project understood that a rigorously applied evidence-based approach would be resource intensive and take more time then a methodology-based upon expert consensus. However, Cedars-Sinai already had several individuals in the Center for Applied Health Services Research with practical hands-on experience in using evidence-based guidelines to improve economic and clinical outcomes. The medical staff appeared receptive to these early efforts. The rationale behind evidence-based care through guidelines and pathways is presented in more detail in Chapter 18. Reasons to use this rigorous approach for the resource management project included the following:

- **Guidelines and pathways should encode optimal medical practice rather than usual practice.** Cedars-Sinai had already attempted to implement consensus-based guidelines and pathways in a previous program. They tended to prescribe current practice or to make recommendations too vaguely worded to implement.
- **EBM empowers all members of multidisciplinary care team to shape guidelines and pathways.** A genuine concern expressed by many health care providers was that the multidisciplinary teams would be dominated by a few very vocal and dogmatic members who would attempt to encode their practice rather than be open to the recommendations of other team members. Requiring the use of rigorous literature searches and critical appraisal would hopefully remove the personal agenda issues and help level the playing field. Therefore, at the initial meeting of each multidisciplinary team, a team "guideline" stating that the best scientific clinical evidence would be used was presented and agreed upon.
- **EBM provides the maximum opportunity to change practice.**
  A natural result of the agreement to use an evidence-based approach is the opportunity to encode optimal practice which may often represent a dramatic change from the current baseline. Rather than incremental (evolutionary) change, dramatic (and perhaps revolutionary) change in practice can be encoded if new and compelling scientific clinical research emerges. The agreement to use the most recent and best literature represents a unique "contract" between all of the health care providers.
- **Most likely to improve patient outcomes.** Perhaps the most important result of an evidence-based approach is the implicit understanding that encoding the best literature (from which improved outcomes have been demonstrated) is most likely to improve patients' health. If the clinical studies can be faithfully translated into guidelines, the probability of demonstrating improved outcomes is high.
- **Avoids micromanaging those aspects of care that may not affect outcomes.**
  Another important reason to use an evidence-based medicine approach is to avoid

the temptation to micromanage multiple aspects of care that are unlikely to impact outcomes. Collecting and analyzing process variables is expensive and time consuming. If there is no literature supporting a particular intervention, it may not be important in determining patient outcomes. If consensus exists that an element of care has significant *potential* to change outcomes, however, then measurement can proceed as clinical investigation rather than the tracking of supportable state-of-the-art care.

Why Should We Not Use an Evidence-Based Medicine Approach to Resource Management?

A number of questions were raised about the use of evidence-based medicine as a foundation for this project. These included the following:

- What is evidence-based medicine?
- Does it really make a difference?
- Are there important articles in the clinical literature that would change current practice or is Cedars-Sinai already practicing the best medicine?
- Won't this expensive and time-consuming process just slow the project down and cause it to lose momentum?
- Does Cedars-Sinai have the required resources to practice evidence-based medicine?
- Other institutions are not using this approach, why should we?

These concerns and questions were addressed early and, once the decision was made to proceed using an EBM approach, the necessary resources including medical librarian time and physician and nurse education in the principles and tools of EBM were provided. The library staff was overwhelmingly enthusiastic and supportive of the project and approximately 10,000 pages of articles were pulled and duplicated in the first several months of the project.

Using Guidelines and Pathways to Improve Outcomes

The resource management project uses an eleven-step approach to improving clinical and economic outcomes. Chapter 18 provides an overview of these eleven steps in **Table 19.1**, along with a detailed explanation of the nuances of literature searching and critical appraisal. The present chapter focuses on developing a clear problem statement, the practical challenges of writing guidelines and pathways, and the challenges of measuring and reporting process variation and outcomes. In addition, the chapter discusses the important issue of implementation in depth. The following sections describe Cedars-Sinai's application of this eleven-step process.

1. **Formulate a clear problem statement**. At this early phase the resource management team identified a variety of conditions as candidates for process and outcome improvement. It was agreed that each clinical department should organize multidisciplinary teams to clearly define the patient population, gather background economic and clinical information, define the problem, and add other members to each team to be sure that all "stakeholders" were involved at the initiation of the team's efforts. For example, a team from the department of medicine was formed to develop guidelines and a pathway for patients with

stroke. The team reviewed information suggesting that non-hemorrhagic stroke was the most common clinical presentation of all stroke patients and that a large number of patients (about 300) were admitted annually with this diagnosis. Length of stay data demonstrated wide variation and no process was in place to aggregate these patients in one particular area of the hospital. One of the stroke guideline group's first responsibilities was to review its membership. The team added several "opinion leaders" and soon included a neurologist and an internist as co-chairs, an emergency department physician, a physiatrist, a speech therapist, an occupational therapist, a physical therapist, a nurse, a quality management coordinator, and an analyst from resource management.

Another important early step is to identify the important elements of care for which a process outcome link had been demonstrated or is probable based upon the knowledge of team members. These "candidates" for guidelines are then the subject of formal literature searches. The importance of this initial step in the process cannot be overemphasized. This step is the equivalent of correctly identifying the chief complaint. If the condition to be addressed is unclear, the team membership is incomplete, or the goals for improvement are not shared, the project is unlikely to succeed. In addition, team members are continually reminded to consider implementation, even at this early stage of development. Thus, the team remains focused on the potential realities of making the guidelines and pathways work.

2. **Perform a formal literature search.** At Cedars-Sinai, each team assigned specific topics to members of the guideline group who had an expressed interest in the subject and had familiarity with the clinical content area. These individuals (often a physician, but other clinical group members were also assigned) were scheduled for a one-hour appointment with the medical librarian and together they composed an effective search strategy. The library kept that search strategy on file for review and use in updating the guideline in the future. The combination of a librarian and clinician searching the literature seemed a potent strategy for finding and focusing on relevant, high quality articles. In addition, any member of the team with articles about the specific topic was asked to bring copies for review. On the stroke guideline group, members were assigned topics including appropriate level of care, length of stay, DVT prophylaxis, heparin therapy, outcomes from stroke units, swallowing evaluation, and use of echocardiograms and other diagnostic tests.

3. **Assess the quality of the article(s).** Several practical points emerged during the critical appraisal exercises. These included the need to prioritize the grades of evidence as outlined in Chapter 18 and to give high quality articles greater weight than those of inferior scientific rigor. Often this meant disregarding someone's favorite article or helping them realize the limitations of that publication. This process also clarified the clinical circumstances for which good evidence was not available and, therefore, tempered the strength of recommendations. Finally, the team was forced to deal with conflicting recommendations supported by apparently equal grades of evidence. In all of these situations, the ground rules emphasizing the importance of good science helped level the playing field and avoid encoding unsupported personal opinion.

4. **The multidisciplinary team judges the relative value of the benefits, harms, and costs of the critically appraised interventions.** This is a very important charge to each team.

Teams must understand that their ultimate recommendation will carry considerable weight in shaping care, even though the guidelines are to be recommendations, not rules. The teams also understand that their recommendations will inform decisionmaking for providers and their patients and therefore need to include careful consideration of benefits, harms, and costs. Finally, as they translate the recommendations from the critically appraised articles into guidelines, the groups need to carefully review the inclusion and exclusion criteria and the results of any subset analysis.

5. **Develop clinical practice guidelines for each important element of care.** The multidisciplinary team now faces the task of faithfully translating the evidence into useful clinical practice guidelines. In this effort, the team should keep in mind the caveat that if guidelines are to fulfill the "practical need to translate knowledge into decisions, they must use unambiguous language, define terms precisely, and use easy to follow modes of presentation." [2]

The structure of a resource management guideline as submitted to the clinical pathways committee is shown in **Figure 19.6.** The purpose of this structured format is to assure that the guideline developers have been explicit in their recommendations and definitions of terms. Although this is not the final guideline format, it is the beginning of the approval process and will ultimately be encoded into a guideline and pathway. Note the requirements to define the patient population in general (e.g., neutropenic) and specific (e.g., absolute neutrophil count between 500 and 1,000) terms. In addition, note the explicit description of "if......then" this should be done. Finally, note that the highest grade of evidence supporting the recommendation is presented. Resource management keeps all the guidelines in a database and keeps copies of all bibliographic citations and copies of the articles.

Figure 19.6: The Structure of a Cedars-Sinai Guideline

Title: Empiric Antibiotic Recommendations in Patients with Neutropenic Fever

Number: 94-051-G

Patient Population:

1. 18 years of age or older.
2. Has history of neoplastic disease.

Explicit Criteria:

1. Has Chemotherapy induced neutropenia with an absolute neutrophil count (ANC) of <500 to 1000.
2. Has a fever (>38.0C).
3. Does not have culture proven infection.

Intervention:

1. Begin Ceftazidine 2gm IV q eight hours if no evidence of severe sepsis (i.e., hypotension). Recommend addition of empiric aminoglycoside if there is suspicion of Pseudomonas or initial ANC <100.
2. If no improvement in fever or clinical condition at Day 2, then add empiric amino glycoside and Vancomycin or change to single agent imipenem.
3. If no improvement in fever or clinical condition at Days 5-7, and on multiple broad spectrum antibiotics, then begin Amphotericin B.
4. Adjust antibiotic regimen as needed for positive cultures.

Grade of Evidence-A

6. **Place guidelines to form the backbone of a clinical pathway.** **Figure 19.5** shows the placement of two of the guidelines that eventually formed the backbone of the upper GI bleed pathway. The final version of this pathway actually included ten guidelines developed from formal literature review and critical appraisal. As the guidelines are placed on the pathway, it is important to look for potential interactions between them. For example, in the development of the pathway for management of acute myocardial infarction (AMI), both B-blockers and ACE inhibitors were recommended. It was important for the team to consider the potential additive side effects of this combination and carefully review the relevant articles. Fortunately, ISIS-4, a large multicenter, randomized controlled trial, studied many patients on this combination and actually found an additive beneficial effect.[3]

7. **Develop a systematic approach to process measurement and reporting.** With each guideline and pathway, the developers are required to recommend measures of compliance with the recommended processes of care. The guideline groups are reminded that measurement is expensive and that they should therefore choose those measures for which the literature searches have demonstrated a process-outcome link. In addition, the team is requested to identify process measures for aspects of care about which there is controversy regarding best practice.

In addition to identifying process measures, the team, in conjunction with the staff of resource management, develops a tracking mechanism that includes data collection tools and assignment of responsibility for collection of each piece of data. For example, data to be collected by the nursing staff, case managers, and from the hospital's information systems is identified. **Figure 19.7** is the data collection tool used by the unit manager and/or clinical nurse specialist for tracking process measures for the total knee replacement pathway. Note the emphasis on prophylactic antibiotic administration (and duration of therapy), and DVT prophylaxis. These are items that are difficult to collect from any hospital information system. They are also items with good evidence supporting the guideline and, therefore, would warrant an intervention with the attending physician to determine whether the recommendation is appropriate for the patient.

Figure 19.7: Total Knee Replacement Data Collection Sheet

		Guidelines											
	Guideline	95185-G	95184-G	95184-G		?	?						
	Grade of Evid	B	A	A	?	?	?						
		Guideline Criteria											
		1	Y	Seq or Both	N	1	1						
	Admit/OR Date	Doses Abx	Received DVT Prophlx.?	Type DVT Prophylax. Rec'vd	Had a DVT?	PO Day PT Start	PO Day Foley Out	Pathway Start Date	D/C Date	D/C Destination	LOS	Comments
1	5/16/95	6	Y	Seq		1	1	5/16/95	5/22/95	SNAC	6	SNAC bed
2	5/22/95	3	Y	Both		2	4	5/22/95	5/30/95	SNAC	8	diabetes
3	5/22/95	3	Y	Seq		1	2	5/22/95	5/25/95	SNAC	3	
4	5/22/95	6	Y	Seq		1	2	5/22/95	5/25/95	SNAC	3	
5	5/25/95	9	Y	Both		1	2	5/25/95	5/29/95	ECF	4	
6	5/25/95	3	Y	Both		1	2	5/25/95	5/29/95	SNAC	4	
7	5/26/95	9	Y	Seq		1	2	5/26/95	6/6/95	SNAC	11	hemostasis
8	5/31/95	6	Y	Seq		1	1	5/31/95	6/3/95	SNAC	3	
9	6/2/95	6	Y	Both		1	2	6/2/95	6/10/95	Home	8	hemostasis
10											0	not on pathway
11											0	
	Met Guideline	0%	100%	100%	0%	89%	22%				0.5	

8. **Develop a systematic approach to outcomes measurement and reporting.** In addition to collecting process information, the resource management project developed a comprehensive outcomes measurement and reporting system. The department worked with the Cedars-Sinai's Center for Applied Health Services Research to measure multiple economic and clinical outcomes. The center had extensive experience in outcomes measurement over an eight-year period of guideline development and implementation. Each pathway had general and specific outcomes measured by either resource management or the center. For about fifteen pathways, baseline outcomes information was collected prior to pathway implementation. Outcomes measured include the following:

- **Economic outcomes:**
  - Length of stay
  - Direct cost per patient
  - Post-hospital physician and emergency department visits (usually within thirty days).

- **Clinical Outcomes:**
  - Inpatient mortality
  - thirty day post-hospital discharge mortality
  - thirty day post-hospital complication rate
  - Readmissions within thirty days post discharge
  - Functional status: measured by SF-36.™ Items that are specific for the condition being studied are analyzed in depth. For example, pain and physical function are a focus of the hip and knee replacement pathways. Functional status is often measured before surgery and sequentially over the year post discharge.

- **Patient Satisfaction:** measured by the National Consulting Group (NCG) instrument.

Analysis of outcomes measures and reporting are coordinated between resource management and the Center for Applied Health Services Research. An example of a report format (using real and mock-up data) is shown in **Figure 19.8.**

9. **Implement guidelines and pathways.** Now the real work begins. Cedars-Sinai developed a formal approval and implementation process.

- **Approval Process.** An overview of the approval process, placed within the overall context of the resource management project is demonstrated in **Figure 19.9.**

Figure 19.8: An Example of Length of Stay

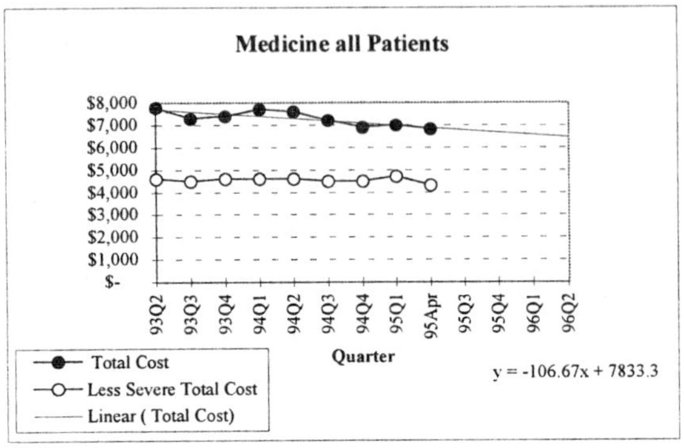

Analysis:

Most significant declines in estimated cost per care are in Nephrology, Pulmonary, GI and ID.

NOTE: All Cost are shown from Trendstar cost accounting system. This system assumes that incremental costs decline as utilization declines. Costs are usually not this flexible in the short run.
Normal newborns excluded.

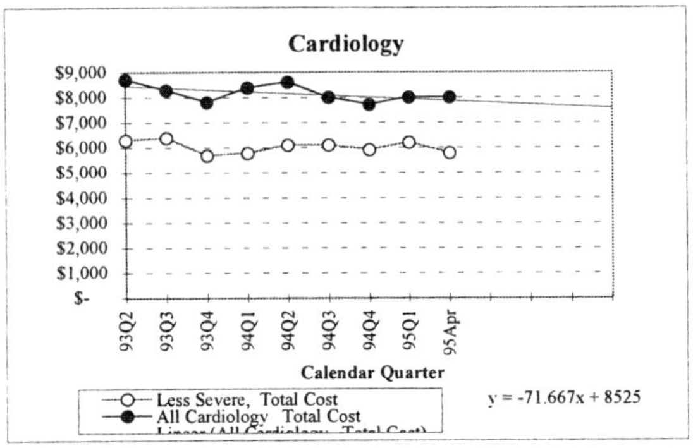

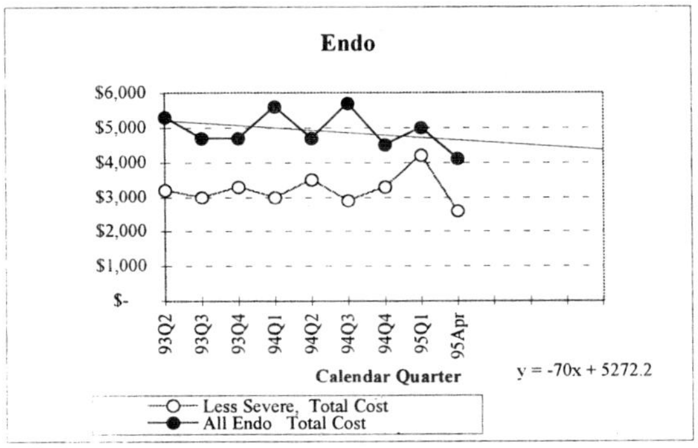

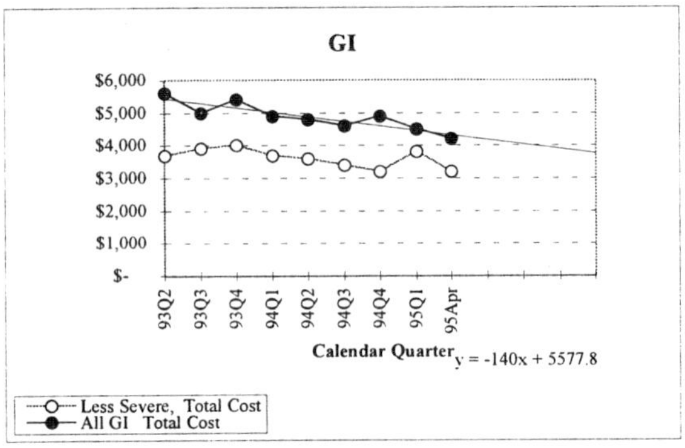

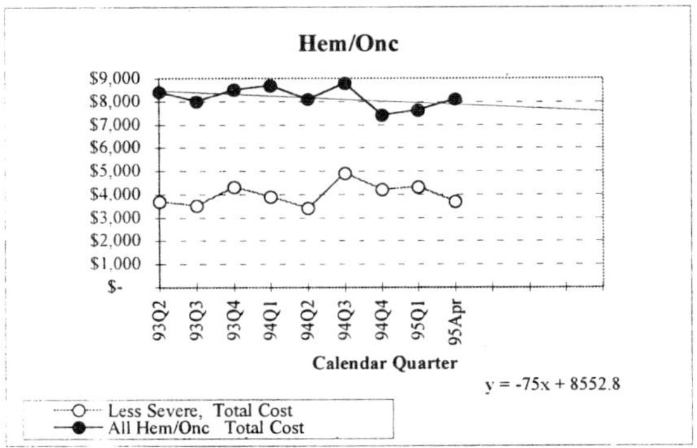

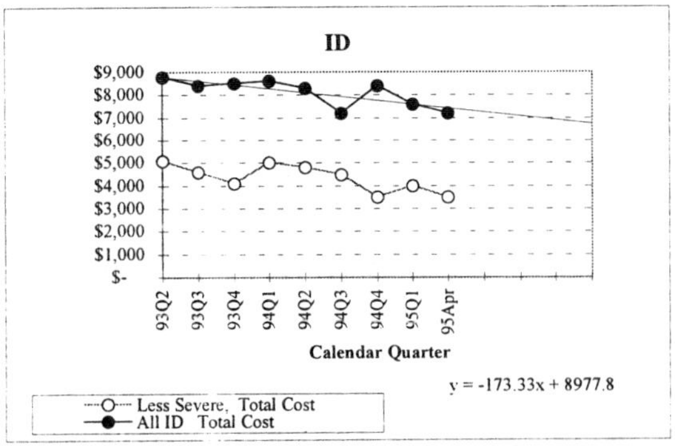

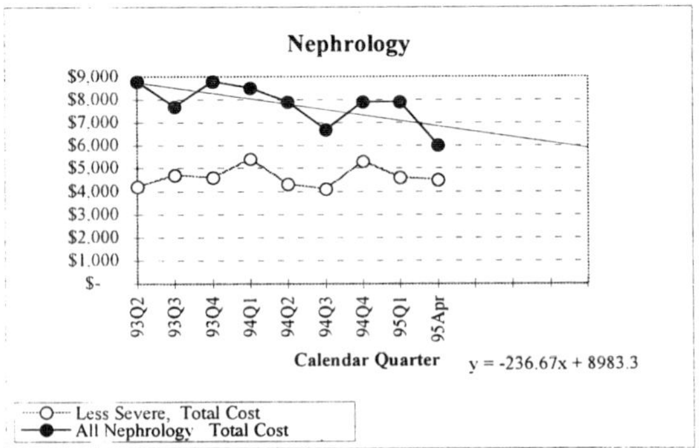

Figure 19.9: Cedars-Sinai Approved Process

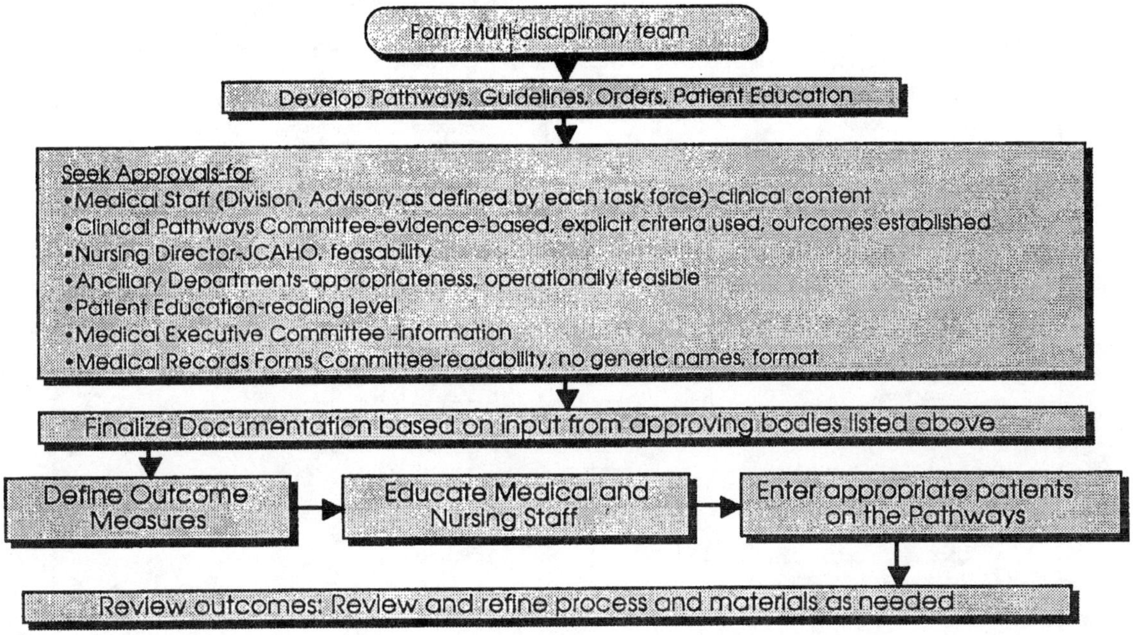

The reasons for the elaborate approval process include the desire to coordinate across departments, obtain broad buy-in, and educate as many of the caregivers as possible. Project staff felt sure that failure to obtain this buy-in would result in resistance later in the implementation process. In addition, support was obtained from various opinion leaders throughout the institution. A step-by-step guide (checklist) was developed to assist teams (see **Figure 19.10**).

Figure 19.10

STEP-BY-STEP GUIDE TO IMPLEMENTING GUIDELINES AND PATHWAYS
rev. 2/5/95

TASK	RESPONSIBILITY	SCHEDULED START DATE	SCHEDULED COMPLETION DATE	COMPLETED
Complete all documentation tools				
_pathway (include definition of population, outcomes)				
_guidelines				
_standing orders				
_patient education				
Obtain all necessary approvals				
_Clinical Pathways Committee				
_Patient Education Committee				
_Division				
_Nursing Director				
_Ancillary Departments				
Imaging				
Lab				
Pharmacy				
other_____				
other_____				
other_____				
Finalize documentation tools; submit to Terry Chamorro for formatting, printing and submission of standing orders to Forms Committee (allow 3-4 weeks)				
Bring Finalized Documentation back to Guideline Group for Review				
Education: (Policy &Procedures, Clinical Aspects of Guidelines and Pathway, Working with Case Managers)				
Identify groups to educate				
Develop training/education materials				
Conduct classes				
Measure				
Identify outcomes to measure				
Determine methodology for data capture				
Define mechanism for reviewing results.				
addressing issues to ensure appropriate change				

Implementation "Go-Live" Date (first use of a pathway):

AVAILABLE REFERENCE MATERIALS
Format/content requirements of the Medical Records/Forms Committee
Format/content requirements of the Patient Education Committee
Schedule of meetings: Forms Comittee, Patient Education Committee, Advisory Committees, Clinical Pathways Committee
Example of educational materials used for implementing Total Hip Replacement pathway and guidelines
Data which can be tracked by Resource Management
Samples of existing pathways and guidelines

- **Documentation.** The documentation tools included the following:

  * **An algorithm.** The asthma algorithm is included as **Figure 19.11.**
  * **A pathway:** One page of the asthma pathway is included as **Figure 19.12.**
  * **Guidelines:** One page of the asthma guidelines is included as **Figure 19.13.**
  * **Standing Orders:** The asthma pathway admission standing orders are included as **Figure 19.14.**
  * **Patient Education:** A version of the pathway is written specifically for the patient and family members. It uses understandable language, explains what happens on each day (or phase) of the hospital stay, and re-emphasizes outcomes and expectations, encouraging the patient to be an active participant in his/her care.

Figure 19.11

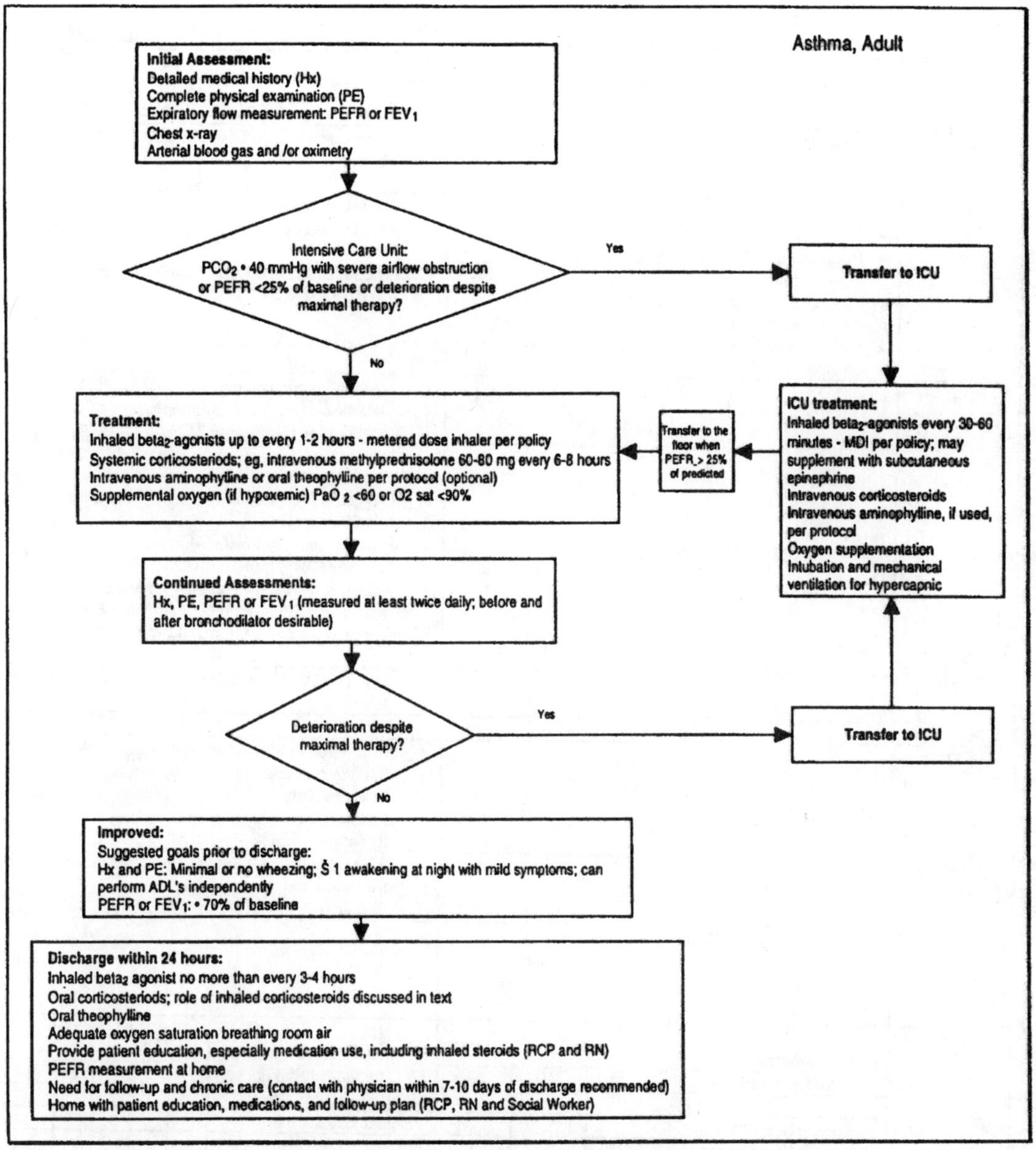

Asthma, Adult
Initial Assessment:
Detailed medical history (Hx)
Complete physical examination (PE)
Expiratory flow measurement: PEFR or FEV1
Chest x-ray
Arterial blood gas and /or oximetry
Intensive Care Unit:
PCO2 • 40 mmHg with severe airflow obstruction or PEFR <25% of baseline or deterioration despite maximal therapy?
Yes
Transfer to ICU
No
Treatment:
Inhaled beta2-agonists up to every 1-2 hours - metered dose inhaler per policy
Systemic corticosteriods; eg, intravenous methylprednisolone 60-80 mg every 6-8 hours
Intravenous aminophylline or oral theophylline per protocol (optional)
Supplemental oxygen (if hypoxemic) PaO 2 <60 or O2 sat <90%
Transfer to the floor when PEFR > 25% of predicted
ICU treatment:
Inhaled beta2-agonists every 30-60 minutes - MDI per policy; may supplement with subcutaneous epinephrine
Intravenous corticosteroids
Intravenous aminophylline, if used, per protocol
Oxygen supplementation
Intubation and mechanical ventilation for hypercapnic
Continued Assessments:
Hx, PE, PEFR or FEV1 (measured at least twice daily; before and after bronchodilator desirable)
Deterioration despite maximal therapy?
Yes
Transfer to ICU
No
Improved:
Suggested goals prior to discharge:
Hx and PE: Minimal or no wheezing; Š 1 awakening at night with mild symptoms; can perform ADL's independently
PEFR or FEV1: • 70% of baseline
Discharge within 24 hours:
Inhaled beta2 agonist no more than every 3-4 hours
Oral corticosteriods; role of inhaled corticosteroids discussed in text
Oral theophylline
Adequate oxygen saturation breathing room air
Provide patient education, especially medication use, including inhaled steroids (RCP and RN)
PEFR measurement at home
Need for follow-up and chronic care (contact with physician within 7-10 days of discharge recommended)
Home with patient education, medications, and follow-up plan (RCP, RN and Social Worker)

Figure 19.12

	PRE-ADMISSION. DATE ___/___/___	22 ACUTE PHASE DATE ___/___/___
LEVEL	• Emergency Department **(GUIDELINE 2)**	• General Care Area **(GUIDELINES 3 & 4)**
DIAGNOSTIC TESTS/ PROCEDURE	• Detailed Medical History • Complete Physical Exam • PEFR or FEV_1 2 times daily, before and after bronchodilators • Arterial Blood Gas (ABG) and/or Oximetry **(GUIDELINE 2)** • Peak Expiratory Flow Rate (PEFR), or Forced Expiratory Volume (FEV_1)	• Complete Physical Exam • PEFR or FEV_1 2 times daily, before and after bronchodilators • Arterial Blood Gas (ABG) and/or Oximetry **(GUIDELINE 2)**
MEDICATIONS		• Systemic corticosteroids **(GUIDELINE 1)** • Optional: Intravenous aminophylline or theophylline **(Guideline 7)**
TREATMENTS		• Inhaled beta agonists up to every 1-2 hours-MDI **(GUIDELINE 5)** • Oxygen if P_aO_2 <60mm Hg or O_2 Sat <90% **(GUIDELINE 6)** • Provide calm, quite environment • Elevate HOB 40" to facilitate respiratory effort • Assess & document Patient's respiratory status upon admission, throughout shift & PRN • Assess signs & symptoms of bronchodilator toxicity
ACTIVITY		
NUTRITION		• Maintain IV fluids until adequate oral hydration is achieved
ELIMINATION		
EDUCATION		• Instruction in use of Metered Dose Inhaler (MDI) • Explain procedures to family, document level of understanding • Instruct on coughing, deep breathing & relaxation techniques
DISCHARGE PLANNING		• Asses & document D/C planning needs, instructions for follow-up • Initiate referrals as appropriate
OUTCOMES	• Detailed Medical History completed • PEFR or FEV_1 less than/equal 40% baseline • Persistence in marked or diffuse wheezes or shortness of breath	

PROGRESS

See Progress Notes for Patient Status	DATE	
	7AM	7PM
Progress to Next Phase		
Referred to Case Manager		

See Progress Notes for Patient Status	DATE					
	7a	7p	7a	7p	7a	7p
Maintains Pathway Criteria						
Progress to Next Phase						
Referred to Case Manager						

	Signature / Title	Signature / Title

Figure 19.13.

G 0 **PATIENT POPULATION FOR PATHWAY FOR ACUTE EXACERBATION OF ASTHMA IN ADULTS**

95164-G Best Grade of Evidence: C
Population: Adult patients admitted with a primary diagnosis of bronchial asthma.

Purpose: To standardize the approach to adult asthma in order to treat asthma patients in the most efficient, appropriate, and effective way.

Criteria & Recommendations:
Patient is/has:
1. Admitted to CSMC with primary diagnosis of bronchial asthma with an acute exacerbation.
2. 18 years of age or older.
3. History of reversible bronchospasm.
4. Acute exacerbation is defined as episode or progressively worsening shortness of breath, cough, wheezing, or chest tightness or some combination of these symptoms. Respiratory distress is common. Episode is characterized by decreases in expiratory airflow that can be documented and quantified by measurement of lung function (PEFR or spirometry).
5. Has one or more of the following:
   (a) FEV1 or PEFR <40% baseline (predicted or personal best, as determined by the Respiratory Therapist)
   (b) PaO2 <60 mmHg or 02 saturation <90%
   (c) PCO2 > 40 mmHg
   (d) Use of accessory muscles of respiration
6. Exclude if has infiltrate on CXR; exclude the following unstable comorbidities:
   (a) Myocardial infarction (Hx)
   (b) Congestive Heart Failure
   (c) Coronary artery disease (Hx)
   (d) COPD (Hx)
   (e) Sepsis
   (f) Immunosuppression

Date of Clinical Pathways Comm. Review:

G 1 **CORTICOSTEROID THERAPY FOR ASTHMA IN ADULT PATIENTS IN THE EMERGENCY DEPARTMENT (ED)**

94107-G Best Grade of Evidence: A
Population: Adult (<18 years of age) patients admitted to the ED with a primary diagnosis of acute exacerbation of asthma.

Purpose: To standardize the approach to corticosteroid therapy in adult asthma in the ED.

Criteria & Recommendations:

1. Intravenous methylprednisolone 60-80 mg every 6-8 hours.

2. Convert to oral corticosteriods: when minimal or no wheezing: <1 awakening per night with mild symptoms PEFR or FEV1 >=70% of baseline

Date of Clinical Pathways Comm. Review: 11/18/94

G 2 **ARTERIAL BLOOD GASES (ABGS) FOR ASTHMA IN ADULT PATIENTS IN THE EMERGENCY DEPARTMENT (ED)**

94109-G Best Grade of Evidence: B
Population: Adult patients admitted to the ED with a primary diagnosis of acute exacerbation of asthma.

Purpose: To standardize the approach to obtaining Arterial Blood Gases (ABGs),to diminish potential morbidity from ABGs not indicated.

Criteria & Recommendations:

Arterial Blood Gases (ABGs) may be considered in patients not clinically improving to aggressive therapy who have the following: a PEFR <200 L/min or b. PEFR <25% - 40% predicted.

PEFR % baseline refers to the norm for the individual, established by the clinician. This may be % of standardized norms of % patients personal best.

Date of Clinical Pathways Comm. Review: 11/18/94

Figure 19.14

1. [ ] Activate Acute Exacerbation of Asthma
2. Vital signs Q_____________
3. Diet: a. [ ] Regular [ ] Other_____________
   b. Encourage PO fluids
4. Elevate HOB
5. Chest x-ray _____________
6. [ ] Arterial blood gases _____________ [ ] Oximetry _____________
7. Supplemental oxygen to keep oxygen saturation > 90%: [ ] by mask [ ] NC
8. Before and after bronchodilator peak expiratory flow measurements (PEFR) 2X daily
9. [ ] Methylprednisolone IV push: [ ] 60 mg [ ] 80 mg [ ] Q 6 hr [ ] Q 8 hr
   [ ] Prednisone _______ mg PO Q _____ hours
10. HHN: Albuterol Sulfate (convert to MDI per policy) [ ] 1.25 mg [ ] 2.5 mg
    [ ] Q 1 hr [ ] Q 2 hr [ ] Q 3 hr [ ] Q 4 hr [ ] Q 6 hr
11. MDI: $Beta_2$ Agonist:_____________ # of puffs: _______
    [ ] Q 1 hr [ ] Q 2 hr [ ] Q 3 hr [ ] Q 4 hr [ ] Q 6 hr Instruct patient in proper use of MDI spacer
12. MDI: Inhaled steroids: _____________ # of puffs: _______
    [ ] Q 6 hr [ ] Q 8 hr [ ] BID Instruct patient in proper use of MDI spacer
13. Social Service and discharge evaluation
14. Activity: Progressive ambulation as tolerated
15. Additional orders:
    ____
    ____

● **Implementation Plan.** In addition to the required approvals and documentation, specific educational plans including target groups and teaching materials are developed before actual implementation of the pathway. The process and outcome measurement and analysis systems must also be in place before taking the pathway "live." Finally, the actual implementation plan, including feedback mechanisms, must be ready. For this portion of implementation, the resource management project drew heavily on the previous experience of the Center for applied Health Services Research and articles about changing physician behavior by John Eisenberg and coworkers.[4,5] Options considered for implementation included the following:

* **Education.** Although traditional continuing medical education (CME) has not shown consistent effects, particularly when health outcomes have been measured, the

project used lectures and small group sessions to introduce general concepts and give overviews of specific guidelines and pathways. [6] Traditional CME was considered necessary to achieve buy-in, but not sufficient to change physician behavior.

* **Academic detailing.** Personalized one-on-one sessions, often using pharmacists, have been shown to be effective. [7,8] Although the project did not use this specific intervention, whenever possible small group interactive sessions were conducted to discuss the potential advantages and disadvantages of a particular guideline or pathway. The clinical nurse specialists and unit managers had many one-on-one conversations with physicians about the concepts and use of pathways and guidelines.

* **Opinion Leaders.** Evidence does exist that the early involvement of respected peers is effective in changing physician practice patterns.[9] The project sought to have these individuals lead or at least participate in all guideline and pathway teams to assure that the end product would be acceptable to these critical individuals.

* **Feedback.** Based upon previous experience and the literature, a method of concurrent feedback by nurses, case managers, and physicians (when necessary) was selected to assure prompt compliance with guideline recommendations or delineate the reasons for lack of compliance and attempt to facilitate the care process. [10, 11] Although retrospective feedback may be an option for certain guidelines (such as preventive services), the need for a timely reaction to recommendations for inpatient pathways influenced the selection of concurrent mechanisms.

* **Provide Incentives.** No incentives for pathway compliance were provided to physicians. However, as payers begin to drop physicians with seemingly high cost practice patterns from provider panels and capitated care becomes more prevalent, the "external" incentives will be quite powerful.

* **Remove Disincentives.** The providers of care are always searching for ways in which efficient care can be expedited. For example, if a patient appropriately needs a treadmill for evaluation of a patient with chest pain before discharge, a nurse or case manager will assist in scheduling the test or obtaining timely results.

* **Administrative Rules.** This type of intervention was specifically avoided. Previous guideline implementation has shown concurrent feedback combined with educational programs to be effective in obtaining a compliance rate of about 70%.[10] Further improvements were not likely to be attained by rules or sanctions, but by further improving feedback systems and efficiency.

* **Sanctions.** Like administrative rules, sanctions such as reporting physicians to peer review committees were also avoided. Nevertheless, the medical staff has agreed that if an individual is consistently noncompliant with guidelines and pathways (without clinical reasons) they are willing to make it a peer- review issue.

* **Medical/Legal.** Again, these extreme types of measures have not been necessary.

* **Combinations of Strategies to Change Behavior.** For all pathways and guidelines the project elected to use a combination of strategies for implementation. Evidence from the literature would suggest that such an approach is most likely to be successful in implementation.[5] For almost all pathways these strategies include education, use of opinion leaders early in the development process, concurrent feedback, and removal of disincentives.

It is obvious that Cedars-Sinai has focused significant resources on implementation, including approval processes that involve stakeholders, extensive documentation support, in-depth education of providers, and the use of multiple methods shown to change physician behavior. Many of the guidelines are currently supported by laptop computer tracking systems and explicit risk-stratification programs for length of stay guidelines. In the near future, all guidelines and pathways will be placed on a Local Area Network (LAN) and on a local web server so that all providers will have easier access to the documentation and tracking tools and the evidence behind the guidelines. Since a fundamental principle of implementation is to make things easier for all caregivers and particularly patients, computerization should have a significant impact.

10. **Measure and report process variation and clinical and economic outcomes.** Steps 7 and 8 outlined in some detail the process and outcome measures to be collected and analyzed. Chapter 18 also discusses the subtleties of these measurements. This chapter will simply highlight a few important concepts and questions.

- The interpretation of compliance with guideline recommendations must include consideration of clinical subtleties, accuracy of the feedback message (Was the patient really low risk and therefore ready for discharge?), and hospital efficiency (Was the service delivered promptly as ordered by the physician?).[4]
- Was the data collection complete? Were all patients on the pathway studied? How many patients were actually on the pathway? Are there significant missing data points?
- For outcomes the analysis should include the percentage of patients lost to follow-up and low response rates must raise flags about the validity of the data.
- Both process variation and outcomes must be reported using rigorous statistical analysis. Was the change in practice associated with the guideline or pathway clinically and statistically improved?
- If the process and outcome measures have been rigorously collected and scientifically analyzed, the resulting reports must be usable by the pathway team in its efforts to further improve performance. It is reasonable to have the pathway team work with the analysts to assure usable information.

11. **Use process and outcomes measures with updated literature searches and appraisals to continually improve the care of the target population.** This step essentially closes the loop and begins the process again. All three elements (process variation, outcomes, and updated literature reviews) are necessary for optimal practice. Without accurate process information (e.g., the percentage of patients undergoing total hip replacement who received effective DVT prophylaxis), the pathway team cannot interpret outcomes and will not know which processes of care can be improved. Without outcomes information, including patient satisfaction, the team is again unable to evaluate its processes of care. Finally, since medicine is a rapidly changing field, a guideline or pathway which is not continually updated with the most recent scientific literature is no longer state-of-the-art. Since more sophisticated outcomes studies with excellent designs are appearing, failure to update clinical recommendations is difficult to justify.
These literature updates should use the same rigorous methods discussed in the

Chapter 18. There are multiple ways to continually update the scientific underpinnings of guidelines and pathways. One method is to retain and reuse the literature search strategies which yielded high quality articles for the original guideline development. Another is to have team members routinely review journals which are relevant to the pathway condition. Finally, team members should be encouraged to read high quality journal summary newsletters. Within internal medicine these include *Journal Watch* published by the *New England Journal of Medicine* and *ACP Journal Club* published by The American College of Physicians. Team members should be encouraged to bring forward any high quality articles for consideration by the pathway team. Cedars-Sinai's guidelines automatically expire on the anniversary of their initial approval by the clinical pathways committee. Authors will be notified three months in advance to allow time for review of process and outcome measures, updated literature searches, and medical staff approvals.

Analytic and Administrative Support

The resource management project mobilized significant resources within the Cedars-Sinai Health System: These include the following:

- **Lead Analysts.** Six lead analysts act as process managers for the six task forces. These individuals help task force leaders plan effective meetings, insure appropriate departmental involvement, coordinate the work of guideline group analysts, and attend the project team meetings to update management on task force progress and issues. Typically these analysts have previous experience in the patient-focused care project or in resource management.
- **Guideline Group Analysts.** The guideline group analysts provide support for clinical process redesign up front or as process managers behind the scenes for the guideline groups launched by each of the six task forces. They are data analysts who have been educated to use Trendstar ®, the medical center's principal database, and are able to locate and structure the data required for each group to move forward.
- **Department Analysts.** Department analysts are staff members from ancillary departments whose focus is identifying and quantifying cost reduction opportunities within their respective departments.
- **Special Support Analysts.** In addition to the analysts described above, two or three other analysts perform special behind-the-scenes work such as:
  - Assistance for team members with difficult analyses
  - Hard to get computer analyses
  - Observational Studies
  - Chart Reviews
  - Linking Data Sets
  - Coordinating and tracking project activity for task forces, guideline groups, and departments
- **Quality Management (QM) Coordinators.** The QM coordinators are the main link to the medical staff formal approval process for issues involving changes in physician practice or for issues that require tracking and oversight by a medical staff committee. They coordinate the writing and approval of clinical guidelines for

guideline groups and task forces, provide early assistance in getting guidelines to meet the standards of the Clinical Guidelines and Pathways Committee, ensure that the several dimensions of quality are addressed, and that work is not duplicated within the medical staff committee system.

- **Medical Librarian.** A half-time medical librarian and several other hospital librarians dedicate their time to sit with guideline group members to guide literature searches. Having a librarian available saves considerable time in reviewing abstracts and ensures that literature searches do not omit important relevant information.

- Departmental co-chairs and members of guideline and pathway committees developed and implemented guidelines and pathways.

Project Status

By July 1995, approximately one year following the inception of the project, the following has occured:

- Over 10,000 pages of articles have been photocopied and reviewed, with most articles formally appraised by team members
- Over 200 guidelines have been drafted based on this research.
- Over 150 guidelines have been approved by the Clinical Pathways Committee, with approximately eighty of these reviewed and approved by the medical staff.
- Over forty-five pathways have been built around these guidelines and details filled in.
- Over twenty-three pathways have been approved by the Clinical Pathways Committee and the medical staff.
- Thirteen pathways and guidelines have been implemented, with process and outcome measures being collected. An additional twenty will be implemented by Fall 1995.

Summary

The goal of the resource management project is to improve clinical appropriateness and effectiveness. This approach complements hospital efficiency efforts such as patient-focused care. Although changing the clinical practice of a large academic medical center is difficult and complex, by setting appropriate goals, providing clear project definition, developing an organizational structure, and supplying process and analytic support significant progress has been made in one year.

Although the Cedars-Sinai Health System has had significant success with guidelines developed and implemented through the Center for Applied Health Services Research, the resource management project does not yet have economic and clinical outcomes information to judge the success or failure of the program. Since most of the principles learned in the health services research projects have been directly applied to resource management, the project team is cautiously optimistic. The use of a formal evidence-based medicine approach, multidisciplinary teams, vigorous implementation strategies, and sophisticated systems of process and outcomes measurement should provide the necessary foundation for success. The resource management team remains optimistic and awaits the evidence.

References

1. Field MJ , KN Lohr eds. Clinical Practice Guidelines: Directions for New Program (Summary), Washington, DC, National Academy Press: 1990.

2. Field MJ , KN Lohr eds. Clinical Practice Guidelines: Directions for New Program (Summary) Washington, DC National Academy Press: 1990.

3. ISIS-4 (Fourth International Study of Infarct Survival) Collaborative Group. "ISIS-4: A Randomized Factorial Trial Assessing Early Oral Captopril, Oral Monoitrate, and Intravenous Magnesium Sulphate In 58 050 Patients With Suspected Acute Myocarial Infarction. *Lancet* 345 1995: 669-85.

4. Ellrodt AG, et al. "Measuring and Improving Physician Compliance with Clinical Practice Guidelines: A Controlled Interventional Trial. *Annals of Internal Medicine* 122(4) 1995: 277-282.

5. Greco PJ, JM Eisenberg. "Changing Physicians' Practices." *New England Journal of Medicine* 329(17) 1993: 1271-1274.

6. Davis DA, et al. "Evidence for the Effectiveness of CME: a review of 50 Randomized Controlled Trials." *Journal of the American Medical Association* 268 1992: 111-7.

7. Soumeria SB, J Avorn. "Principles of Educational Outreach ('Academic Detailing') to Improve Clinical Decision Making." *Journal of the American Medical Association* 263 1990:549-56.

8. Schaffner W, et al. "Improving Antibiotic Prescribing in Office Practice: A Controlled Trial of Three Educational Methods." *Journal of the American Medical Association* 250 1983: 1728-32.

9. Lomas J, et al. "Opinion Leaders vs. Audit and Feedback to Implement Practice Guidelines: Delivery After Previous Cesarean Section." *Journal of the American Medical Association* 265 1991:2202-7.

10. Weingarten, SR, et al. "Practice Guidelines and Reminders to Reduce Duration of Hospital Stay for Patients with Chest Pain: An Interventional Trial." *Annals of Internal Medicine* 120 1994: 257-263.

11. Tierney WM, SL Hui, CJ McDonald. "Delayed Feedback of Physicians Performance Versus Immediate Reminders To Perform Preventive Care: Effects On Physician Complaince." *Medical Care* 24 1986: 659-66.

Chapter 20

The Quality of Well-Being Scale: Overview and Applications

Robert M. Kaplan, PhD
Peter N. Rosen, MD

The Quality of Well-Being Scale (QWB) is a general, utility based measure of health related quality of life that was designed for a variety of purposes. This paper reviews the QWB and the General Health Policy Model (GHPM) from which the measurement strategy was derived. After reviewing the validity of the QWB, the chapter considers the need for valid and reliable general measures of health outcomes for a variety of different purposes.

A General Health Policy Model

The QWB is derived from a comprehensive theoretical model of health status that includes several components. The major aspects of the model are mortality (death) and morbidity (health-related quality of life). In several papers, it has been suggested that diseases and disabilities are important for two reasons. First, illness may cause the life expectancy to be shortened. Second, illness may make life less desirable at times prior to death (health-related quality of life). [1-3] A comprehensive model of health status combines morbidity and mortality into a common index.

Over the last two decades, a group of investigators at the University of California-San Diego has developed the General Health Policy Model (GHPM). Central to the GHPM is a general conceptualization of quality of life. The model separates aspects of health status and life quality into distinct components. These are life expectancy (mortality), functioning and symptoms (morbidity), preference for observed functional states (utility), and duration of stay in health states (prognosis).

ROBERT M. KAPLAN, PHD—Department of Family and Preventive Medicine, Division of Health Care Sciences, University of California, San Diego, CA.

PETER N. ROSEN, MD—Department of Ophthalmology, Southern California Permanente Medical Group, San Diego, CA; Department of Family and Preventitive Medicine, Division of Health Care Sciences, University of California, San Diego.

Supported, in part, by Grant PO 1-AR-40423 from the National Institute of Arthritis, Musculoskeletal, and Skin Disorders of the National Institutes of Health

Portions of this paper were presented at the Eighth Conference of European Health Psychology Society, Alicante, Spain, July 13-15, 1994

Mortality. A model of health outcomes necessarily includes a component for mortality. Indeed, many public health statistics focus exclusively on mortality through estimations of crude mortality rates, age-adjusted mortality rates, and infant mortality rates. Death is an important outcome that must be included in any comprehensive conceptualization of health.

Morbidity. In addition to death, quality of life is also an important outcome. The GHPM considers functioning in three areas—mobility, physical activity, and social activity. Descriptions of the measures of these aspects of function are given in many different publications. [1-4] Most public health indicators are relatively insensitive to variations toward the "well" end of the continuum. To give an extreme example, measures of infant mortality provide no information on the quality of life of individuals capable of reading this chapter since the they have lived one year following their births (assuming that no infants are reading this chapter).

Disability measures often ignore those in relatively well states. For example, the RAND Health Insurance Study reported that about 80% of the general populations have no dysfunction. Thus, they would estimate that 80% of the population is well. Our method asks about symptoms or problems in addition to behavioral dysfunction. In these studies, only about 12% of the general population report no symptoms on a particular day.[5] In other words, symptoms or problems are a very common aspect of the human experience. Although unobservable, symptoms are highly correlated with the demand for medical services, expenditures on health care, and motivations to alter lifestyles.

Utility (Relative Importance). Components of morbidity and mortality may not be of equal importance. For example, it is possible to develop measures that detect very minor symptoms. Yet, because these symptoms are measurable, it does not necessarily mean they are important. A patient may experience side effects of a medication but be willing to tolerate them because the side effects are less important than the probable benefit that would be obtained if the medication is consumed. A treatment in which 30 of 100 patients die is not equivalent to one in which 30 of 100 patients develop headaches. The General Health Policy Model attempts to scale the various health outcomes according to their relative importance. This exercise adds the dimensions of quality to health status. In the preceding example, the relative importance of dying would be weighted more than developing headache. The weighting is accomplished by rating all states on a quality continuum ranging from 0 (for dead) to 1.0 (for optimum functioning). These ratings are typically provided by independent judges who are representative of the general population. Using this system it is possible to express the relative importance of states in relation to the life-death continuum. A point halfway on the scale (0.5) is regarded as halfway between optimum function and death. The quality of life weighting system has been described in several different publications.[4-6]

Prognosis. Another dimension of health status is the duration of a condition. A headache that lasts one hour is not equivalent to a headache that lasts one month. Pain that lasts three days is not equivalent to pain that lasts three years. This concept is basic, yet most contemporary models of health outcome measurement completely disregard the duration component. In the GHPM, the term prognosis refers to the probability of transition among health states over the course of time. In addition to consideration of duration of problems, the model considers the point at which the problem begins. A person may have no symptoms or dysfunctions currently but may have a high probability of health problems in the future. The prognosis component of the model takes these transitions into consideration and applies a discount rate for events that occur in the future. Discount rates are used to value resources, and health outcomes differently if the onset is delayed as opposed to immediate. A headache that will begin a year from now may be less of a concern than a headache that will start immediately.

Quality of Well-Being Scale (QWB)

The Quality of Well-Being scale is one of several different approaches for obtaining quality-adjusted life years. [3, 8-9] Using this method patients are classified according to objective levels of functioning. These levels are represented by scales of mobility, physical activity, and social activity. These scales are shown in **Table 20.1**. In addition to classification into these observable levels of function, individuals are also classified by the symptom or problem that bothered them most (see **Table 20.2**). On any particular day, nearly 80% of the general population is optimally functional; however, fewer than half of the population experience no symptoms. Symptoms or problems may be severe such as serious chest pain or minor such as taking medication or a prescribed diet for health reasons. Human value studies have been conducted to place the observable states of health and functioning onto a preference continuum for the desirability of various conditions, giving a "quality" rating between 0 for death and 1.0 for completely well. A quality adjusted life year is defined as the equivalent of a completely well year of life, or a year of life free of any symptoms, problems, or health-related disabilities. The well-life expectancy is the current life expectancy adjusted for diminished quality of life associated with dysfunctional states and the durations of stay in each state. It is possible to consider mortality, morbidity, and the preference weights for the various observable states of function. The model quantifies the health activity or treatment program in terms of the quality adjusted life years that it produces or saves.

A mathematical model integrates components of the model to express outcomes in a common measurement unit. Using information on current functioning and duration, it is possible to express the health outcomes in terms of Quality-Adjusted Life Years (QALYs).

Table 20.1: Quality of Well-Being/General Health Policy Model: Elements and Calculating Formulas (Function Scales, with Step Definitions and Calculating Weights)

Step No.	*Step Definition*	*Weight*
	Mobility Scale (MOB)	
5	No limitations for health reasons	-.000
4	Did not drive a car, health related; did not ride in a car as usual for age (younger than 15 yr), health related, *and/or* did not use public transportation, health related; *or* had or would have used more help than usual for age to use public transportation, health related	-.062
2	In hospital, health related	-.090
	Physical Activity Scale (PAC)	
4	No limitations for health reasons	-.000
3	In wheelchair, moved or controlled movement of wheelchair without help from someone else; *or* had trouble or did not try to lift, stoop, bend over, or use stairs or inclines, health related; *and/or* limped, used a cane, crutches, or walker, health related; *and/or* had any other physical limitation in walking, or did not try to walk as far as or as fast as other the same age are able, health related	-.060
1	In wheelchair, did not move or control the movement of wheelchair without help from someone else, *or* in bed, chair, or couch for most or all of the day, health related	-.077
	Social Activity Scale (SAC)	
5	No limitations for health reasons	-.000
4	Limited in other (e.g., recreational) role activity, health related	-.061
3	Limited in major (primary) role activity, health related	-.061
2	Performed no major role activity, health related, but did perform self-care activities	-.061
1	Performed no major role activity, health related, *and* did not perform or had more help than usual in performance of one or more self-care activities, health related	-.106

Calculating Formulas

Formula 1. Point-in-time well-being score for an individual (W):

$$W = 1 + (CPXwt) + (MOBwt) + (PACwt) + (SACwt)$$

where "wt" is the preference-weighted measure for each factor and CPX is Symptom/Problem complex. For example, the W score for a person with the following description profile may be calculated for one day as:

CPX-11	Cough, wheezing or shortness of breath, with or without fever, chills, or aching all over	-.257
MOB-5	No limitations	-.000
PAC-1	In bed, chair, or couch for most or all of the day, health related	-.077
SAC-2	Performed no major role activity, health related, but did perform self-care	-.061

$$W = 1 + (-.257) + (-.000) + (-.077) + (-.061) = .605$$

Formula 2. Well-years (WY) as an output measure:

$$WY = [\text{No. of persons} \times (CPXwt + MOBwt + PACwt + SACwt) \times \text{Time}]$$

Table 20.2: Quality of Well-Being/General Health Policy Model: Symptom/Problem Complexes (CPX) with Calculating Weights

CPX No.	CPX Description	Weights
1	Death (not on respondent's card)	-.727
2	Loss of consciousness such as seizure (fits), fainting, or coma (out cold or knocked out)	-.407
3	Burn over large areas of face, body, arms, or legs	-.387
4	Pain, bleeding, itching, or discharge (drainage) from sexual organs--does not include normal menstrual (monthly) bleeding	-.349
5	Trouble learning, remembering, or thinking clearly	-.340
6	Any combination of one or more hands, feet, arms, or legs either missing, deformed (crooked), paralyzed (unable to move), or broken--includes wearing artificial limbs or braces	-.333
7	Pain, stiffness, weakness, numbness, or other discomfort in chest, stomach (including hernia or rupture), side, neck, back, hips, or any joints or hands, feet, arms, or legs	-.299
8	Pain, burning, bleeding, itching, or other difficulty with rectum, bowel movements, or urination (passing water)	-.292
9	Sick or upset stomach, vomiting or loose bowel movement, with or without chills, or aching all over	-.290
10	General tiredness, weakness, or weight loss	-.259
11	Cough, wheezing, or shortness of breath, *with* or *without* fever, chills, or aching all over	-.257
12	Spells of feeling, upset, being depressed, or of crying	-.257
13	Headache, or dizziness, or ringing in ears, or spells of feeling hot, nervous or shaky	-.244
14	Burning or itching rash on large areas of face, body, arms, or legs	-.240
15	Trouble talking, such as lisp, stuttering, hoarseness, or being unable to speak	-.237
16	Pain or discomfort in one or both eyes (such as burning or itching) or any trouble seeing after correction	-.230
17	Overweight for age and height or skin defect of face, body, arms, or legs, such as scars, pimples, warts, bruises or changes in color	-.188
18	Pain in ear, tooth, jaw throat, lips, tongue; several missing or crooked permanent teeth--includes wearing bridges or false teeth; stuffy, runny nose; or any trouble hearing--includes wearing a hearing aid	-.170
19	Taking medication or staying on a prescribed diet for health reasons	-.144
20	Wore eyeglasses or contact lenses	-.101
21	Breathing smog or unpleasant air	-.101
22	No symptoms or problem (not on respondent's card)	-.000
23	Standard symptom/problem	-.257
X24	Trouble Sleeping	-.257
X25	Intoxication	-.257
X26	Problems with sexual interest or performance	-.257
X27	Excessive worry or anxiety	-.257

Note: For symptoms marked by x (numbers 24-27) no weight is available at this time. Instead, a standardized weight is used.

The model for point in time Quality of Well-Being is:

QWB = 1 - (observed morbidity x morbidity weight)
- (observed physical activity x physical activity weight)
- (observed social activity and social activity weight)
- (observed symptom/problem x symptom/problem weight)

The net cost/utility ratio is defined as

$$\frac{\text{net cost}}{\text{net QWB x duration in years}} = \frac{\text{cost of treatment-cost of alternative}}{[QWB_2 - QWB_1] \text{ x duration in years}}$$

Where QWB_2 and QWB_1 are measures of quality of well being taken after and before treatment.

Consider, for example, a person who is in an objective state of functioning that is rated by community peers as 0.5 on a 0 to 1.0 scale. If the person remains in that state for one year, he or she would have lost the equivalent of one-half of one year of life. Thus, a person limited in activities who requires a cane or walker to get around the community would be hypothetically rated at 0.50. If he or she remained in that state more than one year, he or she would lose the equivalent of one-half year of life; however, a person who has the flu may also be rated as 0.50. In this case, the illness might only last three days and the total loss in well-years might be 3/365 X 0.50 which is equal to 0.004 well-years. This may not appear as significant an outcome as the disabled person. But suppose that 5,000 people in a community get the flu. The well years lost would then be 5,000 x 0.004 which is equal to 20 years. Now suppose that a vaccination has become available and that the threat of the flu can be eliminated by vaccinating the 25,000 people in the community. The cost of the vaccine is \$5.00 per person or \$125,000. The cost/utility of the program would be

$$\frac{\$125{,}000 \text{ (cost)}}{20 \text{ years (utility)}} = \$6{,}250/\text{QALY}$$

Validity of QWB

The QWB has now been used in a wide variety of different studies. The validity evidence will be reviewed briefly and the reader is referred to the specific papers. The QWB has been used in both population and clinical studies. **Figure 20.1** summarizes QWB scores, estimated from the U.S. National Health Interview Survey, in relation to three problems, sinusitis, diabetes, and chronic lung disease. In each of three age groups, sinus disease is shown to be a less serious problem than diabetes which, in turn, has less impact than emphysema. [10] **Figure 20.2** shows how the method might be used to estimate the impact of an illness such as cystic fibrosis. According to this analysis, cystic fibrosis causes the loss of about fifty-two QALYs each year. The total area under the curve shows total QALYs for the U.S. population. The area under the second curve shows life expectancy for people with cystic fibrosis. The third curve shows the Quality-Adjusted Life

Figure 20.1

Sinus Disease, Diabetes, and Emphysema in the General Population

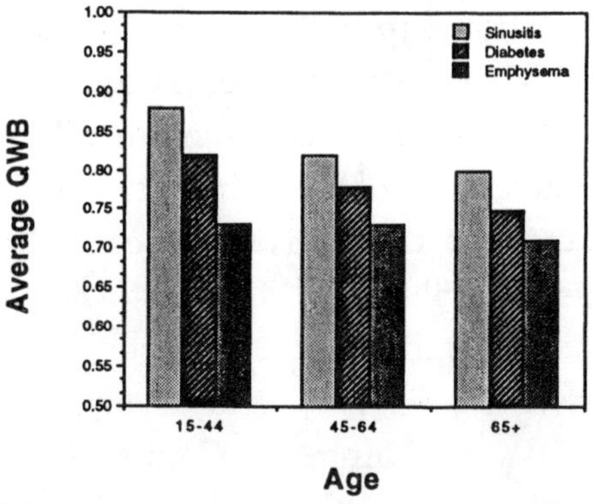

Source: Comparison of estimated QWB for patients with sinusitus, diabetes millitus, and emphysema at different ages. (Data for the National Health Interview Survey adapted from Erickson et al).[10]

Figure 20.2

Treating Cystic Fibrosis (Ornstein & Kaplan 1991)

Estimated CF Treatment Benefit

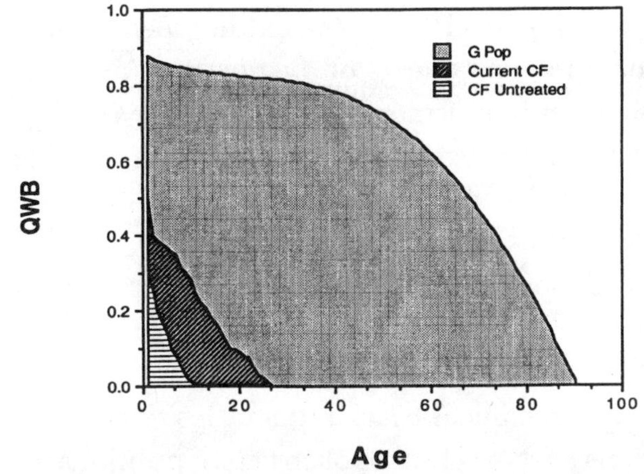

Area under curve in Cystic Fibrosis. Top curve is the estimated U.S. Quality Adjusted Life Expectancy. Middle curve is the estimate for patients with cystic fibrosis. The bottom curve is the estimate for Cystic Fibrosis 25 years of age.(Adapted from Orenstein & Kaplan).[11]

Source: Orenstein DM, RM Kaplan. "Measuring the Quality of Well-Being in Cystic Fibrosis and Lung Transplantation. The Importance of the Area under the Curve." Chest 100 1991: 1016-1018.

Figure 20.3

QWB by Level of Cognitive Impairment in Alzheimer's

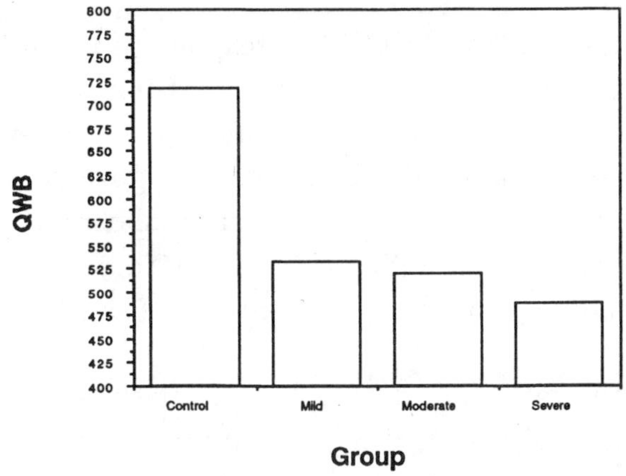

Source:QWB scores by levels of cognitive impairment for patients with Alzheimer's disease. (From Kerner et al.)[12]

Expectancy for people with cystic fibrosis twenty-five years ago. The area between the second and third curves shows the advances in cystic fibrosis treatment within the last quarter century. The area between the first and second curves describes the distance that must be traveled in order to reduce the impact of this disease.[11]

Figure 20.3 summarizes the relationship between the QWB and measures of cognitive impairment for patients with Alzheimer's Disease. Those with disease are significantly lower on the QWB and the degree of illness is systematically related to QWB score.[12] A variety of studies have evaluated the relationship between QWB and HIV disease. A series of studies was conducted at the University of California at San Diego HIV Neurobehavioral Research Center (HNRC). These studies evaluated the relationship between neurocognitive impairment, disability, and the QWB. **Figure 20.4** summarizes some of the relationships between the QWB, and a variety of outcomes. When QWB scores were broken down by HIV grouping, the Centers for Disease Control (CDC) IV group was significantly lower (0.661) than the CDC II/III groups (0.755) and the control groups (0.802) (upper left panel). The differences between the Class IV and Class II/III is about 0.10 units of well being, suggesting that individuals lose one-tenth equivalents of well years of life for each year they are in the AIDS category in comparison to the asymptomatic groups. In comparison to the uninfected controls, this would equal a one year of life loss for each ten infected individuals. The QWB was shown to be significantly associated with CD4+ lymphocytes ($p<0.001$) (upper middle), Beta-2 Micro globulin quartile ($p < 0.03$) (upper right), neurologists ratings of dysfunction ($p<0.001$) (lower left), clinician ratings neuropsychological impairment ($p<0.04$) (lower center), future vital status ($p< 0.05$) (lower right) and several psychiatric variables including POMS scores for vigor ($p<0.001$) and dejection ($p<0.001$). Multivariate models demonstrated high covariation between predictors of QWB. These results suggest that the QWB is a significant correlate of biological, neuropsychological, neurological psychiatric, and mortality outcomes for male HIV infected patients.[13]

The QWB has also been used in clinical trials and studies to evaluate medical and surgical thearapies in conditions such as chronic obstructive pulmonary disease, AIDS, cystic fibrosis, diabetes mellitus, atrial fibrillation, lung transplantation, arthritis, cancer, and several other conditions.[14-22] Further, the method has been used for health resource allocation modeling and has served as the basis for an innovative experiment on rationing of health care by the state of Oregon.[22-23]

Studies have also demonstrated that the QWB is responsive to clinical change in a variety of conditions. **Figure 20.5** compares QWB scores for patients undergoing sinus surgery versus a control group that did not receive surgery. Patients who undergo this difficult surgery achieve significant QWB benefits.[24] **Figure 20.6** offers a comparison between small groups of patients who were in the original clinical trial evaluating zidovudine for the treatment of patients with AIDS. Here, there was a very large clinical impact of the treatment, although the benefit lasted only a short time.[15]

Some evidence supports the validity of the QWB in studies of mental health. One recent study evaluated the validity of the Quality of Well-Being Scale (QWB) as an outcome

Figure 20.4

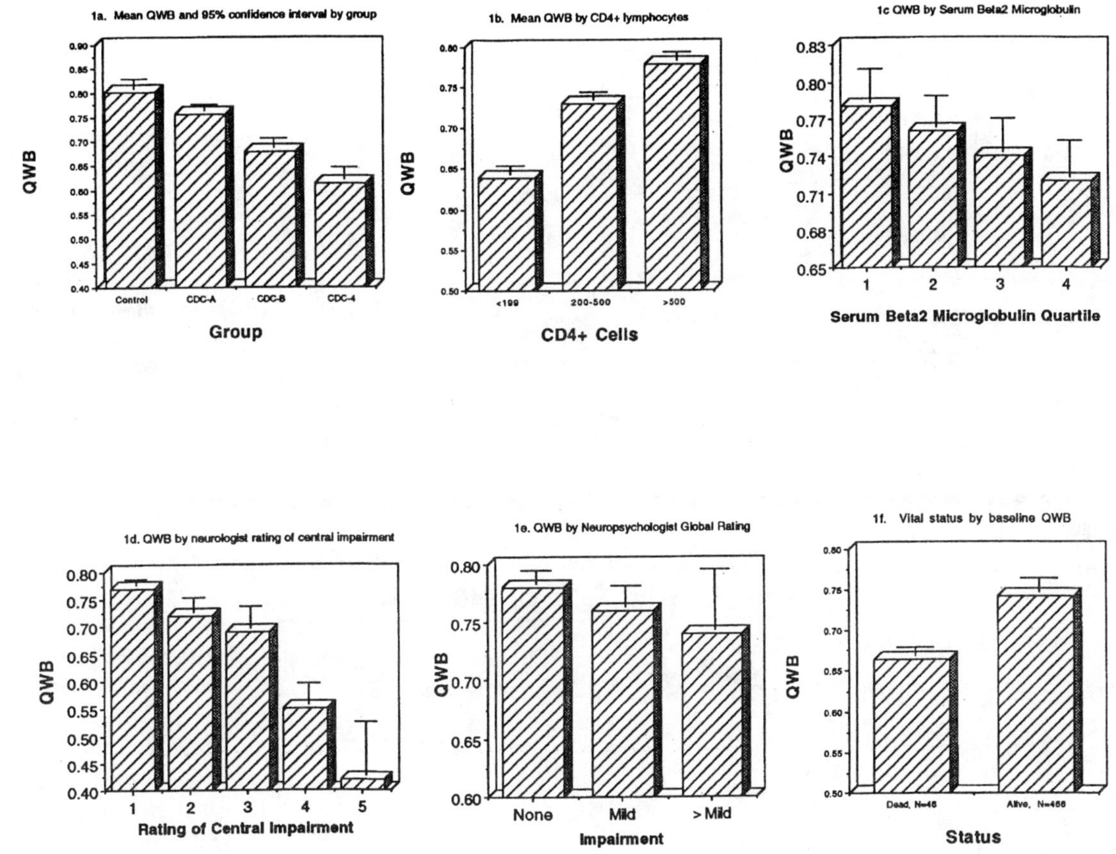

Comparison of mean QWB by CDC class (upper left), CD_4 + lymphocites (upper middle), Beta-2 Micro-Globulin quartile (Upper right), neurologists integrative clinical ratings (lower left), neuropsychological test summary scores of impaired and unimpaired (lower center), and future vital status (lower right) (From Kaplan et al.)[13]

Source: Kaplan RM, JP Anderson, TL Patterson, J Chandler, I Grant." Validity of the Quality of Well-Being Scale for Persons with HIV Infection." Psychomatic Medicine 57 1995: 138-147.

Figure 20.5

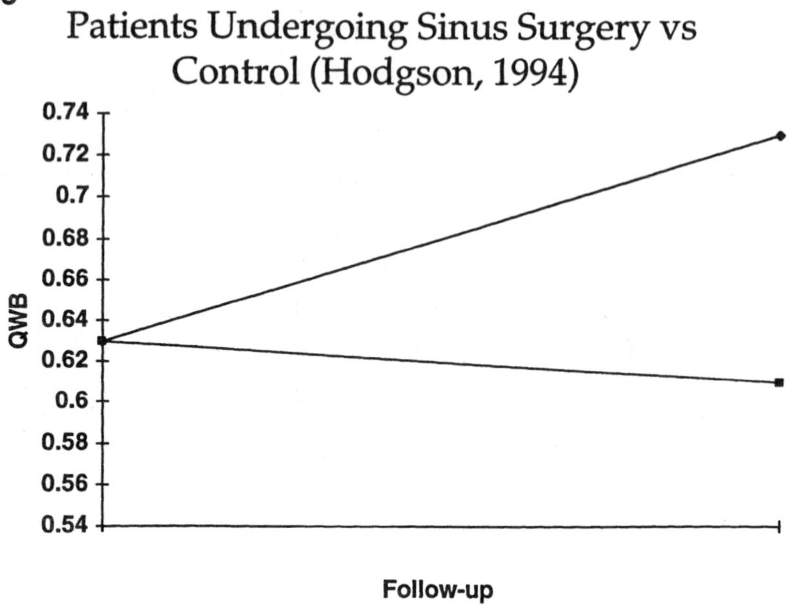

Source: QWB scores for those undergoing sinus surgery in comparison to controls. (Adapted from Hodgkin.) [24]

Figure 20.6

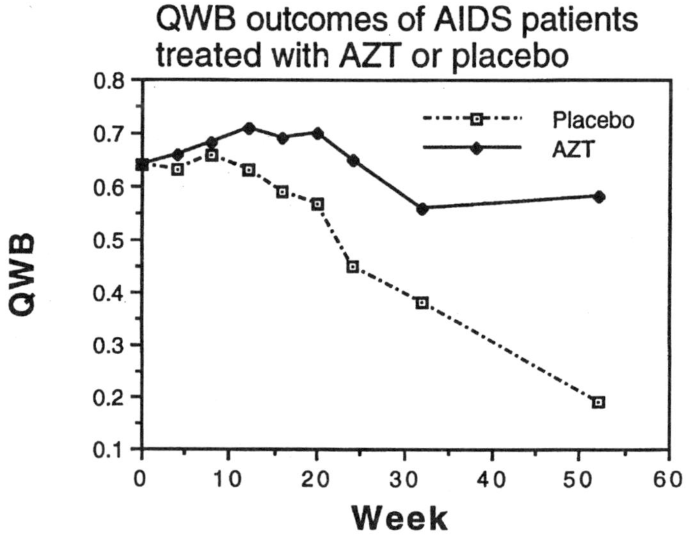

QWB outcomes of AIDS patients treated with AZT or Placebo and followed 52 weeks. (Adapted from Kaplan et al.) [15]

Source: Kaplan RM, JP Anderson, AW Wu WC Mathews, F Kozin, D Orenstein. "The Quality of Well-Being Scale Applications in AIDS, Cystic Fibrosis, and Arthritis," Medical Care 27 1989: S27-S43.

measure for older psychotic patients. Seventy-two psychotic patients and twenty-eight matched controls from the San Diego Veterans Affairs Medical Center completed the QWB, the SCID, SAPS, SANS, and Global Severity Index (GSI) from the Brief Symptom Inventory (BSI). The QWB correlated with the SANS -0.52 ($p<0.001$) with the SAPS -0.57 ($p<0.001$) and with the GSI -0.62 ($p<0.001$). Patients and controls were significantly different on the QWB, and there was a linear relationship between QWB and severity of illness (as classified by the SANS and the SAPS). In addition, component scores of the QWB (i.e., mobility, physical activity, social activity, and worst symptom) were significantly lower among patients as compared to controls, and declined systematically as psychiatric symptoms increased.[25]

Using the GHPM, it is possible to estimate the benefit of any health care intervention in terms of the Quality-Adjusted Life Years the treatment produces. Suppose, for example, that a treatment for anxiety elevates patients from a level of 0.65 to a level of 0.75. Suppose further, that this treatment benefit lasted for one year. Each patient would gain 0.1 QALY (0.75 - 0.65 = 0.10 X 1 year = 0.1 QALY) for each year the benefit was observed. The treatment benefit would be expressed in terms of general QALY units. The productivity of the providers could be compared with providers in other aspects of health care. All providers in health care use resources. Dividing the cost of a treatment by the QALY productivity provides the cost/utility ratio. Measuring mental health productivity in QALY units would allow the assessment of investments in mental health services to be compared directly to those in other aspects of health care.

The QWB-SA 1.0

One of the major concerns about the QWB is that it must be administered by a trained interviewer. Although it is still believed that the interviewer administered QWB is the optimal way to collect health outcome information, a self-administered form, which is known as the Quality of Well-Being Self-Administered (QWB-SA) version 1.0, has recently been developed. The self-administered form can be completed in about ten minutes and can be machine scored. Validity and reliability data on the QWB-SA 1.0 is expected to released in the near future.

In summary, the general QWB measure has evidence for validity in a variety of different specific diseases. It has shown to be responsive to change and its application has been found to be feasible in a wide variety of different populations.

Why is a Valid and Reliable Measure of Health Status Necessary?

There are many different reasons why a valid and reliable measure of health status is necessary. This chapter will explore the four primary reasons. They are the following: 1) to determine whether a treatment produces a benefit, 2) to allocate scarce health care resources, 3) to determine effects of policy changes, and 4) to help patients and providers make informed choices.

Determination of Treatment Benefit

Traditional measures of health status have emphasized mortality or measures of disease process. Fowler reviewed some of the major conditions requiring surgery in the United States. [26] These included transuretheral resection prostatectomy (TURP) for patients with benign hyperplasia of the prostate, cataract extraction with intraocular lens replacement, joint arthroplasty for osteoarthritis, and hysterectomy for diseases of the uterus. It is difficult to evaluate the value of these procedures using traditional outcome measures that focus on life expectancy, because none of these common operations have a significant impact on mortality. In each case, however, the surgery may lead to improvements in functioning or the reporting of symptoms. For example, TURP may reduce the symptom of urinary frequency in men. Cataract extraction may help older patients function better with reading, night driving, or other activities of daily living. Joint arthroplasty may increase mobility for older patients. For most of these cases, traditional physiological measures are limited as outcome assessments.

For example, there is no correlation between visual acuity and patient perceptions of their satisfaction or trouble with vision.[27] Further, there is little or no correlation between visual acuity in the worse eye and measures of visual function (reading and driving) after cataract surgery in one eye alone.[27] However, improvements in visual functioning, but not in binocular visual acuity, were significantly greater after cataract surgery on the second eye. This suggests that the ability to perform vision dependent activities is related more to vision in the better eye, that surgery in both eyes improves visual function better than in one eye alone, and that visual acuity alone is an insensitive indicator of improvement when compared with measures of visual functioning. Lastly, improvements in visual functioning are associated with significant improvements across nonvision-related health dimensions and have been linked to the blunting and occasionally reversal of some progressive functional degenerations in the elderly population. [28-31]

Similarly, there are substantial discrepancies between studies of x-ray evidence of osteoarthritis and performance of usual activities. Studies on back pain help illustrate some of these issues. Radiographic studies show that an estimated 57% of Americans age sixty or older have ruptured discs or spinal stenosis; however, these patients often report little or no pain. Surgery to correct the spinal stenosis may be of little value if the patient is not impaired to begin with. Conversely, pain is often reported by patients who have no abnormalities on x-ray. According to traditional measures, these patients have no problem. Nevertheless, they remain impaired using standardized outcome measures. [32]

In summary, traditional measures of clinical status, including x-rays or clinical tests do not tell the whole story with regard to health benefit. A valid and reliable index of health status is required in order to demonstrate the benefits of treatment from the patient's perspective.

Allocation of Scarce Resources

Health care resources are severely limited. The Medicare Trust Fund is estimated to run out of resources by the year 2001. In order to avoid this catastrophe, either health care costs will need to be cut in half, or payroll taxes will need to be doubled.[33] Valid and reliable measures of health status may help direct difficult resouce allocation decisions. Perhaps the most controversial proposal to allocate resources on the basis of the expected outcome of procedures came from the state of Oregon. [34]

In 1989, Oregon passed three pieces of legislation, including the controversial Senate Bill 27, which mandated that health services be prioritized using a process similar to the GHPM. The justification for the prioritization was to eliminate services that did not provide benefit. The process of creating the prioritized list was an extremely difficult one. The commission began by creating a prioritized list of all health services. It soon became apparent, however, that this was an impossible task. Thus, the commissioners began searching for combinations of conditions and treatments that could be lumped together. For example, the problem of rectal prolapse was paired with the treatment partial colectomy while osteoporosis is paired with "medical treatment" which was a generic term for treatment with medication.

A major portion of the commissioners activity was to evaluate services using the Quality of Well-Being Scale from the GHPM. The commissioners could not possibly have conducted clinical trials for each of the many condition-treatment pairs. Further, estimation of treatment benefit using the QWB cannot be left to laymen. So, the commission formed a medical committee which had expertise in essentially all specialty areas and had the participation of nearly all of the major provider groups in the state. Working together, the committee estimated the expected benefit of 709 condition-treatment pairs.

The QWB, which was used to estimate the effect of services, requires subjective judgments to score the importance or desirability of health states. These weights are not medical expert judgments and should be obtained from community peers. The Oregon citizens were particularly concerned about using weights from California in order to assign priorities in their state. Thus, 1,001 Oregon citizens participated in a separate weighting experiment. The weights were obtained in a telephone survey that was conducted by Oregon State University. In 1990, the commission released a draft copy its first prioritized list. Unfortunately, many of the rankings seemed counter intuitive and the approach drew serious criticism in the popular press. As a result, the system was reorganized according to three basic categories of care: essential, very important, and valuable to certain individuals. Within these major groupings there were seventeen subcategories. The commission decided to place greatest emphasis on problems that were acute and fatal. In these cases, treatment prevents death and there is full recovery. Examples include appendectomy for appendicitis and non-surgical treatment for whooping cough. Other categories classified as essential included maternity care, treatment for conditions that prevent death but do not allow full recovery, and preventive care for children. There were nine categories classified as essential. Listed as very important were treatments for non-fatal conditions that would return the individual to a previous state of health. Also included in this category were acute non-fatal one time treatments that might improve quality of life, such as hip replacements and cornea transplants. At the bottom of the list were treatments for fatal or non-fatal conditions that did not improve quality of life or extend life. Aggressive treatments for the end stages of diseases such as cancer and AIDS or care for conditions in which the treatments were known not to be effective.

In other words, services that did not help people live longer or function better were given low priority. In the revised approach, the commission decided to ignore cost information and to allow their own subjective judgments to influence the rankings on the list. Unfortunately, the final exercise in Oregon resulted in many deviations from the GHPM. The exercise, however, demonstrates an attempt to resolve the health care crisis on the basis of health outcome. After nearly five years of debate, a revised Oregon plan was implemented on February 1, 1994.

Although the Oregon experiment was very controversial, others have suggested that health outcomes can be used to allocate scarce resources and to evaluate whether treatment is not only possible but also advisible. [30,35-37]It can be related to assessing risk and predicting utilization, thereby controlling costs and improving care.[37] Reimbursement mechanisms in fee-for-service and managed care are currently tied to the delivery of service and covered lives. Functional outcomes can help differentiate which results are important to the patient and link payment to the provision of benefit rather than the provision of service. [36,38] Appropriate manpower needs and provider mix ratios (specialist vs. primary care), assessing health risk and demand for service, identifying at-risk or underserved populations (poor, elderly, women, children), and developing practice guidelines are additional uses of functional health status measures in allocating scarce resources. [27, 29, 38, 39, 40]

Determination of the Effects of Policy Changes

It is commonly argued that health care reform will cause significant harm. Allocation schemes, such as that proposed in Oregon, have not been formally evaluated; however, many provider groups assert that allocation schemes will result in significant damage to population health status. In addition to allocation by service, other dramatic health policies have been proposed. For example, Fisher and colleagues argue that excess hospital capacity leads to unnecessary health service utilization.[41] They report that Medicare beneficiaries in Boston who have been admitted to the hospital have a 64% higher chance of being re-admitted within one year than patients in New Haven, CT. The major difference between Boston and New Haven is that Boston has an excess number of hospital beds. Fisher and colleagues also considered hospitalizations in the state of Oregon.[43] They discovered that there was wide variability in the number of patient days for discretionary admissions in different parts of the state. If the rate of discretionary hospital admissions was equal to that in the state capital of Salem, Oregon, significant savings would accrue. Salem has a ceiling of 218 days per 1,000 residents. Using this rate as the state-wide ceiling, 238 beds could be closed in 20 Oregon hospitals and service areas.

This would result in an estimated savings of $47.3 million. Such savings may reduce the need to ration specific medical services.

Allocation schemes based either on specific services, numbers of hospital beds, or number of discretionary admissions all have the potential to have either positive or negative effects on population health status. Unfortunately, there are not accurate and sensitive measures to determine whether these policies do good or harm. Thus, another rationale for developing valid and reliable general health outcome measures is to determine the impact of public health policy. It has been proposed that government agencies, such as the National Center for Health Statistics, keep and report measures of population health status. Such efforts were called for in the Healthy People 2000 Report. [43]

Informed Patient Decisionmaking

Measures of health-related quality of life may also have some clinical application. To illustrate this issue, consider the problem of prostate cancer in older men. Prostate cancer is an extremely common cancer for men age seventy years and older.[44] The treatment of this disease varies dramatically from country to country and within regions of the U.S. For example, surgical removal of the prostate gland is done nearly twice as often in the Pacific Northwest as it is in New England. Yet, survival rates and deaths from prostate cancer are no different in the two regions.[45] The traditional approach to the treatment of prostate cancer was to identify the tumor and to get rid of it through either surgery or radiation therapy. Success is defined either through improved life expectancy or through evidence that the man is tumor free. Formal analysis using QALYs can shed different light on these decisions.

There are three main options for the treatment of prostate cancer—radical prostatectomy (surgical removal of the prostate gland), external beam radiation therapy, and "watchful waiting." Both radical prostatectomy and radiation therapy carry high risks of complications which may reduce life satisfaction. For example, there are significant increases in the chances of becoming impotent or incontinent. Watchful waiting, on the other hand, does not require therapy, but only evaluation and supervision by a physician. The watchful waiting option has been used least often because it does not treat the cancer.

One recent analysis estimated QALYs under these three options. The analysis assumed a cohort of sixty-eight year old men and used published studies to estimate outcomes under different treatment options. For men diagnosed at this age, the risk of distant metastases is relatively rare: these outcomes occur in five of each hundred patient years of observation. The median time to metastasis is fourteen years, and during this period 58% of the men would be expected to die of other causes. For those men who do develop metastases, hormonal therapy is available and can efficaciously delay disease progression until a larger percentage of the men die of other causes. [44] **Figure 20.7** summarizes quality adjusted life expectancy (QALE) under the three treatment options for men with moderately-differentiated tumors at different ages. As the figure shows, the quality adjusted life expectancy is essentially equivalent under the three options. The small differences between approaches are not statistically significant.[44] The traditional view emphasizes tumor eradication and aggressive treatment. This analysis suggests that the alternatives are equivalent and that the choice should be a matter of patient preference.

Patient preference is especially important since the relationships between physiological variables, symptoms, functional health status, and general health perceptions is not clear. Interventions aimed at biological and physiological factors alone will not relieve symptoms or improve functioning in predictible ways. [37] Further, when symptoms do occur, tolerance and interference with functioning is highly variable among different patients. Treatments themselves can produce symptoms and reductions in quality of life, most notably in silent diseases (hypertension, glaucoma, hypercholesteremia). Understanding patient preferences, therefore, has additional value in shared decisionmaking particularly when functioning can be improved, but may be accompanied by side effects. By making explicit hidden assumptions and alerting the decisionmakers to unexpected and unintended results, functional outcomes can serve as a decicision support aide.[35] Decision support outcomes databases can be used to enlarge the individual clinician's clinical and financial awareness, and allow patients and families to understand what is unchangeable, what is beyond the control of the system, and what both the doctor and the patient can jointly address. [28, 36]

QWB Applications in Managed Care

To date the QWB has primarily been used in clinical studies and public policymaking. Each of the applications described above (i.e., determination of treatment benefit, allocation of scarce resources, determination of whether policy changes do good or harm, and informed patient decisionmaking) can play a potentially powerful role in a managed care environment. In addition, there are numerous other potential uses to benefit patients, providers, and health care organizations. **Figure 20.8** details some of these applications and the primary and secondary beneficiaries. The following section discusses some of these applications in greater detail.

Quality Improvement and Work Redesign

Across the United States, health care providers are embarking on work redesign and quality improvement projects and implementing clinical guidelines and pathways. These efforts are designed to streamline care processes and reduce costs, as well as to ensure the provision of appropriate, high quality clinical care. In order to measure the results of these projects, providers must have tools to compare current patient outcomes with past practices. More specifically, valid and reliable measures are needed to determine whether the new care delivery processes and/or treatments are of benefit to the patient, provide equal or better outcomes while making appropriate use of scarce resources, and make provision for informed provider and patient decisionmaking. Furthermore, as competition for managed care contracts increases, providers must be able to supplement cost data with information on plan member health status, clinical

Figure 20.7: Quality adjusted life expectancy for moderately differentiated postate tumors under three options.

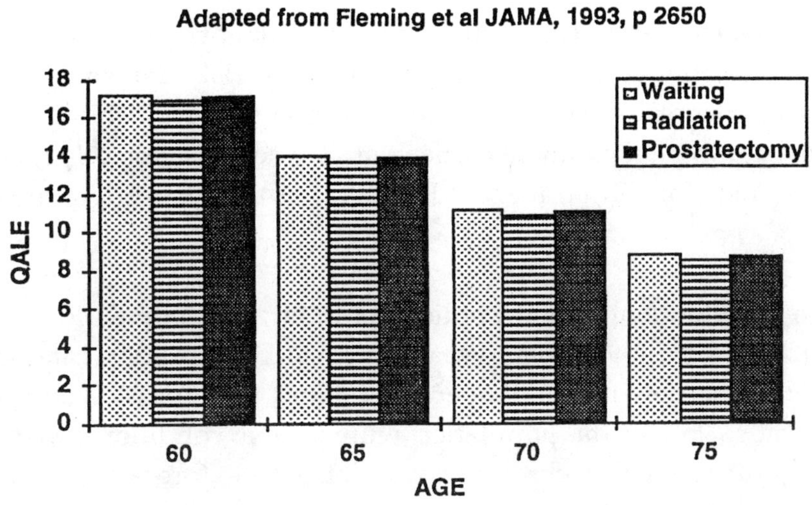

Source: Quality adjusted life expectancy (QALE) under the three treatment options for men with well-differentiated tumors at different ages (data from Fleming et al.).[44]

Figure 20.8: QWB Application Matrix

Application	Patient	Beneficiary Provider	Organization
Practice management	O	O	X
Resource allocation	O	O	X
Manpower needs	O	O	X
Provider-mix ratios	O	O	X
Cost-effectiveness analysis	O	O	X
Cost-utility analysis	O	O	X
Applied research	O	X	X
Outcomes	X	X	O
Practice guidelines	X	X	O
Regulatory compliance	O	O	X
Quality assurance (CQI)	X	X	O
Risk assessment/adjustment	O	O	X
Forecasting/rate making	O	X	X
Patient communication	X	O	O
Provider communication	X	O	O
Patient decisionmaking	X	O	O
Informed consent	X	O	O
Provider decision support	O	X	O
Patient/staff education needs	X	X	X

X = primary beneficiary O = secondary beneficiary

changes as a result of procedures and treatments. The QWB may be useful for documenting these outcomes.

Risk Assessment, Abatement, and Cost Reduction

The QWB can also be used to identify risk in the general population and in targeted subsets of the population. For the general population, unbiased risk assessment models, using health status as a measure, have been used to identify enrollee health care needs in order to set and justify health plan payments (dues rates). These risk models have been shown to be powerful predictors of permanent health states and the propensity to use health services.[38]

The QWB can also be used to identify and predict risk in targeted populations such as the elderly frail, diabetes, cardio-vascular disease, stroke, HIV, cancer, cataract, hip replacement, depression, and new health plan enrollees. Risk identification and prediction are important because 25% of the population with chronic conditions account for 80% of the cost of care. Information on clinical risk is often used to forecast financial risk, important information for organizations who derive most of their income from capitated contracts.

Risk assessment alone, however, tells us little about the outcomes, quality, and cost-effectiveness of care. Health status assessment can be used to translate risk identification into a strategy for risk abatement and cost reduction. By using the QWB to measure outcomes and cost-effectiveness, it can serve as a metric for the practice management side of the risk-cost model. This will differentiate risk from benefit (outcome), and it may also demonstrate how risk reduction leads to better patient outcomes.

By extending the use of health status (QWB) to prevention, outcomes, quality assessment, and cost-effectiveness, the cost of data gathering can be amortized over a number of applications and departments, thereby increasing its return on investment, adding longevity to its life cycle, and decreasing the performance burden on any one use. In addition, health status surveys have been shown to be effective for getting data unavailable by other means, data that is more cost-effective and reliable than data linked to episodic doctor office visits alone, less subject to misinterpretation than diagnostic labels, and of interest to benefits managers. As additional valid uses for health status are identified, more data will be available to enhance the predictive power of risk models. Lastly, surveys can be conducted outside the system of health care, revealing potential unmet needs and patient dissatisfaction with care.

Practice Management

The QWB can also be used for practice management outcomes and cost-effectiveness analysis. Linking structure and process measures to health outcomes will allow us to differentiate the provision of benefit from provision of service (cost). Adjustments in manpower needs, provider-mix ratios, lengths of stay, and access to care are important manipulations. Using health status will provide new ways to demonstrate quality of care for regulatory compliance (JCAHO, NCQA), and to identify patient and staff educational needs. For patients with comorbidities, whose care cuts across many departments, health status scores can be the co-management thread that integrates care where continuity and coordination can affect outcomes.

Because the QWB provides a single global score expressed as a quality adjusted life year (QALY), it can be used for cost utility analysis (CUA). Important comparisons for individual and group clinical and administrative decision making can be made. For example, evaluating alternative treatment plans within single diagnostic groups, across diseases or departments and benchmarking to other practices or health plans is possible with the QWB. Risk and outcome assessment, when combined with patient satisfaction data, can provide a powerful core data set that has benefits to the patient, the provider, the organization and the payers of health care.

Summary

A GHPM may have applications in many different areas of health services research. One component of the model, known as the Quality of Well-Being Scale (QWB) is used to measure health-related quality of life. Evidence supports the validity of this measure in population studies and in clinical investigations involving numerous different patient groups. A valid and reliable health status indicator may have value in estimating treatment benefit, allocating scarce health care resources, estimating the impact of public policy changes, and in helping patients and providers make informed choices. At present, there have been few applications of outcome measurement in health care. We encourage continued research and application of these models.

References

1. Anderson JP, RM Kaplan, JW Berry, CC Bush, RG Rumbaut. "Interday Reliability of Function Assessment for a Health Status Measure. The Quality of Well-Being Scale." *Medical Care* 27 1989; 1076-1083.

2. Kaplan RM, SJ Coons, JP Anderson. "Quality of Life and Policy Analysis in Arthritis." *Arthritis Care and Research* 5 1992;173-183.

3. Kaplan RM, JP Anderson. "An Integreted Approach to Quality of Life Assessment: The General Health Policy Model." In B. Spilker (ed.), *Quality of Life in Clinical Studies.* New York: Raven, 1990; 131-149.

4. Kaplan RM. "The Ziggy Theorem: Toward an Outcomes-Focused Health Psychology." *Health Psychology* 13 1994; 451-460.

5. Kaplan RM, JW Bush, CC Berry. "Health Status: Types of Validity and the Index of Well-Being." *Health Services Research* 11(4) 1976; 478-507.

6. Kaplan RM, JW Bush, CC Berry. "The Reliability, Stability, and Generalizability of a Health Status Index." American Statistical Association, Proceedings of the Social Status Section 1978; 704-709.

7. Kapla RM, JW Bush, CC Berry. "Health Status Index: Category Rating Versus Magnitude Estimation for Measuring Levels of Well-Being." *Medical Care* 17 1979; 501-525.

8. Patrick DL, P Erickson. *Health Status and Health Policy: Quality of Life in Health Care Evaluation and Resource Allocation.* Boston: Oxford, 1993.

9. Torrance GW, D Feeny. "Utilities and Quality-Adjusted Life Years." *International Journal of Technology in Assess Health Care* 5 1989; 559-575.

10. Erickson P, EA Kendall, JP Anderson, RM Kaplan. "Using Composite Health Status Measures to Assess the Nation's Health." *Medical Care* 27 1989; S66-S76.

11. Orenstein DM, RM Kaplan. "Measuring the Quality of Well-Being in Cystic Fibrosis and Lung Transplantation. The Importance of the Area Under the Curve." *Chest* 100 1991; 1016-1018.

12. Kerner D, TL Patterson, RM Kaplan. "Validity of the Quality of Well-Being Scale in Alzheimer's Disease." 1994, in preparation.

13. Kaplan RM, JP Anderson, TL Patterson, et al. "Validity of the Quality of Well-Being Scale For Persons with HIV Infection." *Psychosomatic Medicine* 57 1995; 138-147.

14. Kaplan RM, CJ Atkins, R Timms. "Validity of a Quality of Well-Being Scale as an Outcome Measure in Chronic Obstructive Pulmonary Disease." *Journal of Chronic Diseases* 37 1984;85-95.

15. Kaplan RM, JP Anderson, AW Wu, WC Mathews, F Kozin, D Orenstein. "The Quality of Well-Being Scale. Applications in AIDS, Cystic Fibrosis, and Arthritis." *Medical Care* 27 1989;S27-S43.

16. Orenstein DM, PA Nixon, EA Ross, RM Kaplan. "The Quality of Well-Being in Cystic Fibrosis." *Chest* 95 1989; 344-347.

17. Kaplan RM, SL Hartwell, DK Wilson, JP Wallace. "Effects of Diet and Exercise Interventions on Control and Quality of Life in Non-Insulin-Dependent Diabetes Mellitus." *Journal of General Internal Medicine* 2 1987; 220-228.

18. Ganiats TG, LA Palinkas, RM Kaplan. "Comparison of Quality of Well-Being Scale and Functional Status Index in Patients with Atrial Fibrillation." *Medical Care* 30 1992; 958-964.

19. Squier H, RM Kaplan, AL Ries, et al. "Quality of Well-Being Predicts Survival in Lung Transplantation." *American Journal of Respiratory and Critical Care Medicine,* in press.

20. Kaplan RM, F Kozin, JP Anderson. "Measuring Quality of Life in Arthritis Patients (Including Discussion of a General Health-Decision Model)." *Quality of Life and Cardiovascular Care* 4 1988; 131-139.

21. Kaplan RM. "Quality of Life Assessment for Cost/Utility Studies in Cancer." *Cancer Treatment Reviews* 19 Suppl A 1993; 85-96.

22. Kaplan RM. "Application of a General Health Policy Model in the American Health Care Crisis." *Journal of the Royal Society of Medicine* 86 1993; 277-281.

23. Kaplan RM. *Hippocratic Predicament: Affordability, Access, and Accountability in Health Care.* San Diego: Academic Press, 1993.

24. Hodgkin PS. "Health Impact of Endoscopic Sinus Surgery Assessed by the Quality of Well-Being (QWB) Scale." Unpublished paper, University of California, San Diego, 1994.

25. Patterson TL, RM Kaplan, I Grant, SJ Semple, et al. "Quality of Well-Being in Late-Life Psychosis." Submitted for publication, 1995.

26. Fowler FJ, Jr., PD Cleary, J Magaziner, DL Patrick, KL Benjamin. "Methodological Issues in Measuring Patient-Reported Outcomes: The Agenda of the Work Group on Outcomes Assessment." *Medical Care* 32 1994; JS65-JS76.

27. Steiner CA, EB Bass, MA Talamini, HA Pitt, EP Steinberg. "Surgical Rates and Operative Mortality for Open and Laparoscopic Cholecystectomy in Maryland." *New England Journal of Medicine* 330 1994; 403-408.

28. Kane RL. "The Implications of Assessment." *Journal of Gerontology* 48 Spec No 1993; 27-31.

29. Wasson J, A Keller, L Rubenstein, R Hays, E Nelson, D Johnson. "Benefits and Obstacles of Health Status Assessment in Ambulatory Settings. The Clinician's Point of View. The Dartmouth Primary Care COOP Project." *Medical Care* 30 1992; MS42-MS49.

30. Mangione CM, RS Phillips, MG Lawrence, JM Seddon, EJ Orav, L Goldman. "Improved Visual Function and Attenuation of Declines in Health-Related Quality of Life After Cataract Extraction." *Archives of Ophthalmology* 112 1994;1419-1425.

31. Brenner MH, B Curbow, JC Javitt, et al. "Vision Change and Quality of Life in the Elderly. Response to Cataract Surgery and Treatment of Other Chronic Ocular Conditions." *Archives of Ophthalmology* 111 1993; 680-685.

32. Boden SD, PR McCowin, DO Davis, TS Dina, et al. "A Prospective Investigation." *Journal of Bone and Joint Surgery [America]*, 72 1990; 1178-1184.

33. Eddy DM. "What Care Is 'Essential'? What Services Are 'Basic'?" *Journal of the American Medical Association* 265 1991; 782, 786-782, 788.

34. Crawshaw R, MJ Garland, B Hines, C Lobitz. "Oregon Health Decisions. An Experiment with Informed Community Consent." *Journal of the American Medical Association* 254 1985; 3213-3216.

35. Diamond GA, TA Denton, JM Matloff. "Fee-For-Benefit: A Strategy to Improve the Quality of Health Care and Control Costs Through Reimbursement Incentives." *Journal of the American College of Cardiology* 22 1993; 343-352.

36. Diamond GA, TA Denton. "Alternative Perspectives on the Biased Foundations of Medical Technology Assessment." *Annals of Internal Medicine* 118 1993; 455-464.

37. Wilson IB, PD Cleary. "Linking Clinical Variables with Health-Related Quality of Life. A Conceptual Model of Patient Outcomes." *Journal of the American Medical Association* 273 1995; 59-65.

38. Hornbrook MC, MJ Goodman. "Assessing Relative Health Plan Risk with the RAND 36 Health Survey." *Inquiry* 32 1995; 56-74.

39. Sturm R, Wells KB. "How Can Care For Depression Become More Cost-Effective?" *Journal of the American Medical Association* 273 1995; 51-58.

40. Eddy DM. "Clinical Decision Making: From Theory To Practice. Rationing Resources While Improving Quality. How to Get More for Less." *Journal of the American Medical Association* 272 1994; 817-824.

41. Fisher ES, JE Wennberg, TA Stukel, SM Sharp. "Hospital Readmission Rates for Cohorts of Medicare Beneficiaries in Boston and New Haven." *New England Journal of Medicine*, 331 1994; 989-995.

42. Fisher ES, HG Welch, JE Wennberg. "Prioritizing Oregon's Hospital Resources. An Example Based on Variations in Discretionary Medical Utilization." *Journal of the American Medical Association* 267 1992; 1925-1931.

43. U.S. Dept. of Health and Human Services, Public Health Service. Healthy People 2000: National Health Promotion and Disease Prevention Objectives: U.S. G.P.O., [1991 Series title: DHHS publication; no. (PHS) 91-50213.

44. Fleming C, JH Wasson, PC Albertsen, MJ Barry, JE Wennberg. "A Decision Analysis of Alternative Treatment Strategies for Clinically Localized Prostate Cancer. Prostate Patient Outcomes Research Team." *Journal of the American Medical Association* 269 1993; 2650-2658.

45. Lu-Yao GL, JA Baron, JA Barrett, ES Fisher. "Treatment and Survival Among Elderly Americans with Hip Fractures: A Population-Based Study." *American Journal of Public Health* 84 1994; 1287-1291.

Section IV

Case Studies

Section IV rounds out the book by providing seven case studies illustrating outcomes measurement and the implementation of clinical guidelines and pathways. The first chapter examines the medical rehabilitation model of outcomes measurement and management for its applicability and potential lessons to be learned as other acute care service lines move towards health care team models and a focus on patient outcomes. Chapter 22 describes a Cedars-Sinai project in which practice guidelines and physician reminders were used to reduce the length of hospital stay for patients with chest pain. Chapter 23 builds upon information about the organization's resource management effort (Chapter 19) by providing examples of the implementation and interim outcomes of several of the clinical pathways developed as part of the resource management project. Chapter 24 moves to women's care and addresses methods for setting an appropriate institutional target for vaginal birth after cesarean (VBAC). The project combines consideration of the literature, national benchmarking, and chart reviews of Cedars-Sinai patients to establish a VBAC target specific to the Cedars-Sinai population. Chapter 25 describes a study to determine the cost and health outcomes of two methods of delivering bronchodilators—updraft nebulizer (UDN) and metered dose inhaler (MDI). Findings showed that MDI, when used with a slightly higher dosage, was equally effective. The use of MDI when appropriate also resulted in significant cost savings. Chapter 26 details the department of pharmacy's involvement in the development of a number of clinical pathways. The chapter provides evidence for the pharmacological guidelines developed and patient and cost outcome information. Chapter 27 presents the findings of a study that combined literature review with a prospective research project to establish appropriate guidelines for the monitoring of patients with epidural or intrathecal morphine for postoperative pain. Finally, in Chapter 28, we provide some thoughts for the future in the book's conclusion.

Chapter 21

Outcomes Measurement and Management: The Medical Rehabilitation Model

Harriet Udin Aronow, PhD
Joan Sanders, MA
Pamela Erhardt, PhD
Patricia Gomavitz, PT
Eugene Richards, MD

The purpose of this chapter is to present the model of program management and evaluation based on patient outcomes used in the field of Physical Medicine and Rehabilitation. The chapter will lay out a brief history of the field, the development of multidisciplinary teams and product line programs, and the measurement of patient outcomes. The chapter also will present a case study of team management from the acute rehabilitation unit at Cedars-Sinai Medical Center. Its focus will be on recognizing the strengths of medical rehabilitation as a model and the lessons that other medical specialties can learn.

A Brief History of Medical Rehabilitation

While some methods of physical medicine (e.g., hydrotherapy, massage) were present in ancient times, the crippling injuries resulting from World Wars I and II and the development of military medicine drove the emergence of the modern field of Physical and Medical Rehabilitation. [1] In contrast to the physician who practiced independently with his or her preferred tools of trade (i.e., scalpels or pills), physical and occupational therapists tools were a team of care providers (including physician, nurse, therapists, and the patients' families). The necessity of a team intervention was due to the very nature of the orthopedic and neurological impairments treated. These impairments typically

HARRIET UDIN ARONOW, PhD—Research Associate, Nursing Research and Development, Cedars-Sinai Medical Center; Assistant Researcher, University of California-Los Angeles, Department of Medicine.

JOAN SANDERS, MA—Education Coordinator, Physical Medicine and Rehabilitation, Cedars-Sinai Medical Center.

PAMELA ERHARDT, PHD—Assistant Director, Physical Medicine and Rehabilitation, Cedars-Sinai Medical Center.

PATRICIA GOMAVITZ, PT—Director, Physical Medicine and Rehabilitation, Cedars-Sinai Medical Center.

EUGENE RICHARDS, MD—Medical Director, Physical Medicine and Rehabilitation, Cedars-Sinai Medical Center.

involved multiple organ systems and bodily functions; required physical assistance and re-education in basic daily self-care needs such as eating and bathing; and put the patient at increased risk of secondary complications (e.g., pneumonia, dermal ulcers, etc.).

In the latter half of the twentieth century, advances in emergency and acute medical technology resulted in increased survival rate of persons with catastrophic illness and injury. This success at the beginning of the treatment process (or continuum of care) radically increased the demand later in the treatment process for rehabilitative care of persons with sustained and chronic functional impairments. [2] The rapid growth of rehabilitation programs in the last twenty-five years has attested to the concern for health and well-being and loss of productivity associated with increasing numbers of persons living with disability.

Rehabilitation in the Continuum of Health Services

The goal of medical rehabilitation is to maximize the reintegration of a person into the community at the highest quality of life and level of independent function possible while minimizing the cost to patient, family, and society of long-term care and dependence. Rehabilitation has succeeded when patients are functioning at the highest possible level in the home and community setting and maintaining health in the context of chronic illness and impairment. The place of rehabilitation at the transition from acute care to the community and the relationship of rehabilitation to the rest of health care as a tertiary care service directed towards the minority of persons who have chronic or acute catastrophic care needs have resulted in the field being marginalized from the mainstream of acute medical services. Yet, the treatment model of rehabilitation has been slowly emerging in all of acute episodic health services as the focus of health services shifts from illness to wellness and from the process of health care services to the outcomes. Paul Elwood, MD, who is credited with the development of the concept of "health maintenance organization" and is board certified in both pediatrics and physical medicine, once stated that if the health care system functioned as it should, rehabilitation as a separate field of medicine would disappear and become the underlying model for all health care interventions (personal communication).

The Medical Rehabilitation Treatment Model

The medical rehabilitation treatment model focuses on outcomes of an episode of care in response to illness or injury and its resulting functional impairments. A patient's functional status, the level of independent performance of social roles and activities of daily living, is the standard measurement for rehabilitation outcomes. Carl Granger, MD, a long-time proponent of the standardization and use of functional assessment in medical rehabilitation, describes the use of functional assessment as a "method for integrating data on diagnostic descriptions of pathological conditions and impairment status with data related to limitations of residual abilities in the performance of social roles. By constructing a set of data that profiles the whole person, it becomes possible to understand better how a person with a disability functions." [3] With the data, the individual patient's continued intervention and care needs could be planned and evaluated. With the same data in the aggregate, treatment programs could be monitored and evaluated. The transition from the use of functional status assessment for treatment planning to the use of functional status data for program evaluation and planning occurred in the late 1960s and early 1970s when the growth of rehabilitation hospitals and units permitted the concentration of patients with similar diagnoses, treatment needs, and outcome into multidisciplinary treatment programs.

Development of Treatment Programs

Just as patient-focused restructuring today uses the reaggregation of patients with similar needs as an enabler, diagnostic-based treatment programs in medical rehabilitation afforded the opportunity to design team treatment interventions; train generalist therapists in specialized applications; and develop treatment programs that tailored service mix, duration, and settings to best meet the needs of patients. These specialized treatment programs with teams of providers using and sharing functional data on patients were a natural setting in which to develop programs with specific patient-centered goals and objectives.

The Commission on Accreditation of Rehabilitation Facilities (CARF)

By the mid 1960s, when Medicare had been implemented as a payment mechanism for the elderly and disabled, rehabilitation had begun to emerge as a recognized presence in the continuum of acute and chronic health services. The trade organizations representing medical and vocational rehabilitation recognized the need to set their programs apart, convince the health services market of the value of rehabilitation services, and secure a referral base among the physicians and other providers upstream in the continuum of levels of care. The Commission on Accreditation of Rehabilitation Facilities (CARF) was founded in 1966 in response to a request from the trade organizations for an independent commission to set standards and to apply them in a voluntary accreditation process.

In 1967, the first accreditation awards were presented. The field of rehabilitation professionals and the payers (led by the Insurance Rehabilitation Study Group) provided input into the development of standards. There was growing awareness among this group of the importance of rehabilitation services demonstrating its effectiveness. By 1973, the standards had evolved to include patient/client outcomes as a critical element in evaluating the quality of treatment programs. For the next twenty years rehabilitation facilities using the CARF standards implemented program evaluation systems that focused in part on the clinical outcomes of patients, initially on the basis of outcomes at discharge from the rehabilitation program; and later, on new standards requiring follow-up assessments in the community.

A National Uniform Data System

The formidable task of developing data collection methods and information systems capable of following patients after discharge and reporting outcomes fell on individual facilities and rehabilitation systems. The national Uniform Data System for Medical Rehabilitation (UDSMR) was developed in 1983 to offer a standardized data collection and reporting method. This would enable facilities to compare and combine data on patient mix and outcomes for use in marketing and policy research as well as program planning. The UDSMR system, currently located at The Buffalo General Hospital and State University of New York at Buffalo, is endorsed by several national rehabilitation organizations. Over 400 rehabilitation hospitals and units are official participants in the data system, and several others independently use components within their facilities. The Functional Independence Measure (FIM), a validated and reliable functional assessment scale that can be administered by any trained health professional or interviewer, is a cornerstone of the UDSMR. The complete data set was designed to facilitate treatment program monitoring and management, quality assessment, analyses of cost-effectiveness, and policy analyses and decisions.

Use of Outcome Measurement for Management

Like so many other organizational change efforts, the technical side of change—data collection and reporting systems—has generally been implemented satisfactorily. On the other hand, the use of outcome data to make decisions about implementing, adapting, and discontinuing programs has been more problematic. In January 1994, CARF gathered a national leadership and consumer panel to review the effects of the program evaluation standards on the field of rehabilitation. As a result of the panel discussions, new CARF standards have been developed that will further promote outcome measurement and management, and the use of quality, cost, and outcome information at all levels of an organization (Christine MacDonell, National Director, Medical Rehabilitation Division, personal communication).

Case Study - Cedars-Sinai Medical Center

Acute Medical Rehabilitation Unit

Cedars-Sinai Medical Center is a community-based teaching hospital in Los Angeles, CA. Within the medical center there is a thirty-two bed acute licensed rehabilitation unit. The unit serves the hospital and community, with about 65% of its patients referred from within Cedars-Sinai. Diagnoses typically treated in 1994 on the acute rehabilitation unit included strokes (43%), orthopedic diagnoses (27%), and traumatic and nontraumatic brain injuries (14%). Cedars-Sinai also runs a twenty-eight bed hospital-based sub-acute and skilled nursing unit, where the majority of older orthopedic patients and medical and cardiac surgery patients receive rehabilitative services as needed.

The acute rehabilitation unit is organized into four multidisciplinary teams that include physical and occupational therapists, nurses, physician, social worker, psychologist, and speech pathologist. A supervisor from physical or occupational therapy performs a mentor role, supervising less experienced team members and coaching treatment planning. The whole team meets twice weekly to plan patient care and coordinate team activities.

The four teams are supported administratively by an inpatient (admissions) coordinator and a service-line director. The teams are partially specialized diagnostically, although the size of the unit requires considerable flexibility and cross-training among therapists.

Multidisciplinary Team Management

Team management occurs on three levels—patient care management, treatment team management, and service line management. Patient care disciplines have separate lines of management. The matrix model of management is one in which a single treator reports to the team, the program (or service line), and the discipline-specific supervisor. Traditionally, disciplines have been responsible for professional development and continuing education, hiring, promotions, counseling, and terminations. With demands for cost reductions have come management staff reductions, and the lines between disciplines have become more blurred and management responsibilities more shared. While discipline division heads remain at Cedars-Sinai, many management responsibilities have shifted into program (service line) administrative accountabilities.

Figure 21.1 displays the change in the inpatient rehabilitation unit management structure before and after PFC restructuring. In the "Before" management hierarchy, the matrix of discipline and service line management intersected at each discipline's division manager position. Under the division manager were supervisors for each service line—acute inpatient, rehabilitation inpatient, skilled nursing/sub acute unit, and outpatient rehabilitation. Only the rehabilitation inpatient unit is shown. The supervisors from each service line reported to their own discipline manager. The division managers reported to the administrative director and the director's assistant. After restructuring, the administrative hierarchy has become interdisciplinary. All therapists report to a service line manager who may or may not be of the same professional discipline. The service line managers of acute inpatient, inpatient rehabilitation, etc., report to the administrative director. The discipline leadership role now focuses on clinical competence, recruitment, retention and continuing education; the service line managers role now focuses on the day-to-day operations of the unit.

Rehabilitation physicians, nurses, social workers, do not report through the same administrative hierarchy as do the other rehabilitation disciplines. In the current organizational structure, physicians do report through the medical director of Physical Medicine and Rehabilitation and then up into the department of Medical Affairs. The administrative director reports to the medical director but has administrative accountability through clinical care services hierarchy. Nursing services has its own administrative hierarchy in clinical care services, but the nurse manager on the rehabilitation unit meets regularly with the administrative director of Physical Medicine and Rehabilitation. Social workers have their own administrative hierarchy, so that clinical team meetings are the focal point of communication and accountability with the rehabilitation team.

Two groups meet regularly to complete a participatory form of service line governance and provide opportunities for program evaluation, monitoring, and change. The full staff meets monthly. The format of meetings provides opportunities for staff education, review of monitoring and evaluation data, staff updates, and brainstorming sessions. Because of the sheer numbers of staff that are able to attend meetings regularly, staff meetings are often dominated by physical and occupational therapists. If the full staff meeting is like the House of Representatives with representation determined by population, the Rehabilitation Operations Committee (Rehab Ops) is like the Senate. Rehab Ops includes equal numbers of members from each discipline, and therefore it has a more even balance of power by discipline. This group meets weekly and is a treatment oversight and problem solving group. About 50% of a meeting is spent on specific patient care problems and about 50% on programmatic management.

Role of Administration

In a system where multidisciplinary teams are managing patient care and program development and adaptation, the role of administration, in the position of service line manager, represents the organization, or system, point of view. The focus of patient care staff is inclined toward examining individual patient needs and away from the programmatic or aggregate patients' needs. The service line manager represents central administration demands for productivity, financial accountability, and quality care. The service line manager develops and promotes programmatic treatment approaches, including team models of cross preparation and intermixing discipline activities and clinical pathways and guidelines. The service line manager also is involved in continuing education for staff, converting discipline treatments learned in professional schools into collaborative team interventions and reinforcing multidisciplinary treatment models.

Multidisciplinary coordination and interdisciplinary cross preparation and cross-treatments are the reality of team treatment in medical rehabilitation, yet many young professionals have little or no experience in this kind of a treatment setting during their formal training. The service line manager's role has been to reduce isolationism in the disciplines and to create the experience of the "discovery" that patient recovery is enhanced by multidisciplinary team treatment.

As patient length of stay has dropped and management resources been reduced, there has been less opportunity for therapists to learn multidisciplinary and interdisciplinary approaches to rehabilitation. Diagnostic-specific clinical pathways should continue to provide the structure to shape and reinforce the multi- and interdisciplinary approach to rehabilitation. This chapter's appendix displays a portion of the clinical pathway for stroke developed by the interdisciplinary rehabilitation treatment team under the direction of the inpatient rehabilitation service line manager. In parentheses are initials for the discipline responsible for assessing and communicating each piece of information about the patient and his or her progress through the therapeutic program. Each performance area has shared accountability with at least two disciplines.

Figure 21.1: Organizational Structure Before and After Reorganization and Downsizing

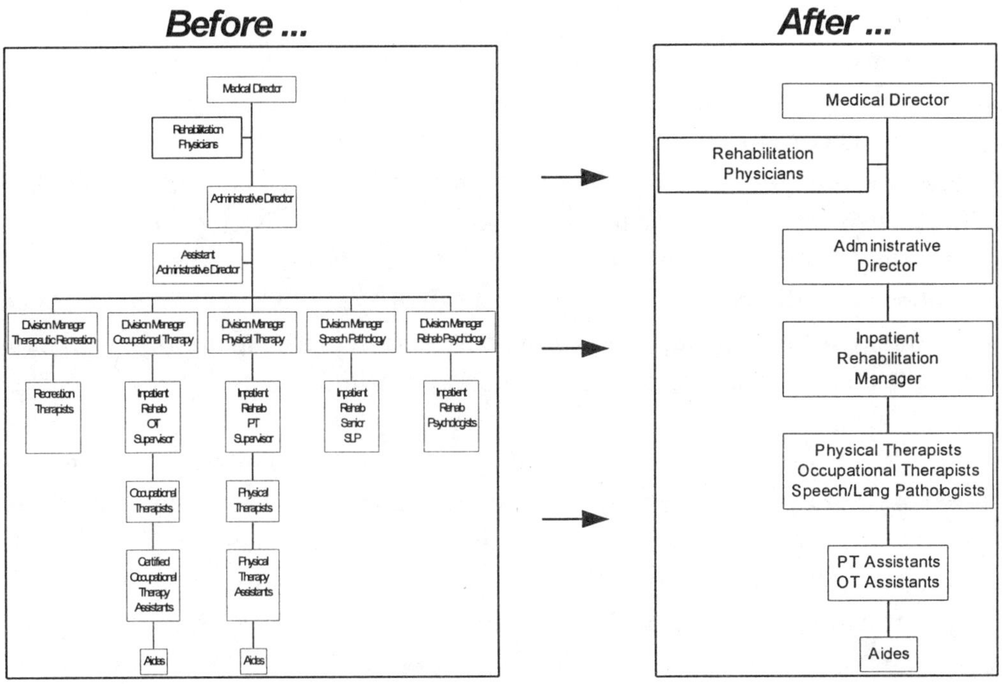

Program Evaluation System

The acute rehabilitation unit at Cedars-Sinai received its first CARF accreditation in 1989. The acute rehabilitation unit has been on the UDSMR for over two years and now has reliable data through post-discharge follow-up for one full year. However, the history of developing and using evaluation data to manage programs dates back to 1986. The role of evaluator grew out of the education coordinator, whose initial responsibility lay in monitoring staff licenser and mandatory training. In the rehabilitation team approach to treatment, care providers come from multiple sets of discipline training requirements. The role of evaluator has been linked to the evolution of multiple accreditation requirements—some within discipline and hospital-based (JCAHO) and some programmatically or service line based (CARF). With only the slim promise in the future that these multiple bases of evaluation may join to share a common format for information collection, reporting, and management use, the current job of education director and evaluator is a full time responsibility. Currently, information is processed with more than one focus, including the staff (e.g., continuing education, and credentialing), the patient (e.g., functional status outcomes), and the process (e.g., hours of treatment provided). Each focus or approach requires a different kind of data processing and reporting format, as does each accrediting organization.

The demand for evaluation results began with the accrediting organizations' requirements, and it has a lengthy history. Demand for evaluation results by program staff and team management has been less well organized. Program evaluation information has traditionally been "for them," not "for us." "They" had formal reports, but "we" had patients to treat. As a result, service line administrative staff assumed the role of advocate of the use of these data to represent organization's point of view.

"Stats" Meeting. Once a month the management group meets to a review of program statistics. The meeting includes the administrative staff responsible for treatment program finances, patient intake, continuing education and evaluation, and service line management. Intended to integrate program evaluation and cost data and program development initiatives, this group has until recently been supplied with only process and productivity statistics such as trends in admissions, deferrals, treatments, lengths of stay, and intensity of therapy. Discharge destination was the only outcome variable discussed. As more outcome data become available, this will be the group that will review and assess evaluation information and make recommendations for implementing program adaptations.

Reliable data on patient mix, admission functional status, functional outcomes at discharge and three months post-discharge, and acute inpatient charges have recently become available for management review and action on a regular basis. In addition, the UDSMR offers reliable comparative data for the region and the nation for patient mix, length of stay, and functional outcomes. An example of program evaluation data is displayed in **Figure 21.3.**

Figure 21.3: Sample Program Evaluation Report

Physical Medicine & Rehabilitation
Program Evaluation Report

Patients Discharged First Quarter, 1994

Total 110 cases:	Living	Premorbid	Post Discharge
56 Stroke	Environment:	100%	68%
31 Ortho	Home	(50%)	(22%)
8 Brain Injury	(Alone)	(50%)	(46%)
5 Neurology	(With others)	0	21%
5 SCI	SNF		
4 Amputee			
1 Arthritis			

Population	Age	Average Length of Stay	Admission FIM Score	Discharge FIM Score	Follow-Up FIM Score
Total Discharges	71 years	18 days	64.9	85.2	106.3
Stroke (n=56)	74 years	20 days	57.9	78.7	101.1
Orthopedic (n=31)	74 years	14 days	74.8	95.6	115.4
Brain Injury (n=8)	55 years	21 days	61.4	77.5	108.8

The outcomes management group might review the regional data from UDSMR that suggest that Cedars-Sinai rehabilitation patients are older and have a shorter average length of stay than similar facilities in the West. With the average age of all patients at seventy-one years, management must assure that the treatment program responds to special geriatric rehabilitation concerns, such as general physical deconditioning, community mobility, social networks and community supports, other chronic diseases and disabilities, and medications. Does the discharge rate of 21% to Skilled Nursing Facilities (SNF) represent difference in patient mix? Shorter acute rehabilitation stay? Appropriate use of sub-acute services post-acute rehabilitation? Or failure of the treatment program to meet discharge functional needs? High follow-up FIM scores suggest that patients are recovering to a high level of functional independence by the time of the ninety-day post-discharge follow-up. Once trend data are established, the group will develop program objectives with expected peformance levels as part of an ongoing process of improving organizational performance.

Informational reports are presented once monthly to the "Stats" meeting, the "Rehab Ops" meeting, and the Physician CQI meeting. The "Rehab Ops" report is forwarded to the director of quality management for Cedars-Sinai annually. Data are presented on occasion to the full rehabilitation unit staff in an educational format. The administrative director of physical medicine and rehabilitation is updated in regular standing meetings.

The central administrative staff, in this case the education coordinator and the inpatient rehabilitation service line manager, receive and process all the data for outcomes management. They extract and summarize the data. They then feed it back into the management process. Data summaries may occasionally be paired with suggested alternative actions. The staff have creative and effective ideas for program innovations, but little time to process and understand data.

Two factors have contributed to the outcomes management process being valued and used increasingly in the inpatient rehabilitation team management process. The first factor is the development of functional status assessment into reliable and common scales that span treatment to home settings. Having a common language to understand functional recovery has permitted treators to understand and evaluate their position in the sequence of interventions in an episode of acute illness and disability. The second factor is the development and availability of external referent data (regional and national UDSMR data) for patient functional status outcomes. The UDS FIM data provide a patient outcome benchmark by which the rehabilitation program can compare its effectiveness within commonly defined diagnostic categories.

Lessons Learned from Medical Rehabilitation Restructuring

Costs Associated with Outcomes Measurement and Management

The full matrix management structure of a multidisciplinary team, in which each care provider is accountable to multiple discipline, administrative, and program authorities, costs more than traditional management structures. The additional costs at Cedars-Sinai included management level individuals (usually senior and supervisory treatment staff) and administrative support staff for both disciplines and programs or service lines. As cost reduction became an institution-wide imperative, the number of management staff in medical rehabilitation was reduced by 50%. With fewer people to plan, supervise, coach, and perform management activities, some disciplinary lines have blurred. On the one hand, this has benefited the movement to interdisciplinary treatment and multidisciplinary program management. On the other, it has created a challenge by reducing the overall time available for outcomes based management.

Production of outcomes data is another cost associated with outcomes management. Costs include therapists' time to reliably assess patient functional status, clerical time to complete and check data forms, data processing and post-discharge follow-up costs, and staff time to summarize and interpret the results and support the process of outcomes management. Therapists would be rating patients' functioning as part of patient care, so the added costs are only marginal to educate and maintain reliable rating skills among these staff. It takes approximately 0.25 of a full-time equivalent (FTE) of clerical support and 0.25 FTE of the education coordinator to support the UDSMR system. Data processing and follow-up data collection cost the rehabilitation unit approximately $7,000 per year.

Regular annual costs for data collection, processing, reporting, and outcomes management can be anticipated when the health care system transitions from demonstration/research on patient outcomes to operational measurement of all or a truly representative sample of all patients. However, in return, one can expect to have informed managers making more cost-effective decisions, rational organizational change, and valid data for marketing to referral sources and payers.

Data Collection and Reporting Cycles—Expertise, Control, Reliability

While program evaluation and outcomes management have been part of the organizational environment of medical rehabilitation for several years, few decisions will be based on outcomes data unless the users have confidence in its quality and accuracy. During the five years between first CARF accreditation and production of reliable post-discharge outcomes data, Cedars-Sinai experimented with in-house methods of functional assessment and data collection. The organizational structure was set up to use outcomes data for management purposes, but there was no confidence in the data because there was too much unreliability in the assessment and collection processes. Becoming a participant in UDSMR and using the central follow-up data collection service has produced the first full year of data that staff feel are reliable.

Once quality of the data is assured, two additional factors emerge as being especially important to the multidisciplinary team outcomes management process—timeliness of the reporting cycle and ownership of the process of organizational change.

Timeliness. The service line manager and evaluator rely on education to establish the relevance of data that reflect the aggregate outcome of groups of patients and the validity of using outcome measures that are removed physically (in the community) and temporally (three-months post-discharge) from the treatment setting. With a time lag of three to four months between the episode of care and the reporting of the outcome of that care, care team members find it difficult to relate how they organized patient care to the results. Information on cost of care, on the other hand, can be managed both in a short and long feedback loop. Just as functional status assessment is used clinically to give feedback to therapists, the patient, and family on progress in treatment; direct operating costs can be used to give immediate feedback on alternative choices of treatment. In the aggregate, when the functional outcomes of patients post-discharge are known, cost can be rolled up and reported as measures of cost-effectiveness of care. The goal of management would then be to help staff begin to see the cost implications of their individual actions. Presented in an economic analysis of the "trade-off" between one treatment and another, cost-outcomes can be an equally powerful instrument of organizational behavior change.

Ownership of Change. Ownership of the process of change in participatory team management has several necessary ingredients. Regular participation in management meetings and accountability for the outcomes are two of the most important. At Cedars-Sinai, in a fast-moving and downsized organizational environment with care providers operating on varied work schedules, the first requirement is not always met satisfactorily. Physicians' and nurses' schedules are determined by patient demand (e.g., census, acuity, medication and ancillary scheduling), while the therapeutic disciplines maintain a schedule of individual and group appointments. The appointment schedule is more conducive to attendance at regular management meetings. Irregular attendance has led to the perception of physicians and nurses being less invested in team management and less accessible or accountable to the organizational change process being created in the team and outcome management process.

There have always been competing authorities in hospital organizations. Typically nurses, physicians, and ancillary services report through different supervisory channels. In the medical rehabilitation unit, the multidisciplinary team organizational structure has been maintained through the ancillary services administrative hierarchy. At Cedars-Sinai physicians, nurses, and social workers have each had reporting hierarchies separate from the physical therapists, occupational therapists, speech pathologists, psychologists, and recreational therapists. These latter ancillary therapy groups make up a majority of the patient care teams and have a single reporting hierarchy. All care providers work collaboratively as a team on the unit. However, the process of multidisciplinary decisionmaking and programmatic change is made more inefficient by the separation of accountabilities and authority. The people at the top levels of management do not always share immediate organizational priorities and strategies, despite strong agreement on overall mission and organization goals and objectives.

Pace of Organizational Change

At Cedars-Sinai, as elsewhere, it is difficult to locate, let alone implement, an orderly planning and evaluation cycle in the hurricane of organizational change being brought about in the health care industry at present. When one does find an outcomes management system, the rate of change from cyclical review of outcome data may be disappointingly slow compared to the rate of change being demanded by other external market forces. On the other hand, having an outcomes-based information system established in the acute rehabilitation unit will permit management to evaluate the impact of the major changes occurring in the organization of health services, including shortening inpatient length of stay and use of step-down programs and the continuum of levels of care, down-sizing, and skill mix reorganizations. In addition, if one could engineer the adoption of a standatd functional status outcomes measures, like the FIM, across treatment settings one could fully manage the episode of acute and chronic disease in which the acute rehabilitation admission occurred.

Medical Rehabilitation Model Generalizability

Functional Status Measures

Functional status, a person's ability to perform the roles and activities of daily life, is a powerful tool to measure recovery from the impairments and disabilities caused by acute life-threatening illness. If there were agreement on measurement methods, functional outcomes could be the *lingua franca* of acute hospital services outcomes. As current trend for acute care hospitals to divert patients who are younger, less acutely ill, and with fewer chronic diseases to outpatient treatment, functional status becomes a more relevant outcome.

Since functional status outcomes cross all levels of care, its use would sensitize staff to the patient experience of the continuum of care provided for the acute life-threatening illness or injury. Major advances in the prevention of medical complications in patients with catastrophic immobilizing illnesses have been made by introducing rehabilitation principles of early mobilization into intensive care models and acute care settings. Much is yet to be learned and could be fostered with an acute care management model that used functional status as a measure of outcome.

The field of medical decisionmaking has recently been advanced significantly by the introduction of functional status outcomes as a part of a method to establish the value of a service to patients. If patients can be informed about the likely functional outcomes of alternative treatments and the costs of those treatments, patients will be more likely to understand the trade-offs in medical decisionmaking. Patients will also be a more informed and an equal participant in the health care.

Case Management

Medical case management is the process by which a person's health care resources (financial, social, and personal) are coordinated and the settings and levels of care organized to achieve the best health and functional outcome possible. The process, which is becoming more common in acute hospitals as managed care and risk contracts are increasing demand for efficiencies, grew out of the medical rehabilitation model in the catastrophic insurance industry combined with the long-term community care model. Case management in the acute medical center manages the patient's recovery by placing the patient in the best setting to promote recovery, based on patient progress in recovery of medical stability and independent functional status. While case management has been an intervention adapted from a medical rehabilitation model, it has no standardized outcome assessment methodology by which its intervention can be evaluated.

Patient-Focused Care

Aggregation of patients with similar needs and formation of multidisciplinary and cross-prepared (interdisciplinary) care teams are characteristics of both medical rehabilitation care models and patient-focused care models. Using unlicensed trained staff as extenders of licensed staff has been the model of rehabilitation. With the formation of teams in rehabilitation, much attention has been focused on promoting successful teamwork. Acute hospital medical care has traditionally been multidisciplinary, but the model of care delivery has been one of independent practitioners or discipline groups working in parallel treatment streams. [4] This care model becomes a team care model when its collective sum of practitioners establish a communication process that (1) engages in patient-centered problem solving beyond each discipline's knowledge base; (2) develops trust and obligations among disciplines and between licensed and unlicensed patient care staff; (3) meets regularly to plan for patient care and programs. [5]

The current trend for creating patient-focused, multidisciplinary teams of licensed and unlicensed care providers in acute care settings mirrors the process that has taken place in medical rehabilitation over the past fifty years. While there is little research or theoretical literature on the subject, the field of medical rehabilitation has fostered several thoughtful articles that will help to direct the attention of planners to team building issues in the implementation of patient-focused care models in acute hospital health services. [6,7,8,9] For example, Halstead and his colleagues at The Institute for Rehabilitation and Research identified changes in the participation rates of team members during patient rounds after implementation of a team building experiment. They found that physician members decreased and patients increased their proportion of participation.[10] Experimental team members rated their group environment more egalitarian, open and innovative, and less leader dominated than control group teams in the same hospital.

Summary

Throughout the hospital care industry, outpatient and post medical/surgical services are being substituted for acute inpatient hospital days. Shortened acute hospital stays for many severe acute diagnoses are sensitizing acute care providers to the issues of patient reintegration into community and shifting the rehabilitative goals of the treatment episode into acute care management. While this will blur the distinction between levels of care, it will ultimately lead to increased sharing of programmatic material and management styles between medical rehabilitation and acute inpatient services. The medical rehabilitation model of organizing and evaluating care is a valid model to use to guide the organizational change process in areas of acute care hospital services where there are patients with chronic disease or functional disability.

For more information on the UDSMR, inquiries can be directed to The UDSMR Data Management Service (232 Parker Hall, SUNY - South Campus, 3435 Main Street, Buffalo, NY 14214-3007).

For more information on CARF, inquiries may be directed to the Commission on Accreditation of Rehabilitation Facilities, 101 North Wilmot Road, Suite 500, Tucson, Arizona

References

1. DeLisa JA, GM Martin, DM Currie. "Rehabilitation Medicine: Past, Present, and Future." in DeLisa JA, Gans BM (eds.) *Rehabilitation Medicine: Principles and Practice*. 2nd Edition. Philadelphia: J.B. Lippincott, Co. 1993.

2. Aronow HU. " Rehabilitation Effectiveness with Severe Traumatic Brain Injury: Translating Research into Policy." *Journal of Head Trauma Rehabilitation.* 2 1987:24-29.

3. Granger CV. "Health Accounting – Functional Assessment of the Long-Term Patient" in Kottke FJ, Lehmann JF (eds.), *Krusen's Handbook of Physical Medicine and Rehabilitation.* Fourth Edition. Philadelphia: W.B. Saunders, 1990: 274.

4. Diller L. "Fostering the Interdisciplinary Team, Fostering Research in a Society in Transition." *Archives of Physical Medicine and Rehabilitation.* 71 1990:275-278.

5. Halstead LS, DH Rintala, M Kanellos, et al. "The Innovative Rehabilitation Team: An Experiment in Team Building." *Archives of Physical Medicine and Rehabilitation*. 67 1986:357-361.

6. Schmitt MH, MP Farrell, GD Heinemann. "Conceptual and Methodological Problems in Studying the Effects of Interdisciplinary Geriatric Teams." *The Gerontologist.* 28 1988:753-764.

7. Keith RA. "The Comprehensive Treatment Team in Rehabilitation." *Archives of Physical Medicine and Rehabilitation.* 72 1991:269-74.

8. Purtilo RB, Meier RH. "Team Challenges: Regulatory Constraints and Patient Empowerment." *American Journal of Physical Medicine and Rehabilitation.* 72 1993:327-330.

9. Strasser DC, JA Falconer, D Martino-Satzmann. " The Rehabilitation Team: Staff Perceptions of the Hospital Environment, the Interdisciplinary Team Environment, and Interprofessional Relations." *Archives of Physical Medicine and Rehabilitation*. 751994:177-82.

10. Halstead LS, DH Rintala, M Kanellos, et al. 1986.

Appendix: Portions of the Rehabilitation Care Path for Stroke

CSMC Rehab Care Path: CVA					
Admission Date:	Time:		Primary Diagnosis:		
Estimated DC:			Onset:		
Actual DC:			Secondary Diagnosis:		
Team #					
Path Status:	**On** **Off**		**On** **Off**		. . .
Performance Areas	First 48 Hours Date:	FIM G A	Week 1 Date:		. . .
Medical/Surgical Stability	Medical Status (MD)	[ ][ ]	Medical Status (MD)	[ ]	. . .
	Bladder Mgmt (RN)	[ ][ ]	Bladder Mgmt (MD)	[ ]	
	Bowel Mgmt (RN)	[ ][ ]	Bowel Mgmt (RN)	[ ]	
		Date		*Date*	. . .
	b. Advanced directive discussed (MD)	__/__	*b. Establish B&B program (RN)*	__/__	
	c. Admission completed (RN)	__/__	*c. Establish nutrition program (RN)*	__/__	
	d. Fall precautions (RN)	__/__	*d. Meds teaching initiated (RN)*	__/__	
	e. Bowel/Bladder assessment (RN)	__/__	*e. Skin care training (RN)*	__/__	
	f. Medication assessment (RN)	__/__	*f. Initiate pt/caregiver training (RN)*	__/__	
	g. Skin assessment (RN)	__/__			
	h. Nutrition assessment (RD)	__/__			
Mental Status/ Coping/ Communication	Social Interaction (SW)	[ ][ ]	Social Interaction (SW)	[ ]	. . .
	Adaptation (SW/PSY)	[ ][ ]	Adaptation (SW/PSY)	[ ]	
	Family Support (SW)	[ ][ ]	Family Support (SW)	[ ]	
	Problem-solving (SLP*)	[ ][ ]	Problem-solving (SLP)	[ ]	
	Memory (SLP)	[ ][ ]	Memory (SLP)	[ ]	
	Comprehension -visual (SLP)	[ ][ ]	Comprehension -visual (SLP)	[ ]	
	Comprehension -audio (SLP)	[ ][ ]	Comprehension -audio (SLP)	[ ]	
	Expression -vocal (SLP)	[ ][ ]	Expression -vocal (SLP)	[ ]	
	Expression -non-vocal (SLP)	[ ][ ]	Expression -non-vocal (SLP)	[ ]	
	a. Safety assessment (TM)*	__/__	*a. Safety plan reviewed (TM)*	__/__	. . .
	b. Environment/stimulation plan (TM)	__/__	*b. Envir/Stim plan review (TM)*	__/__	
	c. ID coping mechanisms (PSY/SW)	__/__	*c. SLP evaluation completed (SLP)*	__/__	
	d. SLP evaluation initiated (SLP)	__/__			
	e. Psych eval if indicated (PSY)	__/__			
Functional Status/ Endurance/ Self Care	Bed, Chair, W/C Transfer (PT)	[ ][ ]	.		
	Toilet Transfer (OT)	[ ][ ]	.		
	Tub, shower transfer (OT)	[ ][ ]	.		
	Locomotion -walk (PT)	[ ][ ]			
	Locomotion - wheelchair (PT)	[ ][ ]			
	Stairs (PT)	[ ][ ]			
	Eating (OT/SLP)	[ ][ ]			
	Grooming (OT)	[ ][ ]	.		
	Bathing (OT)	[ ][ ]			
	Dressing - upper body (OT)	[ ][ ]			
	Dressing - lower body (OT)	[ ][ ]			
	Toileting (RN/OT)	[ ][ ]			
	Community integration (TR*)	[ ][ ]			
	a. Mobility plan complete (PT)	__/__			
	b. CSMC wheelchair issued (PT)	__/__			
	c. Bed/W/C positioning (PT/OT)	__/__			
	d. Self-care plan completed (OT)	__/__			
	e. Swallow eval complete (OT/SLP)	__/__			
	f. Out of bed 3 meals/day (RN)	__/__			
Continued Care Planning	*a. Evaluation initiated (SW)*	__/__	.		
	b. Caregivers contacted (SW)	__/__	.		
	c. Orientation to Rehab (RN/SW)	__/__	.		
	d. Patient goals defined (MD)	__/__			
	e. Referring MD contacted (MD)	__/__			
	f. Payor/Case Mgr contacted (IC)*	__/__			
	g. Info submitted to Case Mgr (IC)	__/__			

****SLP = Speech/Language Pathologist; TM = Rehab Team (coordinated by Social work) ; TR = Therapeutic Recreation; IC = Inpatient** Coordinator*

Chapter 22

Practice Guidelines and Reminders To Reduce Duration of Hospital Stay for Patients with Chest Pain

An Interventional Trial

Scott R. Weingarten, MD, MPH; Mary S. Riedinger, RN, MSN; Laura Conner, RN; Thomas H. Lee, MD, MSc; Irwin Hoffman, MD; Betty Johnson, RN; and A. Gray Ellrodt, MD

Objective: The acceptability, safety, and efficacy of practice guidelines have rarely been evaluated. Moreover, despite the recent development of guidelines and decision aids for patients admitted to coronary care and intermediate care units, few have been tested in clinical practice.
Design: A prospective, controlled clinical trial with an alternate-month design.
Setting: A large teaching community hospital.
Patients: Patients admitted to coronary care and intermediate care units with chest pain who were considered at low risk for complications according to a practice guideline (n = 375).
Intervention: Physicians caring for patients with chest pain who were at low risk for complications received concurrent, personalized written and verbal reminders regarding a guideline that recommended a 2-day hospital stay.
Results: Use of the practice guideline recommendation with concurrent reminders was associated with a 50% to 69% increase in guideline compliance ($P < 0.001$) and a decrease in length of stay from 3.54 ± 4.1 to 2.63 ± 3.0 days (0.91-day reduction, 95% CI, 0.18 to 1.63; $P = 0.02$) for all patients with chest pain considered at low risk for complications. The intervention was associated with a total (direct and indirect) cost reduction of $1397 per patient (CI, $176 to $2618; $P = 0.03$). No significant difference was found in the hospital complication rate between patients admitted to the hospital during control and intervention periods, and no significant difference was noted in complications, patient health status, or patient satisfaction when measured 1 month after hospital discharge.
Conclusion: These results suggest that implementation of this practice guideline through concurrent reminders reduced hospital costs for patients with chest pain considered at low risk for complications. Further study of the guideline is warranted.

Ann Intern Med. 1994;120:257-263.
From the Cedars-Sinai Medical Center, Los Angeles, California; and Brigham and Women's Hospital, Boston, Massachusetts. For current author addresses, see end of text.

Thirty years ago coronary care units (CCUs) were developed to care for patients admitted to the hospital with acute myocardial infarction (1-3). The number of patients admitted to CCUs has increased substantially, but now more than 70% of patients admitted to the CCU for chest pain do not have acute myocardial infarction (4-13). In fact, acute myocardial infarction is ruled out in at least 1.5 million patients admitted to U.S. hospitals each year (4, 5). The rapidly increasing costs of acute cardiac care, the growing suspicion that unnecessary CCU care may harm patients (14-16), and the pressing need to reduce unnecessary medical care led investigators to design practice guidelines to decrease inappropriate use of the CCU.

Practice guidelines "are systematically developed statements to assist practitioner and patient decisions about health care for specific clinical circumstances" (17). During the past decade, many published studies described the potential benefits of applying guidelines and decision aids to patient care (4-13, 18-24). Millions of dollars have been spent on the development of practice guidelines on national and local levels (25, 26). Despite these efforts, however, the effect of the use of guidelines on clinical practice and patient care remains largely unknown.

In this study, we examined the benefits, risks, and costs of implementing a practice guideline promoting a 2-day hospital stay for patients with chest pain who were considered to be at low risk for complications and in whom the diagnosis of acute myocardial infarction was dismissed. The study differs from our previous studies because it examines the acceptance of an early-discharge practice guideline by private practitioners rather than by physicians employed by a health maintenance organization, and it examines the effects of early discharge on hospital costs, patient outcome, and patient satisfaction (22, 23, 27-29). We hypothesized that feedback of guideline recommendations would substantially reduce the cost of acute hospital care without compromising quality of care. Moreover, we theorized that these benefits could be achieved through voluntary use of the guideline by physicians in private practice.

Methods

Setting

We did the study at Cedars-Sinai Medical Center, a teaching community hospital that serves West Los Angeles; it has an 18-bed CCU and a 32-bed intermediate care unit. Although a CCU director, cardiology faculty members, cardiology fellows, residents, interns, and medical students care for patients admitted to the CCU, most final hospital discharge decisions are made by private practitioners.

Patients

Men and women older than 30 years who were admitted to the CCU or intermediate care unit with chest pain between 1 September 1991 and 31 August 1992 were eligible for the study. Utilization review coordinators trained to interpret the guideline identified study patients. An earlier version of the guideline was developed by others (20, 21). We modified the guideline through the consensus of local experts and validated the guideline in several of our previous studies (22, 23, 27-29). Patients who satisfied any single criterion from the following criteria within 24 hours after hospital admission were not eligible for enrollment in the study: 1) acute myocardial infarction, 2) recurrent chest pain, 3) previous cardiac intervention, 4) a planned cardiac intervention, 5) a previous significant complication, 6) an ongoing intervention, and 7) an unstable comorbid condition. Absence of all seven criteria during the hospital stay defined low risk.

The Intervention

We evaluated the effects of providing to physicians a practice guideline that recommends consideration of early hospital discharge for patients with chest pain who are considered to be at low risk for complications. The study had an alternate-month time series design. During intervention periods, physicians received a structured message posted on patients' charts the day after admission that conveyed risk information and the guideline recommendation (Appendix Table 1). Physicians caring for patients at low risk who remained in the hospital more than 24 hours after admission were contacted by a utilization management physician via telephone. A structured interaction message was used to deliver the risk information and guideline recommendation (Appendix 1). During control periods, no physician contact was made. A 3-day "washout period" corresponding to the last 3 calendar days of each month was maintained to minimize contamination of control patients. There were 12 study periods (6 control and 6 intervention).

All patients who were admitted to the CCU or intermediate care unit with chest pain during the study period were reviewed concurrently by utilization review coordinators (n = 1531) (Table 1). Retrospectively, research nurse reviewers (who were not blinded to the original judgments of the utilization review coordinators) determined the correct risk classification according to the guideline based on complete information available in the medical record. The consensus of the two research nurses served as the ``gold standard" for risk determination.

The utilization review coordinator classifications were correct for 88% of patients (Table 1). Of the 13% of patients who were misclassified, 9% of patients were truly not at low risk for complications according to the guideline, yet the utilization review coordinators classified them as being at low risk (yielding false-positive results). Another 4% of patients were at low risk for complications yet they were not concurrently identified by the utilization review coordinators as being at low risk, and thus the intervention was not done (yielding false-negative results). Analyses were done and included all 375 patients with chest pain who were considered to be at low risk and who were admitted to Cedars-Sinai Medical Center during the study period (including patients with true-positive and false-negative results).

Table 1. Effectiveness of Utilization Review Coordinators in Concurrently Identifying Patients with Chest Pain Who Were Considered To Be at Low Risk.

Patient Truly at Low Risk According to the Guideline*	Utilization Review Coordinator Judged the Patient To Be at Low Risk According to the Guideline (n = 1531)	
	Yes (%)	No (%)
Yes	21 (n = 320)*	4 (n = 55)*
No	9 (n = 137)	67 (n = 1019)

* Patients included in the analysis.

Information regarding severity of illness was collected at the time of admission. A time-insensitive predictive instrument served as the study's severity-of-illness measure (5, 30). Charlson and associates' comorbidity index was used to quantify the number and severity of patients' comorbid diseases (31).

Patients were categorized as having either acute myocardial infarction, unstable angina, noncardiac chest pain, or unknown diagnoses. Acute myocardial infarction was defined as at least one creatine kinase MB enzyme determination of 3.5% or more.

The primary physician was the physician of record; this was usually the physician who cared for the patient before admission. One hundred fifty-five physicians served as the primary physician for the 375 study patients. Frequently, a combination of physicians was involved with the care of individual patients; combinations usually included at least one primary physician (frequently with a covering partner) and often a consulting cardiologist (often with a covering partner for weekends). There were 280 physician combinations caring for the 375 study patients. Because patients were cared for by many physician combinations, individual physicians could not be used as the unit of analysis (32, 33).

Outcomes

Patient instability at discharge was determined for patients admitted to the hospital during control and intervention months using the RAND instability-on-discharge measure (34). Patients or patients' families were surveyed 1 month after discharge regarding patient survival, hospital readmission, and other problems that might have occurred after hospital discharge. If confirmation of survival could not be obtained from the patient, Equifax (McLean, Virginia), a large computerized database service, was queried to confirm patient survival or death.

Patients were also surveyed about their health perceptions using a summary item from the Medical Outcomes Study short form (35). In addition, patients were asked to rate the quality of information they received from their physicians at discharge (36).

All cost and charge data were obtained from the hospital's financial database. Charges were based on actual prices charged for services rendered during the hospital stay. Charges were aggregated into routine charges (for example, room rates) and ancillary charges (for example, the price for two acetaminophen tablets). Total costs, which reflected the cost to the hospital for providing a service or good, included indirect and direct costs and were calculated after patient discharge from the hospital (37).

Statistical Analysis

Means are reported $\pm$ SD unless otherwise noted. The primary end points for comparison were total length of hospital stay, total hospital costs, and 1-month complication rates. End points were tested using a type I error of 0.05. Statistical analyses were done using the software packages GB-Stat (38), True Epistat (39), SAS (40), or BMDP (41).

One-month complication rates were chosen to avoid framing issues created by earlier hospital discharge. Complications were compared using a chi-square test or Fisher exact test. Confidence intervals around zero numerators were calculated using the method described by Hanley and Lippman-Hand (42).

Continuous data for the study groups were compared using the Student t-test, the Wilcoxon rank-sum test, or both when the data were notably distributed in a non-normal pattern. An adjusted analysis comparing the two study groups with respect to total costs and length of stay was done using a stepwise regression procedure. An initial model was based on patient entry characteristics (patient age, sex, admission source, preadmission residence, initial disposition, comorbidity index, and probability of acute ischemic heart disease). Factors were selected based on a P-to-enter value of 0.10. After the model was finalized, patient groups (control or intervention) were tested for inclusion in the model using a significance level of $P <= 0.05$. The SAS stepwise regression procedure, "STEPWISE," was used for the analysis (40).

We estimated savings in total costs and length of stay by calculating the difference in these values in the intervention and control groups (including outliers). Because the two study groups were similar and the predictive models had very low coefficients of determination (Appendix Table 2), this method provided a good estimate of savings associated with the intervetion. We had a second approach as well—calculating expected total costs and length of stay for each person in the intervention group, based on the control group models. For each patient in the intervention group, an estimated cost or length-of-stay savings was measured as the difference between his or her observed and expected values. Ninety-five percent confidence intervals were calculated as the mean $\pm$ 1.96 times the standard error of the difference distribution.

Results

During the 12-month study period, 1531 patients were admitted to Cedars-Sinai Medical Center with chest pain who were screened for entry into the study. Ninety-nine percent of medical records were available for retrospective analysis. Eighty-six percent of patients were contacted 1 month after discharge and surveyed about their condition. Information on survival status 1 month after hospital discharge was available for 99.7% of patients.

One hundred eighty-three patients with chest pain who were considered to be at low risk for complications were enrolled during intervention periods (1.12 patients per day), and 192 similar patients were enrolled during control periods (1.04 patients per day). The mean patient age was 67.0 ± 14.3 years. Fifty-four percent of patients were women; 83% of patients were white, 11% were black, and 6% were of other races.

Sixty-three percent of patients were initially admitted to the intermediate care unit and 37% of patients to the CCU. Forty-four percent of these patients were cared for by a cardiologist as the primary physician, 41% of patients were cared for by a noncardiologist as the primary physician in conjunction with a consulting cardiologist, and 15% of patients were cared for by a noncardiologist without a consulting cardiologist.

Final diagnoses for the study patients were noncardiac chest pain for 22% of patients; unknown diagnosis for 33%; angina or ischemia without infarction for 29%; acute myocardial infarction for 0.5% of patients; and other diagnoses for 15% of patients.

Severity of illness was similar for patients in the intervention and control groups (Table 2). Therefore, no significant differences were noted in physicians' admitting practices during intervention and control months.

Table 2. Demographic Characteristics and Severity of Illness in Patients Enrolled During Control and Intervention Periods

Variable	Intervention Period (n = 183)	Control Period (n = 192)	P Value
Patients with chest pain, %	25.4	23.7	>0.2
Patient age, *y*	66.6 ± 14.2	67.3 ± 14.3	>0.2
Sex, *% female*	54	54	>0.2
Admission source, *% from emergency department rather than physician office*	91.8	91.1	>0.2
Preadmission residence, *% from a nursing home*	2.2	1.6	>0.2
Admission location, *% to CCU**	38	37	>0.2
Probability of acute myocardial ischemia, %	33.0 ± 14.3	33.7 ± 14.8	>0.2
Comorbid conditions, *n*	0.90 ± 1.10	1.13 ± 1.35	0.08

* CCU = coronary care unit.

Physician Compliance with Guidelines

Physicians complied with the guideline in 69% of cases during intervention periods and in 50% of cases during control periods ($P < 0.001$). This difference showed that guideline feedback significantly changed compliance with guideline recommendations and physician behavior.

Compliance with the guideline (2-day length of stay for patients with chest pain at low risk) was higher when internists cared for patients (84%) than when cardiologists (58%) or combinations of internists and cardiologists (53%) (P = 0.001) cared for them.

Resource Use Data (Cost and Length of Stay)

The mean length of hospital stay for all study patients was 3.1 ± 3.6 days; length of stay in the CCU was 0.45 ± 1.45 days, and length of stay in the intermediate care unit was 1.62 ± 1.5 days. Use of the guidelines reduced total length of stay by 26% (3.54 ± 4.1 compared with 2.63 ± 3.0 days; 0.91-day reduction, CI, 0.18 to 1.63; $P = 0.02$); CCU length of stay was reduced by 47% (0.58 ± 1.95 compared with 0.31 ± 0.56 days; P = 0.06), and intermediate care unit length of stay was reduced by 28% (1.88 ± 1.68 compared with 1.35 ± 1.23 days; $P < 0.001$). After excluding an outlier in the control group, there was still a significant reduction in total length of stay (3.35 ± 3.1 compared with 2.63 ± 3.0 days; $P = 0.02$). These analyses were done by comparing patients who were at low risk according to the guideline.

A significant reduction in total costs of $1397 per patient (CI, $176 to $2618; $P = 0.03$) was achieved during the intervention period. After excluding an outlier in the control group, the difference was still significant ($898; CI, $172 to $1625; $P = 0.02$). The annual cost reduction was projected to be $550 000 per year.

Had we included all patients who were originally identified by the utilization review coordinators (including false-positive results for patients and excluding false-negative results for patients), a significant reduction in hospital length of stay (3.87 ± 4.27 compared with 3.02 ± 3.58 days; $P = 0.02$) and a reduction in total costs of $1232 ($P < 0.05$) were still achieved for each patient at low risk.

The yearly cost of the intervention was estimated to be $34 400. The total cost savings (direct and indirect costs) afforded by the intervention exceeded the cost of providing the reminder by a factor of 15:1, and the total savings for a 1-year period was approximately $515 000.

Use of cardiac diagnostic tests was examined 1 month after hospital discharge to exclude the possibility that shorter lengths of hospital stay had shifted diagnostic testing from the inpatient to outpatient setting. There was no significant difference in the use of treadmill examinations (17% compared with 12%; $P > 0.2$) and left-heart catheterizations (2.7% compared with 5.4%; $P > 0.2$) between patients in the intervention and control periods.

The effect of the intervention in reducing length of stay appeared to persist with time (Figure 1). Moreover, no significant change in physician compliance with the guidelines occurred during the study periods when reminders were discontinued. The control month with the longest lengths of stay was July (when new housestaff began internships).

Figure 1. Patients' Length of Stay Analyzed with Time.

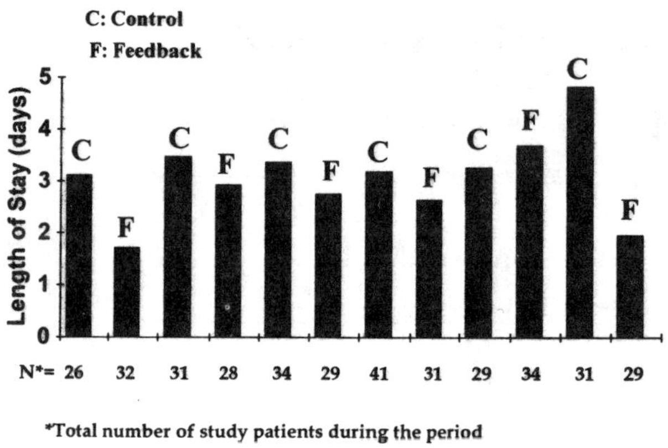

Outcomes

No patients died during their inclusion in either study group (0%; CI, 0% to 0.8%). No significant differences were found in the number of patients who had cardiac complications, in the number of patients who sustained acute myocardial infarctions, in the types of complications, or in the number of patients who required transfer to a higher level of care between intervention and control groups (Table 3). No significant difference was noted between the instability at discharge (0.08 ± 0.29 compared with 0.09 ± 0.29 instabilities; $P > 0.2$) for patients admitted to the hospital during intervention and control periods (34).

Table 3. In-Hospital Clinical Outcomes of Patients with Chest Pain at Low Risk

Outcome	Intervention Period (n = 183)	Control Period (n = 192)	P Value
Death, %	0	0	>0.2
Acute myocardial infarction, %	0.5	0.5	>0.2
Cardiac complications, %	5.5	4.2	>0.2
Iatrogenic complications, %	2.8	3.2	>0.2
Transfer to higher level of care, %			
To coronary care unit	2.8	3.7	>0.2
To intermediate care unit	0.6	1.0	>0.2

No significant difference was found in mortality rates between control and intervention groups when measured 1 month after hospital discharge (Table 4). More patients were readmitted who had been in the control group 1 month after discharge, although no significant difference was noted in the number of patients readmitted because of cardiac conditions.

No significant difference in the overall self-reported health status was noted between the control and intervention groups (Table 4). Also, no significant difference was identified in the number of patients who returned to work, the amount of time before they returned to work, the number who resumed recreational activities, and the amount of time before they resumed recreational activities (Table 4).

Table 4. Post-Discharge Clinical Outcomes of Patients with Chest Pain Who Were Considered To Be at Low Risk For Complications*

Variable	Intervention Period (n = 183)	Control Period (n = 192)	P Value
Mortality, %	0	0.5	>0.2
Acute myocardial infarction, %	0.5	0.5	>0.2
Hospital readmission rate, %	2.5	9.3	0.02
Readmission rate for cardiac conditions, %	1.9	6.8	0.07
Self-reported health at least good, %	66	61	>0.2
Summary health status item (lower is better)	3.04 ± 1.12	3.10 ± 1.17	>0.2
Patient able to return to work, %	90	89	>0.2
Time interval until patient returned to work, *d*	3.6 ± 5.0	3.7 ± 4.2	>0.2
Patient able to resume recreational activities, %	81	80	>0.2
Time interval until patient resumed recreational activities, *d*	4.9 ± 5.6	4.2 ± 5.2	>0.2

* Mean values are expressed ± SD.

Patient Satisfaction

No significant difference was found in patient satisfaction between patients admitted to the hospital during intervention and control periods. A similar percentage of patients would either definitely or probably return to the same hospital (94% compared with 94%; P > 0.2). Most patients in the intervention and control groups thought they stayed in the hospital for an appropriate length of time (77% compared with 76%; P > 0.2).

Statistical Analysis

The regression model for hospital length of stay and total costs is described in Appendix Table 2. The mean difference between the observed and expected length of stay in the intervention group was 0.80 ± 3.1 days (CI, 0.3 to 1.3 days), with the expected length of stay being greater. The mean difference between the observed and expected total costs in the intervention group was $1168 ± $3463 (CI, $662 to $1674), with the expected costs being greater.

We followed the 9% of patients who were misclassified as being at low risk and suitable for the intervention (see Table 1), yet they were not at low risk according to retrospective classification. We found that none of these patients died during the month after hospital admission. The readmission rate for those misclassified patients was not significantly different from that of control patients (8.9% compared with 9.3%; $P > 0.2$).

Two research nurses independently and retrospectively reviewed 82 randomly selected records to determine if the patient was at low risk or high risk according to the guideline. The kappa value was 0.94 ($n = 82$).

Discussion

Our study showed that concurrent feedback of practice guideline recommendations significantly changed physician behavior and resulted in changes in patient care. Feedback of the guideline recommendations resulted in patient care that more closely approximated care outlined by the practice guideline, without adding incentives, threatening sanctions, imposing administrative barriers, or adding other compulsory methods to enforce physician acceptance of guideline recommendations. As a result of this intervention, medical care for patients with chest pain who were considered to be at low risk for complications was provided at a lower cost. Moreover, the reduction in health care costs was accomplished without significantly compromising patient outcome or satisfaction.

Our practice guideline recommended early hospital discharge for these patients. Additional prognostic information is available 24 hours after hospital admission that is not available at admission, and this information can improve the accuracy of physicians' triage decisions. Mulley and colleagues (20) and Lee and associates (21) showed that patients with no evidence of acute myocardial infarction or cardiac complications 24 hours after hospital admission derived little benefit from continued care in the CCU. Earlier discharge of patients at low risk appears to be a promising strategy for safely reducing health care costs for such patients.

Our study contributes to understanding practice guideline implementation and evaluation in CCUs and intermediate care units. First, although many practice guidelines have been developed in the past, few studies describe use of guidelines for patient care (28, 43). The failure of many previously developed practice guidelines to be adopted by physicians is discouraging because the ultimate value of a guideline depends on its effect on patient care (43-46). Despite the vast resources and effort devoted to guideline development, disproportionately few evaluations of their efficacy, safety, and acceptability when used by health care providers in clinical practice are available (46-48). Our investigation is one of the first generation of studies to evaluate the use (or nonuse) of guidelines by physicians in clinical practice.

Second, we measured the effect of shortening length of stay on patient outcomes and satisfaction. By appropriately shortening patient length of stay through implementation of the guideline, we maintained excellent patient outcome and satisfaction that were unchanged from when care was provided without using the guideline.

Third, we examined whether decreasing length of stay would shift diagnostic testing from the inpatient to the outpatient setting. Previous studies documented that some cost-containment programs may have "squeezed the balloon" and shifted costs from the inpatient to outpatient setting without a net reduction in overall costs (49). The cost reduction afforded by our guideline intervention did not appear to be offset by increased outpatient diagnostic testing, although a more rigorous evaluation of outpatient costs after hospital discharge would have been valuable.

Fourth, we measured the efficacy of practice guideline implementation by hospital personnel rather than that of guideline implementation in a research setting (50, 51). As expected, a quantifiable misclassification rate was found when utilization review coordinators implemented medical practice guidelines, even when the guidelines were explicitly defined, extensively tested, and implemented by experienced utilization review coordinators (see Table 1). The misclassification rate of utilization review coordinators with lesser training and expertise may be greater. This study underscores the concern that the effectiveness of guidelines in actual clinical practice may differ substantially from their efficacy as reported in carefully controlled research environments (29).

Fifth, our study showed the possible failure of education alone to sustain substantial changes in physician practice patterns. When direct feedback of guideline recommendations was withdrawn, physician practice reverted to that observed before initiation of the intervention (*see* Figure 1). Even after the reminders were provided for almost 1 year, physicians frequently failed to comply with guideline recommendations when they did not receive direct and concurrent reminders. This observation may support the belief that education alone, and education accompanied by limited periods of feedback, may be relatively ineffective in sustaining long-term changes in physician practice (44, 45). Another possibility is that physicians became accustomed to the discharge reminder when caring for patients with chest pain who were at low risk.

Sixth, after the completion of our study, the Cardiac Advisory and Medical Advisory Committee at Cedars-Sinai Medical Center, which are composed of private practitioners and academic faculty members, approved feedback of the practice guideline recommendations. Feedback of the guideline recommendations has been occurring as part of the operations of the hospital's Utilization Management Department. This extra step of translating research findings to hospital policy would further suggest that practice guideline research could be used by hospitals to control health care costs.

Our study had several important limitations. The guidelines were disseminated at only one community hospital, and therefore the generalizability of our results to other hospitals and health care systems is unknown. The guideline dissemination strategy used in our study was labor-intensive, and not all hospitals have the resources and personnel available to disseminate guidelines in this manner. We found that the cost reduction afforded by the guideline intervention, however, substantially exceeded the cost of the intervention. Also, our study had insufficient power to detect small increases in morbidity, mortality, and readmission rates, as has been the case for many previous studies that investigated less costly strategies of caring for patients with chest pain (10, 11, 13,18, 20-23, 27).

Appendix Table 1. Physician-to-Physician Interaction and Written Physician Reminder To Communicate Practice Guideline Recommendations

For patients who are not discharged within 48 hours after admission and who are at low risk according to the practice guideline:

Your patient * patient name * may be at low risk for serious in-hospital complications. In fact, approximately 98% of patients similar to your patient suffered no serious in-hospital complications after 2 days in the hospital. If your patient continues to have an uncomplicated hospital course without chest pain, please consider if a 2-day stay is appropriate for your patient. If further diagnostic testing is absolutely required before discharge, please let me know if we can help facilitate any test for you. Only you as the primary physician can determine the most appropriate length of stay for your patient. These guideline recommendations have been approved by the Cardiac Advisory Committee and Medical Advisory Committee. Thank you.

Appendix Table 2. Multivariate Model for Lengths of Stay and Total Costs in the Control Group*

Variable	Parameter Estimate	Standard Error	*P* Value
Lengths of stay			
Intercept	3.90	1.82	0.03
Admission source	−3.70	0.97	0.0002
Age	0.045	0.021	0.03
Comorbid condition	0.35	0.21	0.10
Sex	−0.93	0.59	0.12
$r^2 = 0.15$			
Total costs			
Intercept	10243	2039	0.0001
Sex	−2101	1153	0.07
Comorbid condition	669	424	0.12
Admission source	−5944	2003	0.003
$r^2 = 0.08$			

* The independent variables considered in the model were sex (0 = female, 1 = male), age, admission source (0 = physician's office, 1 = emergency room), preadmission residence (0 = home, 1 = nursing home), initial disposition (0 = intermediate care unit, 1 = coronary care unit), comorbidity index, and probability of acute ischemic heart disease.

Another limitation of the study was that there were patients who benefited from hospital care after the second hospital day, and therefore the guideline could not replace careful physician judgment in making discharge decisions. This observation, however, was expected, and it reaffirmed the importance of allowing physicians to over-ride practice guideline recommendations when careful clinical judgment deems this necessary. Because chest pain may be a sign of many different pathophysiologic processes (48), the guideline should be used to complement, rather than replace, physician judgment.

The practice guideline evaluated in this study holds promise for enhancing the efficiency of care and improving health care affordability in the CCU and the intermediate care unit. We found that the practice guideline accompanied by reminders reduced length of stay and health care costs for patients with chest pain judged to be at low risk. Moreover, the reduction in health care costs occurred while maintaining excellent patient outcome, quality of care, and satisfaction. Our results support the future study of the described risk classification strategy and practice guideline at other hospitals and within other health care systems.

Acknowledgments: The authors thank Liz Gaddey, RN, Sylvia George, RN, Donald Hoytt, MD, Alberte Jacobs, RN, Carolyn Sharp, RN, and Vanessa Walker for help with this project.

Grant Support: By a grant-in-aid from the American Heart Association.

Requests for Reprints: Scott Weingarten, MD, Cedars-Sinai Medical Center, Department of Medicine, Becker 146, 8700 Beverly Boulevard, Los Angeles, CA 90048.

Current Author Addresses: Dr. Weingarten, Ms. Riedinger, Ms. Conner, and Dr. Ellrodt: Department of Medicine, Cedars-Sinai Medical Center, Cedars-Sinai Research Instititute, Los Angeles, CA 90048.
Dr. Lee: Department of Medicine, Brigham and Women's Hospital, Boston, MA 02115.
Dr. Hoffman and Ms. Johnson: Department of Utilization Management and the Utilization Mangement Group, Cedars-Sinai Medical Center, Los Angeles, CA 90048.

References

1. Lown B. Intensive heart care. *Sci Am.* 1968;219:19-27.

2. Lown B, Selzer A. The coronary care unit. *Am J Cardiol.* 1968;22: 597-602.

3. Day HW. An intensive coronary care area. *Dis Chest.* 1963;44: 423-7.

4. Fineberg HV, Scadden D, Goldman L. Care of patients with a low probability of acute myocardial infarction. Cost effectiveness of alternatives to coronary-care-unit admission. *N Engl J Med.* 1984; 310:1301-7.

5. Pozen MW, D'Agostino RB, Selker HP, Sytkowski PA, Hood WB Jr. A predictive instrument to improve coronary-care-unit admission practices in acute ischemic heart disease. A prospective multicenter clinical trial. *N Engl J Med.* 1984;310:1273-8.

6. Lee TH, Goldman L. The coronary care unit turns 25: historical trends and future directions. *Ann Intern Med.* 1988;108:887-94.

7. Pozen MW, D'Agostino RB, Mitchell JB, Rosenfeld DM, Guglielmino JT, Schwartz ML, et al. The usefulness of a predictive instrument to reduce inappropriate admissions to the coronary care unit. *Ann Intern Med.* 1980;92:238-42.

8. Fuchs R, Scheidt S. Improved criteria for admission to cardiac care units. *JAMA.* 1981;246:2037-41.

9. Goldman L, Weinberg M, Weisberg M, Olshen R, Cook EF, Sargent RK, et al. A computer-derived protocol to aid in the diagnosis of emergency room patients with acute chest pain. *N Engl J Med.* 1982;307:588-96.

10. Brush JE Jr, Brand DA, Acampora D, Chalmer B, Wackers FJ. Use of the initial electrocardiogram to predict in-hospital complications of acute myocardial infarction. *N Engl J Med.* 1985;312:1137-41.

11. Tierney WM, Roth BJ, Psaty B, McHenry R, Fitzgerald J, Stump DL, et al. Predictors of myocardial infarction in emergency room patients. *Crit Care Med.* 1985;13:526-31.

12. Goldman L, Cook EF, Brand DA, Lee TH, Rouan GW, Weisberg MC, et al. A computer protocol to predict myocardial infarction in emergency department patients with chest pain. *N Engl J Med.* 1988;318:797-803.

13. Young MJ, McMahon LF Jr, Stross JK. Prediction rules for patients with suspected myocardial infarction. Applying guidelines in community hospitals. *Arch Intern Med.* 1987;147:1219-22.

14. Falk RH. Adverse reactions to medication on a coronary care unit. *Postgrad Med J.* 1979;55:870-3.

15. Hackett TP, Cassem NH, Wishnie HA. The coronary-care unit. An appraisal of its psychologic hazards. *N Engl J Med.* 1968;279:1365-70.

16. Sykes DH, Evans AE, Boyle DM, McIlmoyle EL, Salathia KS. Discharge from a coronary care unit: psychological factors. *J Psychom Res.* 1989;33:477-88.

17. Field MJ, Lohr KN; eds. Clinical Practice Guidelines: Directions for a New Program. Institute of Medicine. Washington, DC: National Academy Press; 1990.

18. Eagle KA, Mulley AG, Skates SJ, Reder VA, Nicholson BW, Sexton JO, et al. Length of stay in the intensive care unit. Effects of practice guidelines and feedback. JAMA. 1990;264:992-7.

19. Lee TH, Cook EF, Weisberg M, Sargent RK, Wilson C, Goldman L. Acute chest pain in the emergency room. Identification and examination of low-risk patients. *Arch Intern Med.* 1985;145:65-9.

20. Mulley AG, Thibault GE, Hughes RA, Barnett GO, Reder VA, Sherman EL. The course of patients with suspected myocardial infarction. The identification of low-risk patients for early transfer from intensive care. *N Engl J Med.* 1980;302:943-8.

21. Lee TH, Rouan GW, Weisberg MC, Brand DA, Cook EF, Acampora D, et al. Sensitivity of routine clinical criteria for diagnosing myocardial infarction within 24 hours of hospitalization. *Ann Intern Med.* 1987;106:181-6.

22. Weingarten SR, Ermann B, Riedinger MS, Shah PK, Ellrodt AG. Selecting the best triage rule for patients hospitalized with chest pain. *Am J Med.* 1989;87:494-500.

23. Weingarten S, Ermann B, Bolus R, Riedinger MS, Rubin H, Green A, et al. Early "stepdown" transfer of low-risk patients with chest pain. A controlled inter ventional trial. *Ann Intern Med.* 1990;113: 283-9.

24. Lee TH, Juarez G, Cook EF, Weisberg MC, Rouan GW, Brand DA, et al. Ruling out acute myocardial infarction. A prospective multicenter validation of a 12-hour strategy for patients at low risk. *N Engl J Med.* 1991;324:1239-46.

25. Woolf SH. Practice guidelines: a new reality in medicine. I. Recent developments. *Arch Intern Med.* 1990;150:1811-8.

26. Brook RH. Practice guidelines and practicing medicine: Are they compatible? JAMA. 989;262:3027-30.

27. Weingarten S, Agocs L, Tankel N, Sheng A, Ellrodt AG. Reducing lengths of stay for patients hospitalized with chest pain using medical practice guidelines and opinion leaders. *Am J Cardiol.* 1993;71: 259-62.

28. Weingarten S, Ellrodt AG. The case for intensive dissemination: adoption of practice guidelines in the coronary care unit. *QRB Qual Rev Bull.* 1992;18:449-55.

29. Ellrodt AG, Conner L, Riedinger M, Weingarten S. Implementing practice guidelines through a utilization management strategy: the potential and the challenges. QRB *Qual Rev Bull.* 1992;18:456-60.

30. Selker HP, Griffith JL, D' Agostino RB. A tool for judging coronary care unit admission appropriateness, valid for both real-time and retrospective use. A timeinsensitive predictive instrument (TIPI) for acute ischemia: a multicenter study. *Med Care.* 1991; 29:610-27.

31. Charlson ME, Pompei P, Ales KL, MacKenzie CR. A new method of classifying prognostic comorbidity in longitudinal studies: development and validation. *J Chronic Dis.* 1987;40:373-83.

32. Divine GW, Brown JT, Frazier LM. The unit of analysis error in studies about physicians' patient care behavior. *J Gen Intern Med.* 1992;7:623-9.

33. Whiting-O'Keefe QE, Henke C, Simborg DW. Choosing the correct unit of analysis in medical care experiments. *Med Care.* 1984;22: 1101-14.

34. Kosecoff J, Kahn KL, Rogers WH, Reinisch EJ, Sherwood MJ, Rubenstein LV, et al. Prospective payment system and impairment at discharge. The ``quicker-and-sicker'' story revisited. *JAMA.* 1990;264:1980-3.

35. Stewart AL, Hays RD, Ware JE Jr. The MOS short-form general health survey. Reliability and validity in a patient population. *Med Care.* 1988;26:724-35.

36. Hays RD, Larson C, Nelson EC, Batalden PB. Hospital quality trends. A short-form patient-based measure. *Med Care.* 1991;29: 661-8.

37. Finkler SA. The distinction between cost and charges. Ann Intern Med. 1982;96:102-9.

38. Friedman P. GB-Stat. Version 3.0. Silver Spring, MD: Dynamic Microsystems, Inc; 1991.

39. True Epistat Statistical Software Program. Fourth Edition. Richardson, Texas: Epistat Services; 1992.

40. SAS User's Guide: Statistics, Version 5. Cary, North Carolina: SAS Institute Inc.; 1985.

41. BMDP Statistical Software Manual, Volumes 1 and 2. Berkeley, California: University of California Press;1990.

42. Hanley JA, Lippman-Hand A. If nothing goes wrong, is everything all right? Interpreting zero numerators. JAMA. 1983;249:1743-5.

43. Audet AM, Greenfield S, Field M. Medical practice guidelines: current activities and future directions. *Ann Intern Med.* 1990;113:709-14.

44. Lomas J, Anderson GM, Domnick-Pierre K, Vayda E, Enkin MW, Hannah WJ. Do practice guidelines guide practice? The effect of a consensus statement on the practice of physicians. *N Engl J Med.* 1989;321:1306-11.

45. Kosecoff J, Kanouse DE, Rogers WH, McCloskey L, Winslow CM, Brook RH. Effects of the National Institutes of Health Consensus Development Program on physician practice. *JAMA.* 1987;258:2708-13.

46. Lee TH. Evaluating decision aids: the next painful step [Editorial]. *J Gen Intern Med.* 1990;5:528-9.

47. Selker HP. Coronary care unit triage decision aids: how do we know when they work? [Editorial] *Am J Med.* 1989;87:491-3.

48. Eagle KA. Medical decision making in patients with chest pain [Editorial]. *N Engl J Med.* 1991;324:1282-3.

49. Schroeder SA, Cantor JC. On squeezing balloons. Cost control fails again [Editorial]. *N Engl J Med.* 1991;325:1099-100.

50. Schwartz JS, Ball JR, Moser RH. Safety, efficacy, and effectiveness of clinical practices: a new initiative. *Ann Intern Med.* 1982;96: 246-7.

51. Ransohoff DF, Feinstein AR. Problems of spectrum and bias in evaluating the efficacy of diagnostic tests. *N Engl J Med.* 1978;299: 926-30.

Source: Reproduced with permission from Weingarten SR, Riedinger MS, Connor L, et al. Practice Guidelines and Reminders to Reduce Duration of Hospital Stay for Patients with Chest Pain: An Interventional Trial. Annals of Internal Medicine. 1994;120:257-263

Chapter 23

Implementation of Clinical Pathways: Lessons Learned

Bernice Coleman, RN, MSN, CCRN
Maria Fe M. Mangila, RN, MSN, CCRN
Brigitte Failner, RN, MN

The development of evidence-based guidelines and pathways has been described in Chapter 17, while Chapter 18 provided practical recommendations for implementing clinical guidelines and pathways. Chapter 19 detailed the Cedars-Sinai Resource Management project, including the institution's development and approval process for clinical guidelines and pathways. This chapter presents implementation case studies for a number of surgical clinical pathways. Several clinical guidelines or decision points are also embedded within each pathway. The case studies describe "work-in-progress" and include implementation issues, methods for tracking pathway compliance, interim clinical outcomes, and lessons learned. Each of the pathways discussed in the chapter had already passed through the development and approval processes described earlier in the book. The chapter begins with a general overview of issues in the pathway implementation process and the involvement of each of the stakeholders in the system.

Implementation

Implementing clinical pathways requires deliberate planning, along with intense communication involving all stakeholders. The implementation process is also a time for revision and improvement of the pathway. Prior to implementation, the final versions of all pathway forms (i.e., guidelines, physician orders, pathway documentation forms, patient education materials, etc.) are completed and approved by all appropriate constituencies. Pathway development groups should be prepared and willing, however, to make changes as the forms are introduced to the staff nurses, physicians, and other caregivers who will use them. No matter how carefully the pathway has been developed, refinements will always be necessary. In fact, this refinement process is a valuable part of implementation, for it allows the project to move forward while also making provision for additional input from the professionals who will ultimately use the pathway. The following sections review the important constituencies and their respective roles in implementation.

BERNICE COLEMAN, RN, MSN, CCRN—Clinical Nurse Specialist, Department of Cardiovascular-Thoracic Surgical Nursing, Cedars-Sinai Medical Center.

MARIA FE M. MANGILA, RN, MSN, CCRN—Clinical Nurse Specialist, Department of Surgical Nursing, Cedars-Sinai Medical Center.

BRIGITTE FAILNER, RN, MN—Unit Manager, Orthopedics, Clinical Nurse Specialist, Neuroskeletal and Orthopedic Nursing, Department of Surgical Nursing, Cedars-Sinai Medical Center.

Multidisciplinary Clinical Pathway Framing Team (MCPFT)

The members of the Multidiscipinary Clinical Pathway Framing Team (i.e., the team developing the clinical pathway) are an important resource for reinforcing the concepts of the pathway and should be familiar with the details of the implementation plan before caregivers education begins. Plans for the implementation process, as well as all documents related to the pathway, should be presented to and reviewed by this group. This review also allows another opportunity to incorporate any changes team members may wish to make in the pathway or the documents themselves. If the case manager is not a member of the team, she or he should also be included in this introduction of the final implementation plan and pathway forms.

Departmental Sign-Off

It is also essential to provide a structure that allows all affected departments to have a last minute opportunity to approve the pathways immediately prior to implementation. Since constructing a pathway is a long process, many of the parties who were involved early may require a second chance to review the final pathway. This is particularly important with groups for which practice changes are anticipated. As described in Chapter 19, pathways link the interdisciplinary processes of care, clinical guidelines, and expected patient outcomes. It is essential that each interdisciplinary department "own" the work embedded in the pathways. Obtaining departmental sign-off facilitates this ownership process.

Education of Team Members

Staff Nurses. The major movers and motivators for clinical pathways are the staff nurses, and it is essential to anticipate and plan for the labor intensive time that will be required to help them become comfortable with the pathway process. Cedars-Sinai's experience indicates a need for both group and individual education sessions. Group education is helpful because it provides a forum for the exchange of ideas between nurses. It may change the opinions of some individuals about the pathways, and more importantly, it clarifies the process for those who may be less than enthusiastic about the change. Cedars-Sinai has found that those who usually approach change with an open mind will greet this change in the same manner. Likewise, the group process will identify where further work will be needed with those nurses who prefer things to stay as they were.

It is useful to have nurses who are either informal leaders or champions of new projects to attend the first sessions. This allows for dissemination of the message before all staff nurses attend the education classes. This step is also key, because it allows the presenter to get a sense of how much resistance there might be and identify those nurses opposed to the change. Because staff nurse support is essential to the implementation of clinical pathways, time must be spent in smoothing the process before problems arise.

While classes should be offered over an extended period of time, Cedars-Sinai project staff found that classes, which started one or two weeks prior to the actual implementation, were most useful. A large poster board was placed on each of the units following the unit's education sessions to display the pathway documents, including the pathway and related guidelines, physician orders, patient education materials, and information about the process. This marketing strategy reinforced information from the education sessions and provided a "conversation piece" for all who arrived upon the unit to discuss the planned implementation of the clinical pathways.

Even with the best education plan prior to the implementation of pathways, however, once the process begins a substantial amount of time is required to provide support and assist staff nurses. The need for one-on-one education cannot be overstated. The change is anxiety producing and, until nurses comfortable with the pathway process, some staff nurses may even maintain that they either never attended class or the information now is different from what was taught in class. In most cases, approximately two to four weeks are required for the uncertainty to pass. Once accustomed to using the pathway, however, staff nurses feel empowered by the process and become champions of it.

Physicians. Physician education begins in the pathway development phase and must continue at each patient-physician-health team member encounter. Simultaneous with staff nurse education, mechanisms must be planned to inform the physicians of the implementation process. Although physicians were involved in the creation of the pathway, the implementation plan must include them as well. Any physician with patients on the unit in question, including private physicians, housestaff, and surgeons, should be informed about and involved in the implementation. Successful implementation is dependent upon physician ownership. This was accomplished by identifying physicians to act as implementation champions and provide ongoing one-on-one education to their colleagues. The physician staff meetings, department meetings, and written communication detailing the planned implementation process, including the start date, can also be used to inform physicians. Physicians were invited to view the poster board on the units and voice their commands.

Other Health Team Members. Education of pharmacists, social workers, physical medicine and rehabilitation therapists, respiratory therapists, and others must also take place. Successful methods include one-on-one education at encounter sites, visual materials, and interdisciplinary staff education grand rounds. Health team members must be knowledgeable about the encoded clinical guidelines and the various team members' contribution to monitoring and evaluation of patient outcomes.

Go Live Implications

Actually initiating the pathways requires considerable support on the part of all team members. The major champions for the process at Cedars-Sinai were the clinical nurse specialists (CNSs). CNS efforts were invaluable in assuring that the implementation process went smoothly. The presence of the champion is crucial for answering on-the-spot questions posed by the staff nurses during the early implementation period. Initially, staff nurses are anxious, primarily because the process of delivering care has changed. This change means that the staff nurse may not always know the answer to questions posed by nurse colleagues or physicians. Support regarding how to address these real live questions in a time of uncertainty is essential. Once staff nurses become comfortable with the process, the difficulty eases.

Staff nurses will need to evaluate each patient individually to make an assessment and recommendation for their progression on the pathway. Setting up a process that multidisciplinary team members are allowed to participate and communicate is important. Communication can occur through team rounds, either walking or stationary, but input from physicians as well as all other caregivers is crucial. Typically, it takes about three to six weeks to develop a smooth communication process. Cedars-Sinai found that once the staff nurses were comfortable with their roles, they were excellent advocates for assisting patients toward discharge. Their planning skills improved, and each felt that she or he was making a real contribution to the progression of patient care. A major satisfaction for staff nurses, in fact, was seeing their ideas used to improve the clinical pathway document. Incorporating their input made the institution's commitment to the process more credible in the eyes of staff.

The above observations apply to the clinical pathway implementation process in general, regardless of which pathway is being implemented. The following sections describe the specific implementation experiences and preliminary outcomes for selected surgical pathways, including coronary artery bypass grafts (CABG), total hip replacement, laparoscopic cholecystectomy, mastectomy without reconstruction, and bowel resection.

Cardiac Surgery Pathway (CABG)

Four years prior to the implementation of clinical pathways, the Department of Cardiovascular-Thoracic Surgery (both medicine and nursing) undertook an aggressive and successful exploration of practices to decrease length of stay, with documented improvements resulting from the process. The cardiac surgery pathway for uncomplicated coronary artery bypass grafts (CABG) built upon these efforts and, following a development period, was implemented in March 1995. This section details findings from the first three months following implementation. Outcomes measured during this time period include the time associated with intubation, length of time patients stayed in the ICU, and overall postoperative length of stay for the pathway patients. This pathway was designed to reduce each of these times. Prior to implementation both medical and nursing staff had been primed to work towards these goals. (See Chapter 5 for a discussion of the PFC critical care staffing model and care processes developed to support these goals.)

During the three-month time period following pathway implementation, seventy-three CABG patients were on pathway. Ten (14%) of these were defined as outliers, or patients who experienced prolonged lengths of stays for defined reasons. Five of these patients (50%) had prolonged stays because of the wait required for transfer to an extended care facility (ECF). Other reasons for longer stays included wound infection, two patients (20%); physician preference, one patient (10%); and dysrhythmias, two patients (20%). These data were presented at a housewide oversight committee. The value of this committee is in its ability to plan and implement strategies to address common problems for units undergoing implementation. It is anticipated that additional ECF beds will be available in the future to alleviate this problem.

During the first six weeks of implementation, pathway goals were achieved, with patients on pathway showing reductions in the average time associated with intubation, length of stay in the intensive care unit (ICU), and overall postoperative length of stay **(Figure 23.1)**. The average number of CABG patients during this time period was 7.3 patients per week. The second six weeks saw a drop in the average number of patients to 5.1 patients per week and an increase in lengths of stay. The patients in the second six weeks were also somewhat more sick than in the first six weeks. Week 8, which shows abnormally high lengths of stay, was unique in that all patients were composed of DRG 106 emergent cases and their severity levels increased the overall intubation time and ICU stay. Additionally the length of stay for Week 12 is comprised of two patients.

Overall, findings demonstrated improvement in all of the areas defined above. The improvements, however, also reflect a combination of practice changes implemented prior to the pathway and the contribution of nursing to improved discharge planning and coordination. Observations about the process and lessons learned during CABG pathway implementation included the following:

Figure 23.1: LOS, ICU Stay and Incubation Time (hours)

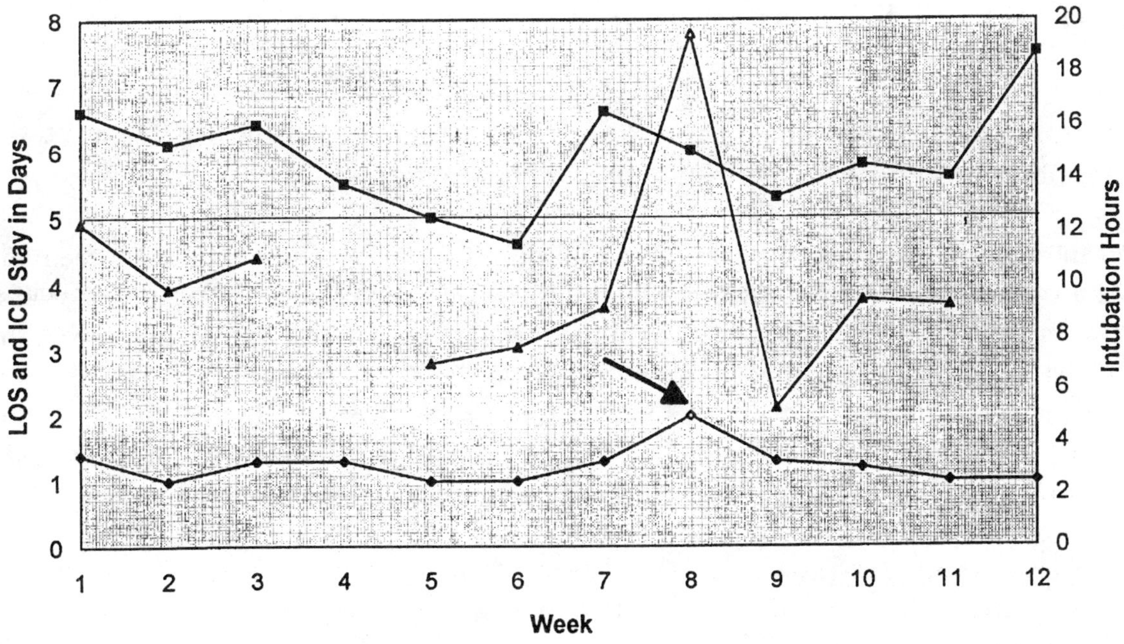

1. Preparation prior to implementation was beneficial in assisting the group in meeting specified goals.

2. During the second six weeks, the major focus was on revising the pathway process and documents and addressing staff nurse concerns. Less time was spent on coordination among the members of the care team. Subsequently, the group returned to the early emphasis on communication, and the team meets briefly each morning to review cases, which require particular attention that day.

3. Having a pathway that operates within a defined service line is valuable. It does, how ever, require a great deal of time to support the staff in the process while monitoring patient progress.

4. Lastly, the pathway implementation process requires a great deal of work, but the out come is positive and the completed pathway provides an organizing framework with in which all nurses, physicians, and other health care providers can work together in assisting the patient and family toward recovery.

General Surgery Pathways

This section presents "work-in-progress" for several surgical clinical pathways and focuses on interim patient care outcomes that were monitored during the first quarter following implementation in the surgical patient population (April-June 1995). The following outcomes will be discussed:

1. average length of stay,

2. the percentage of surgical patients who stayed on pathways vs. those who were taken off the pathway (compliance rate), and

3. practice issues related to the use of clinical guidelines (i.e. antibiotic use for surgical prophylaxis, early diet progression, and pain management).

During the pathway design phase, each multidisciplinary pathway subcommittee identified desired patient care outcomes for their respective patient populations. Baseline data on average length of stay (ALOS) and clinical practice issues, such as antibiotic and DVT prophylaxis, were obtained through chart review, practice review, and community benchmarking. Other outcomes, such as resource utilization, financial targets, and patient satisfaction, are monitored on a service line and housewide basis and discussed in a number of other chapters (e.g., Chapters 16 and 19) in this book.

Average Length of Stay

Length of stay data on three patient populations—laparoscopic cholecystectomy (fifty-one patients), mastectomy without reconstruction (thirty-two patients), and bowel resection (fourteen patients) were collected during the first quarter of implementation. **Figure 23.2** presents average length of stay (ALOS) data for these surgical patient populations against the baseline ALOS data. Three data sets are presented for these populations: a) prior to clinical pathway implementation (Pre-PFC II), b) ALOS for patients on pathways, and c) ALOS for patients who "fell off" the pathway.

Figure 23.3: Average Length of Stay

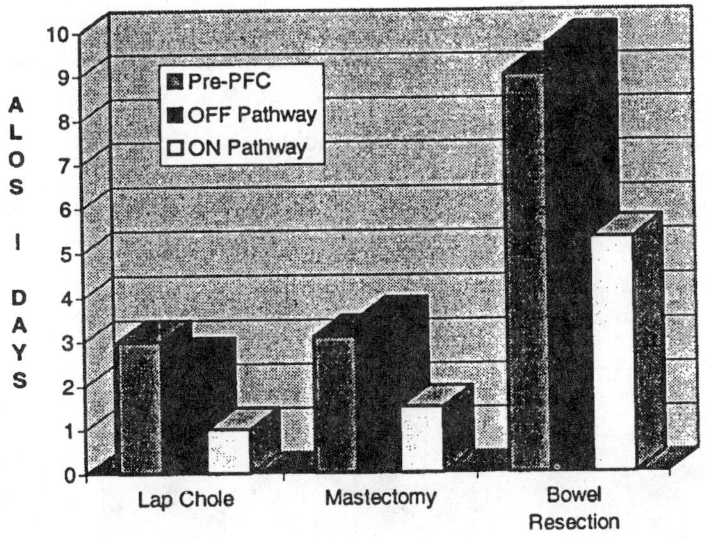

Data show a lower average length of stay for patients who remained on pathways. This decrease is attributed to the use of clinical guidelines. One of the criteria in the discharge guidelines for Lap Chole and Bowel Resection, for example, is the patient's ability to tolerate a clear liquid diet. The feeding guideline for the post-bowel resection was developed to serve as a guide for nurses to assess the patient's readiness for initiation of diet and to progress the patient's diet in collaboration with the surgeon. It is difficult, however, to separate external and internal influences for change and the decrease in LOS may also stem from external changes in health care delivery patterns such as physician practice and/or insurance reimbursement. In some populations (i.e., mastectomy and bowel resection), there was an increase in ALOS for patients who "fell off" the pathway. This increase most likely reflects an overall increase in the acuity level of the inpatient population. Approximately 50% of the bowel resection patients who "fell off" the pathway had lengths of stay only one day longer than that indicated by the pathway. Most of the lap chole patients who remained on the pathway had laparoscopic surgeries. Among both the lap chole and breast surgery patients, most of the uncomplicated (i.e., without comorbidities) cases are done as outpatient surgical procedures or twenty-three hour stay with follow-up support from home health care nurses. Consequently, the inpatient population consists largely of complicated cases, the elderly, and those with comorbidities and a higher acuity status. Other patient care outcomes that will be monitored on a long-term basis include measures such as: a) re-admission rates, b) level of functioning, and c) patient satisfaction.

Compliance to Pathway

Compliance to pathway is determined by the number of patients that stayed "ON" the pathway by meeting all outcome criteria until they are discharged. A patient is deemed "OFF" the pathway when unable to meet the pathway outcome criteria set for a specific day or phase. **Figure 23.3** presents the number of surgical patients who stayed on the pathway and those that "fell-off."

When patients are deemed "off" the pathway, the case manager is notified for follow-up. Then the reason (variance) for taking the patient off the pathway is documented and examined. Data related to variances or reasons for deviation from pathways are collected and examined for areas of improvement or the need for corrective action. **Table 23.1** presents the variances identified in the three surgical patient populations for the patients who "fell-off" the pathway.

Figure 23.3: Pathway Compliance Rate

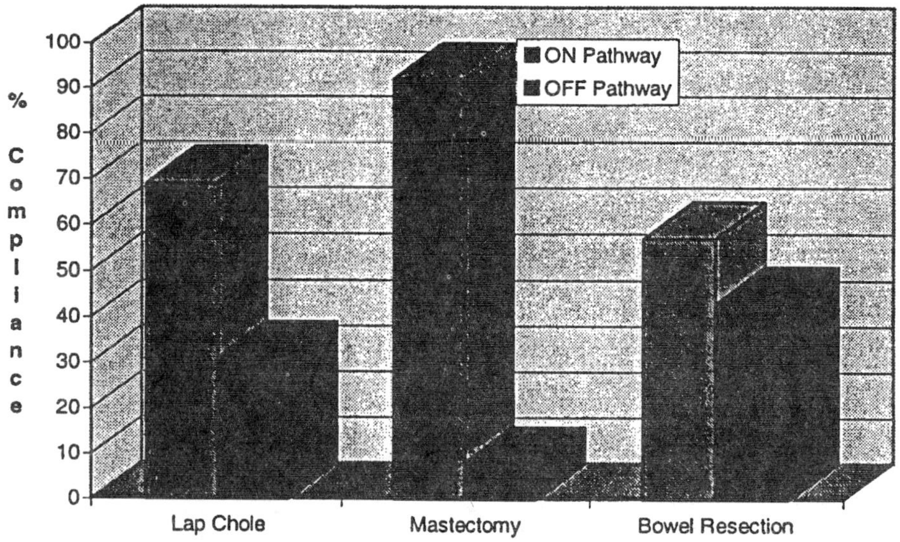

Table 23.1: Occurences of Variances

Patients	Variances	Occurrence
Mastectomy	Delay in testing	1 (50%)
	Low platelet count	1 (50%)
Lap Chole	Nausea/vomiting	4 (27%)
	Slow to progress diet	3 (20%)
	MD (practitioner variance)	3 (20%)
	Existing co-morbidity	2 (13%)
	Dysrhythmia	1 (7%)
	Uncontrolled pain	1 (7%)
	Concurrent lap procedure	1 (7%)
Bowel Resection	Metastatic disease present	2 (33%)
	Existing co-morbidity	2 (33%)
	Nausea/vomiting-partial SBO	1 (33%)
	Slow return of bowel function	1 (33%)

Variances related to the patient's clinical condition and comorbidities were resolved prior to discharge. Pathway revisions will include redefining inclusion and exclusion criteria for patients to be placed on clinical pathways. The main focus for improvement will revolve around further refining clinical guidelines (e.g., pain management guidelines and the use of antibiotics for surgical prophylaxis).

Clinical Practice Outcomes

The use of clinical guidelines has empowered health team members to anticipate and appropriately plan for patient care interventions. For instance, nurses can now take an active role in the patient's diet progression, discontinuation of IV fluids, initiation of DVT prophylaxis, and progression of the patient's activity as prescribed by the pathway. Earlier referral to other disciplines has also resulted from pathway implementation. For example, physical therapists see laminectomy patients in the ICU, and social workers initiate post-discharge referrals for mastectomy patients earlier. Other tools developed to streamline the process of care include the use of preprinted pre- and post-operative orders and population specific patient education materials, which assist patients' and their families' active participation in hospitalization and anticipate discharge needs. The pathway form serves as the interdisciplinary plan of care, which documents what is to be done, when it is done, and by which specific health team member, to achieve the desired patient outcomes.

Total Hip Replacement

The total hip replacement pathway was implemented at Cedars-Sinai in January 1995, following a development period. By July 1995, approximately seventy-five total hip replacement patients had been on the pathway, with complete data available for fifty-seven patients. Of these fifty-seven patients, forty-two (82%) stayed on the pathway, while three patients were not put on the pathway and seven patients "fell off" the pathway. **Table 23.2** provides detailed data on pathway compliance for the 47 patients on the pathway, including pre-operative education, antimicrobial and DVT prophylaxis, physical therapy, foley removal, and length of stay guidelines. **Figure 23.4** shows the actual length of stay for each of the forty-seven patients. Chapter 4 also details the orthopedic PFC care model that supports the physical therapy and other pathway protocols.

Challenges and Lessons Learned

Multidisciplinary buy-in is extremely important and requires time and effort to ensure that nurses, physicians, and other disciplines involved in patient care are fully aware of the clinical guidelines and pathway forms prior to implementation. Mechanisms to address variances in practitioner practices (i.e., peer review committees, division meetings, staff meetings) should be formed and utilized to address clinical issues and barriers to pathway implementation.

Table 23.2: Total Hip Replacement

Number of Patients	Percentage of Patients	
57	100%	Total number of Total Hip Replacement patients for which we have gathered complete data
3	5%	Patients who were not put on the Total Hip Replacement pathway
7	12%	Patients who fell completely off of the pathway due to medical complications

Of the 47 patients (82% of the total) who stayed on the pathway:

	Number of Patients	Percentage of Patients	
			PRE-OP EDUCATION
	13	28%	Patients who attended the Preop Education Class
			ANTIMICROBIAL PROPHYLAXIS
	22	47%	Patients who received the recommended number doses or less of antibiotics for antimicrobial prophylaxis
	25	53%	Patients who received more than the recommended number of doses of antibiotics for antimicrobial prophylaxis
			DVT PROPHYLAXIS
Of these 46 patients:	46	98%	Received one or more of the recommended types of DVT prophylaxis
	16	35%	Received only sequential compression devices
	1	2%	Received only pharmacological prophylaxis
	29	63%	Received both sequential compression devices and pharmacological prophylaxis
			PHYSICAL THERAPY
	45	96%	Started their physical therapy protocol on the recommended day - Postoperative day 1
			FOLEY REMOVAL
	3	6%	Did not have a Foley catheter
Of the 43 pts with a foley:	19	44%	Had their Foley catheter removed on the recommended day - Postoperative day 1
			LENGTH OF STAY
	36	77%	Patients stayed the recommended length of stay or shorter
	11	23%	Patients stayed longer than the recommended length of stay (of these, 9 stayed only 1 day more)

Figure 23.4: Total Hip Replacement Length of Stay Data

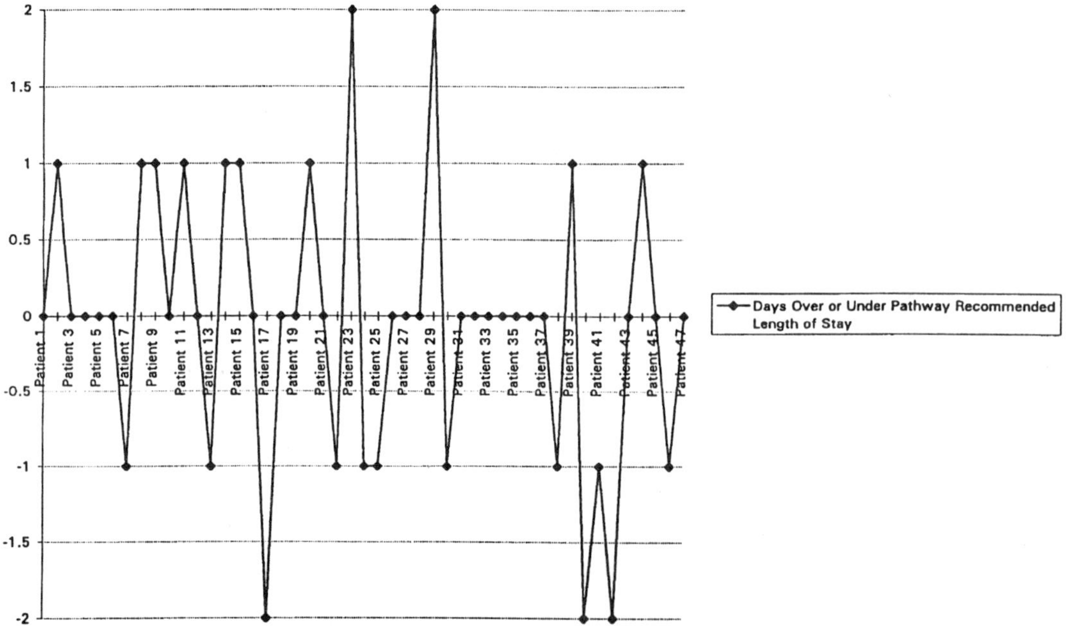

Planning for the patient's care along the pathway should begin prior to the patient's admission from the physician's office and continue through the pre-operative area, operating room, surgical nursing unit, and to discharge home with home health care or to an extended care facility. The challenge lies in ensuring that all these areas are represented, that adequate communication lines are established and maintained, and that the interdisciplinary team effort yields the desired outcomes.

Chapter 24

The Development of Obstetrical Guidelines: Monitoring VBAC Data

Kimberly D. Gregory, MD
Olivia Crookes, MB, BCh, MPH
Ken Fong, MPH
Lawrence D. Platt, MD

There is a well recognized, evidence-based consensus among policymakers that women with a history of prior cesareans should undergo a trial of vaginal birth unless there are medical or obstetric contraindications.[1,2,3] Despite multiple recommendations and endorsements, however, only one-in-five women with a history of cesarean currently undergoes vaginal birth after cesarean (VBAC). [4] Current literature suggests that 70% of women who attempt a trial of VBAC are successful regardless of the reason for the initial cesarean.

This case study was designed to describe the outcome of women in the Cedars-Sinai Medical Center population with prior cesareans in order to develop quality indicators and benchmark the optimal VBAC rate. The study was conducted by the Department of Obstetrics and Gynecology's pathways and guidelines team, which included the director of reproductive health policy, research associates, physician leaders (elected and hospital-based), labor and delivery, nurses, members of resource management, and members of information services. The team's goal was to understand why the Cedars-Sinai's VBAC rate (like the national rate) was low and to identify the ideal VBAC rate.

KIMBERLY D. GREGORY, MD, MPH — Director, Women's Health Policy and Research, Department of Obstetrics and Gynecology, Cedars-Sinai Medical Center and Research Institute; Professor in Residence, University of California-Los Angeles, School of Medicine, Department of OB/GYN.

OLIVIA CROOKES, MB, BCh, MPH — Research Fellow, Department of Obstetrics and Gynecology, Cedars-Sinai Medical Center and Research Institute.

KEN FONG, MPH — Data Analyst, Resource Management, Medical Affairs, Cedars-Sinai Medical Center.

LAWRENCE D. PLATT, MD — Chairman, Department of Obstetrics and Gynecology, Division of Maternal-Fetal Medicine, Cedars-Sinai Medical Center and Research Institute; Professor, University of California-Los Angeles, School of Medicine.

Evaluation of the Problem

The unified hospital discharge database was used to identify all women with a history of prior cesareans based on ICD-9CM discharge code 654.2. A data set was created that included all ICD-9CM procedures and diagnostic codes for each patient.

Women with cesarean section procedure codes 74.0-74.9 were considered to have had a repeat cesarean section. Women without a cesarean procedure code were identified as successful VBACs. Team researchers developed a mutually exclusive hierarchy supported by clinical chart review that separated women into the following categories: [5]

1. successful VBAC	(654.2 + vaginal delivery code)
2. attempted VBAC, unsuccessful (repeat cesarean)	(654.2 + c/s code + ICD-9CM code for dystocia, fetal distress, and cord prolapse)*
3. VBAC not attempted (repeat cesarean, clinically indicated)	(654.2 + cesarean code + ICD-9CM codes for breech and other maternal, medical and obstetrical indications)[6]
4. VBAC not attempted (repeat cesarean, elective)	(654.2 + cesarean section code excludes concurrent ICD-9CM codes in categories 2 or 3 above

* (Submitted elsewhere; details available from author by request.)

The team then looked at successful VBAC, unsuccessful VBAC, and elective cesarean rates and calculated the percentage of successful VBAC relative to all attempted VBAC. Evidence from the literature was used to derive a theoretical optimal benchmark.

Patients

The patient cohort included 854 women with a history of a prior cesarean. The population was racially and culturally diverse: 48% Caucasian, 28% African American, 16% Hispanic, and 8% Asian. The mean maternal age was 31.8 years. The median number of prior pregnancies was three, and the median number of prior births was one. The mean gestational age at delivery was 38.7 weeks, and the mean birth weight was 3,375 grams. Median neonatal Apgar scores were eight and nine at one and five minutes respectively. The patients were distributed amongst the resident service (n=79), staff model HMO (n=206) and the private service (n=569). Eighty-two private doctors were represented by the patient cohort.

Figure 24.1: Flow Diagram of Patient Outcome

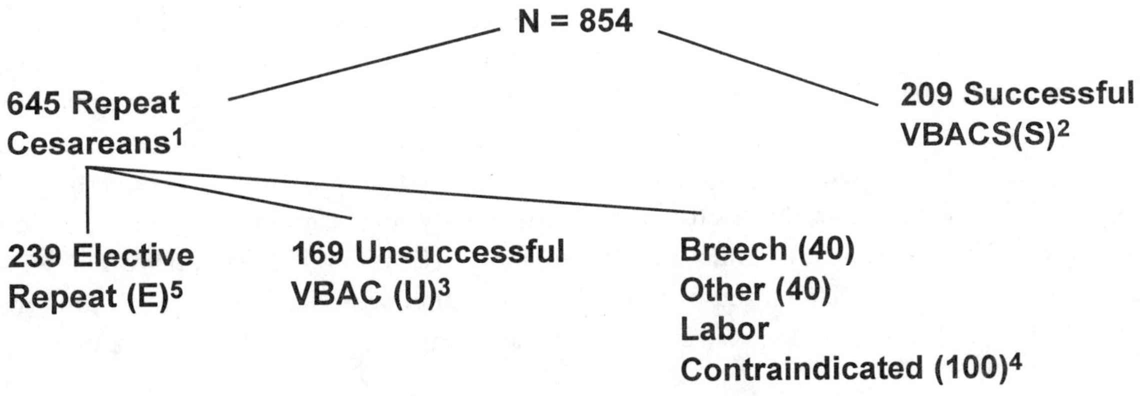

$$\text{Attempted VBAC} = \frac{\text{Successful + Unsuccessful}}{\text{all prior cesareans}}$$

$$\text{Absolute VBAC Success rate} = \frac{\text{Successful VBAC}}{\text{Attempted VBAC}}$$

$$\text{Maximal VBAC Candidates} = (S+U+E)$$

$$\text{Optimal Success Rate} = \frac{(S+U+E)\ (\text{ideal success rate})}{\text{all prior cesareans}}$$

KEY:

1. **Repeat Cesareans - all women who had repeat procedures. Includes patients who attempted VBAC and failed.**
2. **Successful trial of labor after prior cesarean**
3. **Attempted VBAC, but unsuccessful. These women had clinical indications for repeat cesarean**
4. **Clinical contraindication to labor: includes women withprior uterine surgery, classical cesareans, uterine rupture and malpresentation.**
5. **Elective Repeat Cesareans: Did not attempt VBAC, no clinical contraindications to labor, potential VBAC candidates.**

Results: Patient Outcome

Figure 24.1 is a flow diagram of patient outcome. Two hundred and nine women had a successful VBAC for a traditional VBAC rate of 24.5% (209 successful VBAC/854 prior cesareans). One hundred and sixty-nine women had clinical ICD-9CM codes for dystocia or fetal distress. These clinical diagnosis are consistent with attempted trial of labor (or unsuccessful VBAC). An additional 237 women had other indications for cesarean: breech (40), labor contraindicated (100), and other (97). Hence, 47.5% (169+237/854) of repeat cesareans were clinically indicated procedures. Approximately 28% (239/854) of women in the cohort had an elective repeat cesarean without attempting VBAC. This represented 37.1% (239/645) of all repeat cesareans and 28% (239/854) of all women with prior cesareans. The VBAC attempt rate for the hospital was 44.3% (378/854), and the absolute successful VBAC rate was 55.3% (209 successful VBAC/378 attempted VBAC).

Analysis of procedures by doctor revealed variation in attempted VBAC, successful VBAC and elective cesarean rates. Twenty-two physicians had one or less women with prior cesareans. These doctors were excluded from further analysis. Twelve doctors did not attempt any VBACs and had a 100% elective repeat cesarean rate. Twenty-six physicians had variable attempted VBAC rates, but 100% successful VBAC of those patients tried. The remaining twenty-six physicians had variable attempted, successful and elective cesarean rates.

Future Plans

This information is being collected quarterly and sent to physicians via the Department Peer Review Committee. Each report is physician specific and allows the practitioner to evaluate their statistics relative to their colleagues. In addition, physicians who do not attempt any VBACs are being approached individually by elected physician leaders in an effort to encourage compliance with American College of Obstetrics and Gynecology guidelines.

The team is looking at the intrapartum management of labor by different physicians in an effort to understand why some physicians are very successful at VBAC (i.e., 100% success rate) and why others are less successful. More importantly, the absolute success rate (successful VBAC/attempted VBAC) was only 55.3%. This is below the 70% to 80% success rate quoted in the literature. Explanations for this low success rate include suboptimal trials, recurrent obstetric indications, and patients changing their mind and opting for repeat cesareans after a trial of labor has been started.

Figure 24.2: Flow Diagram for VBAC Goal

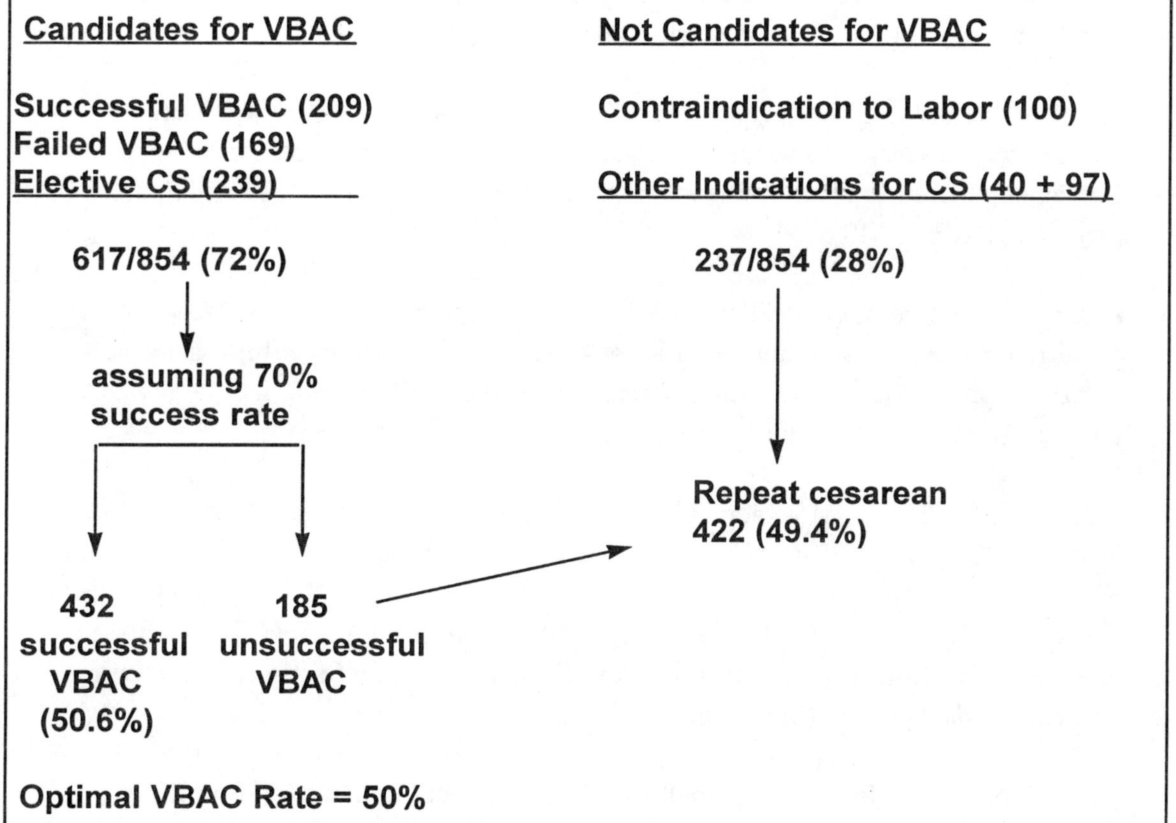

Hypothesis/Benchmarking Goal

The optimal VBAC rate is a function of the successful VBACs, the unsuccessful VBACs and the elective repeat cesareans. Women who fail VBAC (i.e., principal indication for procedure was dystocia or fetal distress) are candidates for process interventions that maximize their potential for vaginal delivery. For example, active management of labor protocols could lower the incidence of cesareans for dystocia. Timing of inductions and use of prophylactic amnioinfusions could lower the incidence of cesareans for fetal distress. Likewise, women who undergo elective cesarean are candidates for VBAC. In the Cedars-Sinai Medical Center patient population, if all the women who had successful VBAC (209) and attempted VBAC (dystocia 129, fetal distress 40) and elective cesareans (239) attempted VBAC, the hospital would have had an attempted VBAC rate of 72% (617/854). Assuming 70% success rate among women who attempt a trial of labor, 432 women would have successful VBACs. This would yield an optimal VBAC rate of 50.6% (432/854). The team has set 50% as the department's goal for an optimal traditional VBAC rate (see **Figure 24.2**). Clinical practice guidelines for cesarean indications are being developed to achieve this goal.

References

1. Cesarean Childbirth. Report of the NICHD Task Force on Cesarean Childbirth. Publication no. 82.2087. Bethesda, Maryland: United States Department of Health and Human Services, National Institute of Health, 1981.

2. Panel of the National Consensus Conference on Aspects of Cesarean Birth. Indications for Cesarean Section: Final statement of the Panel of the National Consensus Conference on Aspects on Cesarean Birth. *Canadian Medical Association Journal* 134 1986; 1348-52.

3. American College of Obstetrics and Gynecologists, Committee on Obstetrics: Maternal and Fetal Medicine. Guidelines for Vaginal Delivery after a Previous Cesarean Birth. ACOG Committee Opinion No.64. Washington, DC: *American College of Obstetrics and Gynecologists,* 1988.

4. Taffel SM, PJ Placek , M Moien , CL Kosary. 1989 "US Cesarean Section Rate Steadies-VBAC Rate Rises to Nearly One in Five." *Birth* 18 1991: 73-7.

5. Henry OA, KD Gregory , DJ Hobel , LP Platt. "Using the ICD-9 Coding System to Identify Indications for Both Primary and Repeat Cesarean Section." *American Journal of Public Health* (in press).

6. Gregory KD, OA Henry , CJ Hobel, LP Platt. "Repeat Cesareans: How Many are Elective." *Obstetrics Gynecology* 84 1994: 574-8.

Chapter 25

Cost-Effective Methods of Delivering Bronchodilators With Equivalent Health Outcomes

Zab Mohsenifar, MD

To control rising health care costs for patients with chronic obstructive pulmonary disease (COPD), investigators have compared the efficacy of bronchodilators delivered by an updraft nebulizer (UDN), which is labor-intensive and costly, to that of the metered dose inhaler (MDI), which is self-administered and less costly. Results show that these two therapeutic modalities have equivalent efficacy; however, the cost of bronchodilators delivered by MDI is one-third of the cost of bronchodilators delivered by the therapist (UDN). This chapter reviews the relevant literature and describes the randomized trail and subsequent audits performed by researchers at Cedars-Sinai Medical Center.

Updraft Nebulizers vs. Metered Dose Inhalers

Single Treatment Outcomes

Between 1980-85, five studies in the literature compared the outcomes of patients who received single treatments with UDN to MDI.[1-5] Stauder and Hidinger compared the effect of Terbutaline delivered by UDN and MDI and concluded that the two modalities were approximately equally effective.[2] Tarala, et al. reported that seven inhalations of Salbutamol delivered by MDI achieved maximal bronchodilation.[3] Even then, however, a subsequent UDN treatment with Salbutamol improved the forced expired volume in one second (FEV1) by a small, but statistically significant, amount. The authors concluded that these two methods of delivery were approximately equivalent; however, two to three inhalations from MDI might not be as effective. The clinical advantage of UDN was discussed by Moss, et al. who, through a double-blind and cross-evaluation of Metaproterenol in patients with acute exacerbation of COPD, demonstrated that improvement in FEV1 was much greater with UDN than MDI.[4] Berenberg, et al. found that these two modalities were approximately the same with respect to their bronchodilatory effect.[5] These studies all compared a single treatment of UDN with MDI.

ZAB MOHSENIFAR, MD— Director, Respiratory Therapy, Cedars-Sinai Medical Center; Professor of Medicine, University of California-Los Angeles, School of Medicine.

MDI With Enhancing Devices

Konig reviewed the use of spacer devices with MDI and identified numerous studies that demonstrated that MDI plus an enhancing device was as effective, or, in some cases, better than delivery by a UDN.[6] Jenkins, et al. investigated the efficacy of Albuterol delivered by MDI in patients with stable chronic obstructive lung disease and found no difference between MDI and UDN with respect to daily peak expiratory flow rates, severity of symptoms, requirement for additional bronchodilator use, and/or follow-up assessment of spirometry, peak flow, and exercise tolerance.[7] Summer, et al. studied thirty-six acutely ill hospitalized patients with chronic obstructive airways disease and found that MDI with a spacer device was the preferred approach if the clinical status of the patient permits its use.[8] The investigators extrapolated their data to their institution and predicted close to $200,000 in savings annually by widespread use of MDI. An interesting feature of the Summer, et al. study was their implementation of MDI during the initial days of hospitalization, in contrast to current practice in most institutions, where the MDI is generally prescribed towards the end of hospitalization.

Kim, et al. compared oropharyngeal deposition of the inhaled bronchodilators with ancillary devices and noted that with the use of delivery enhancing devices, oropharyngeal deposition decreased significantly and that aerosol delivery into the lung was 26% to 62% with the AeroChamber, 34% to 60% with InspirEase, and 31% to 92% with a Nebuhaler.[9] In the study, lung deposition did not improve significantly with small-sized delivery enhancing devices such as AeroChamber, as opposed to large-sized devices such as Nebuhaler. Similar observations were made by Newman, et al.[10] Fairshter demonstrated that the use of delivery enhancing devices increased bronchodilation from MDI; however, the authors concluded that the superior bronchodilatory effect of UDN was only evident on partial expiratory flow volume curves, attributing that observation to airways hysteresis.[11] Therefore, he suggested that physiologic methods that require deep inhalation would be less sensitive in detecting bronchodilation and may not be an appropriate technique for detecting small changes in lung function. Turner, et al. studied a group of patients with acute airways obstruction and found that using a delivery enhancing device could eliminate concerns about the ability of patients to use the MDI effectively, allowing the use of MDI in an acute setting, even in the emergency room.[12]

Interestingly, Turner, et al. felt there was no demonstrable advantage to the use of continuous flow nebulizer over MDI, even in an emergency room setting. Morely, et al. studied the efficacy of MDI in status asthmaticus and compared the spirometric data obtained after the use of MDI to that of UDN.[13] They found that, despite the superiority of nebulizer therapy in the initial phase of hospitalization, the duration of hospitalization and daily rates of spirometric improvement were not significantly different amongst the treatment groups. In addition, the authors concluded that by increasing the number of inhalations by MDI, one could achieve equal efficacy with MDI as compared to UDN. Mestitz, et al. compared Terbutaline administered by UDN and MDI in a double-blind crossover fashion and found that the doses of MDI and UDN chosen produced the same degrees of bronchodilation.[14] The dose of MDI used in the study was approximately one-half of the dose of bronchodilator used by the UDN. These authors felt that the patient preference for UDN reflected a preference for higher doses of bronchodilator delivered by the UDN rather than a preference for the delivery method. They found that 2.5 mg of nebulized Terbutaline produced the same bronchodilation in their patients as 1.25 mg of Terbutaline delivered by MDI (this dose of bronchodilator delivered by MDI is approximately 2½ times the customary dose delivered by MDI). This particular study supported the growing belief that the dose, rather than the delivery method, is the key to response and should contribute to the increasing use of MDI.

Bronchodilator Dosage Effects

Numerous studies have examined the wide range of bronchodilator effects of varying doses nebulized by UDN vs. MDI.[2,15,16,17] Finding from these studies imply that, although nebulizers are less effective than MDI, this lack of efficacy is compensated by the strikingly higher doses of bronchodilators used by UDN. The use of higher doses of bronchodilators through MDI has raised questions of safety, but the dose of bronchodilator delivered by the UDN exceeds that of the bronchodilators delivered by MDI by 50- to 80-fold, and these regimens, in general, have not resulted in any increased cardiac complications or hemodynamic side effects. Many patients with acute exacerbation of COPD are generally tachypneic and this problem, in general, makes the optimal use of MDI difficult. This concern may be one of the main reasons that physicians have resisted using MDIs, at least in the early course of these patients' admissions. Berry, et al. compared the efficacy of bronchodilator delivered by UDN and MDI in acutely ill patients with severe chronic obstructive lung disease.[18] They found a comparable improvement in spirometric indices and Borg scores after administration of bronchodilators via both techniques.[19] It appeared that even severely obstructed patients were able to use MDI with a spacer and might be able to master the technique. Finally, McGuire, et al. compared at the use of UDN with the standard dose of bronchodilator delivered by MDI-spacer and concluded that a standard dosage of Metaproterenol delivered by UDN was somewhat superior to that of the conventional dose of Metaproterenol delivered by MDI-spacer.[20] The authors concluded that the superiority of the UDN was merely due to the fact that the dosage of Metaproterenol delivered by MDI was suboptimal (two puffs each time), and if one increased the dosage of bronchodilator delivered by MDI, one might achieve a comparable or better efficacy than UDN. In this study, McGuire et al. delivered 1.5 mg as opposed to 1.3 mg of Metaproterenol by UDN (two inhalations of Metaproterenol delivered by MDI attached to a spacer device).

Theoretical reasoning predicts better bronchodilation when bronchodilators are used by MDI-spacer rather than by UDN.[21-23] In general, aerosols that are delivered to the bronchial tree are deposited to the bronchial tubes by means of inertial impaction and sedimentation. Inertial impaction generally takes place because of airflow turbulence. Therefore, high inspiratory flow, which is customarily used in UDN, will favor inertial impaction, and bronchodilators, when used via UDN, will tend to be deposited in proximal airways. The second method of bronchodilator deposition is by sedimentation, which usually takes place in the areas of low flow (i.e., peripheral airways). Therefore, bronchodilators used through an MDI-spacer (customarily, the patient takes a deep breath and holds it for a few seconds) should favor deposition of the bronchodilators in peripheral airways and, therefore, more bronchodilatory effect.

The Cedars-Sinai Experience

In 1987, Cedars-Sinai Medical Center performed a randomized trial of aerosolized Metaproterenol delivered either by UDN, which is delivered by therapists, or self-administered MDI with the assistance of a delivery enhancing device, which is less costly.[24] The study used a delivery enhancing device (InspirEase) to facilitate the deposition of the bronchodilators into the bronchi. Nineteen patients were enrolled in each treatment group. The two treatment groups were comparable with respect to age, sex, concurrent medications, Theophylline dose and blood levels, and spirometric indices. Patients were randomized to receive their bronchodilators every four hours either via MDI or UDN. The mean improvement in post-bronchodilator FEV1 was 0.28 + 0.55 liters (mean + 1 SD) in the UDN group, and 0.36 + 0.50 (mean + 1 SD) in the MDI group. The improvement was significant in the MDI group ($p < 0.05$), but not quite significant in the UDN group. The total duration of the hospital stay was 5.8 + 4.2 days (mean + 1 SD) for the UDN group, and 6.2 + 3.7 days (mean + 1 SD) for the MDI group ($p > 0.05$). Examination of patient comorbid conditions and treatments, including history of diagnoses of asthma, past history of smoking, and use of corticosteroids, did not reveal any effects attributable to these factors.

At the time, researchers estimated that at Cedars-Sinai alone, the automatic substitution of MDI for all therapist-administered UDN could save up to $250,000 per year. The study documented the equal efficacy of MDI and UDN. Thus, since May 1987, Cedars-Sinai has implemented an automatic substitution of MDI for UDN in patients who were not in intensive care units. Patients are instructed in the proper use of MDI, and the switch is made only if the patient is able to self-administer the MDI. Patients with poor coordination are instructed to use MDI with the help of a delivery enhancement device such as InspirEase or AeroChamber. A videotape, which can be viewed on the hospital's educational channel, is available to instruct patients on the use of MDI. This policy, an approach designed to reduce expenses while maintaining the quality of care to patients, went into effect in May 1987. Since the implementation of the policy at Cedars-Sinai, a number of hospitals in the country have adopted a similar policy and have used similar protocols as a guide to develop similar cost-containment measures.

Repeated audits of MDI conversion at Cedars-Sinai have revealed that approximately 45% of all patients ordered to receive UDN are suitable for receiving MDI therapy. Those patients who are alert, oriented, understand instruction, and have proper hand-mouth coordination in the use of MDI, are deemed suitable for conversion. Patients may be considered not suitable if they are unable to understand the instructions or are uncooperative, disoriented, and/or mentally obtunded. A recent audit indicated that have approximately 2,600 patients annually were considered suitable for conversion to MDI; of these, only 35% were converted to MDI. Patient and/or physician refusal constituted the main reason for non-conversion in patients whom the respiratory therapist deemed suitable for conversion.

In summary, Cedars-Sinai Medical Center investigators compared the efficacy of different methods of bronchodilators and found the following results:

1. The efficiency of bronchodilators delivered by UDN is similar and, by some accounts, superior to that of conventional doses of bronchodilators delivered by MDI with the help of a spacer (two puffs every four hours).
2. There is no doubt that the efficacy of bronchodilators delivered by MDI at a slightly higher dosage (three to four puffs) is equal to that of the conventional dose of bronchodilators delivered by UDN.
3. There will be significant improvement in cost savings if bronchodilators indicate delivered by MDI. The most conservative estimates are that the cost of delivery of bronchodilators can be reduced by one-third if the bronchodilator is delivered by MDI rather than UDN. Even at Cedars-Sinai, where physicians are able to convert only approximately one-third of the suitable patients to MDI, approximately $100,000-$120,000 in cost savings is achieved annually.

References

1. Pederson JZ, A Bungarrd. "Comparative Efficacy of Different Methods of Nebulizing Salbutamol." *European Journal of Clinical Pharmacology* 25 1983:739-42.

2. Stauder J, KG Hidinger. "Terbutaline Aerosol From a Metered Dose Inhaler With a 750-Ml Spacer or as a Nebulized Solution." *Respiratory* 44 1983:237-40.

3. Tarala RA, BW Madsen, JW Paterson. "ComparativeEfficacy of Salbutamol by Pressurized Aerosol and WetNebulizer in Acute Asthma." *British Journal of Clinical Pharmacology* 10 1980:393-97.

4. Moss K, A McDonald, L Ferrara, D Myles, M Brischetto."Metered Dose Inhaler vs. Compressor Driven Nebulizer in theDelivery of Metaproterenol." *Chest* 88 1985:53S.

5. Berenberg MJ, W Baigelman, LA Cupples, L Pearce."Comparison of Metered-Dose Inhaler Attached to anAerochamber with an Updraft Nebulizer for the Administration of Metaproterenol in Hospitalized Patients." *Journal of Asthma* 22 1985:87-92.

6. Konig P. "Spacer Devices Used with Metered-Dose Inhalers." *Chest* 88 1985:276-84.

7. Jenkins SC, RW Heaton, TJ Fulton, J Moxham."Comparison of Domiciliary Nebulized Salbutamol and Salbutamol from a Metered-Dose Inhaler in Stable Chronic Airflow Limitation." *Chest* 91 1987:804-7.

8. Summer W, R Elston, L Tharpe, LS Nelson, EF Haponik."Aerosol Bronchodilator Delivery Methods: Relative Impact on Pulmonary Function and Cost of Respiratory Care." *Archives of Internal Medicine* 1149 1989:618-23.

9. Kim CS, MA Eldridge, MA Sackner. "Oropharyngeal Deposition and Delivery Aspects of Metered-Dose Inhaler Aerosols." American Review of Respiratory Diseases 135 1987:157-64.

10. Newman SP, D Pavis, SW Clarke. "How Should A Pressurized Beta-Adrenergic Bronchodilator be Inhaled?" *European Journal of Respiratory Diseases* 62 1981:3-21.

11. Fairshter RD. "Evaluation of a Metered-Dose Aerosol Delivery System Using Partial Flow-Volume Curves." American Review of Respiratory Diseases 135 1987:741-3.

12. Turner JR, KJ Corkery, D Eckman, et al.: "Equivalents of Continuous Flow Nebulizer and Metered-Dose Inhaler with Reservoir Bag for Treatment of Acute Airflow Obstruction." *Chest* 93 1988:476-81.

13. Morley TF, E Marozsan, SJ Zappasodi, R Gordon, R Griesback, JC Giudice. "Comparison of Beta-Adrenergic Agents Delivered by Nebulizer vs. Metered-Dose Inhaler with Inspirease in Hospitalized Asthmatic Patients." *Chest* 94 1988:1205-10.

14. Mestitz H, JM Copland, CF McDonald. "Comparison of Outpatient Nebulized vs. Metered Dose Inhaler Terbutaline in Chronic Airflow Obstruction." *Chest* 96 1989:1237-40.

15. Cushley MJ, RA Lewis, AE Tattersfield. "Comparison of Three Techniques of Inhalation on the Airway Response to Terbutaline." *Thorax* 38 1983:908-13.

16. Harrison BA, RJ Pierce. "Comparison of Wet and Dry Aerosol Salbutamol." Australian and New Zealand Jounral of *Medicine* 13 1983:29-33.

17. Weber RW, WE Petty, HS Nelson. "Aerosolized Terbutaline in Asthmatics. Comparison of Dosage Strength, Schedule and Method of Administration." Journal of Allergy and Clinical Immunology 73 1978:116-21.

18. Berry RB, RA Shinto, FH Wong, JA Despars, WA Light. "Nebulizer vs. Spacer for Bronchodilator Delivery in Patients Hospitalized for Acute Exacerbation of COPD." *Chest* 96 1989:1241-6.

19. Borg G. "Physiological Bases of Perceived Exertion." Medicine and Science in Sports and Exercise 5 1982:377-81.

20. Stone D. "Comparison of Hand-Held Nebulizer with a Metered-Dose Inhaler-Spacer Combination in Acute Obstructive Pulmonary Disease." *Chest* 100 1991:1300-5.

21. Newhouse MG, M Dolovich. "Aerosol Therapy for Reversible Airflow Obstruction." *Chest* 91 1987:58S-64S.

22. Newhouse M, M Dolovich. "Aerosol Therapy: Nebulizer Vs. Metered Dose Inhaler." *Chest* 91 1987:799-800.

23. Newhouse MG, MB Dolovich. "Current Concepts: Control of Asthma by Aerosols." *New England Journal of Medicine* 315 1986:870-3.

24. Jasper AC, Z Mohsenifar, S Kahan, et al. "Cost Benefit Comparison of Aerosol Bronchodilator Delivery Methods in Hospitalized Patients." Chest 91 1987:614-18.

Chapter 26

The Department of Pharmacy's Involvement In Clinical Pathway Development

Emmanuel Saltiel, PharmD
Rita Shane, PharmD

Clinical paths (also known as critical paths and care maps) can be defined as a systematic approach to the management of specific diseases, diagnoses, or procedures by defining treatments, diagnostic procedures, monitoring tools and frequencies, and expected outcomes throughout a patient's hospital course from preadmission to post-discharge. The goals of clinical paths are several:[1]

- to increase predictability of demand for patient services;
- to clarify expectations and responsibilities of care team members;
- to facilitate communication between members of the care team;
- to promote the development of better measures of quality of care by strengthening the process-outcome link;
- to decrease documentation time; and
- to reduce expenses.

Many aspects of the development of clinical paths are similar to the development of practice guidelines. Like guidelines, clinical paths are created by expert groups upon careful review of outcome-based data in the medical literature and are used increasingly in health care to help curb rising costs while reducing inappropriate care.[2-5] By reviewing outcomes-based medical literature, benchmarking with other institutions to determine cost-effective strategies, and reducing variances in care which tend to lead to excessive and often unneeded care, clinical paths can reduce institutional expenses while maintaining or improving the quality of care.

EMMANUEL SALTIEL, PHARMD—Clinical Coordinator, Pharmacy Services, Cedars-Sinai Medical Center; Assistant Clinical Professor, University of California and University of the Pacific Schools of Pharmacy; Adjunct Assistant Professor of Pharmacy Practice, University of Southern California School of Pharmacy.

RITA SHANE, PHARMD—Director, Pharmacy Services, Cedars-Sinai Medical Center; Assistant Clinical Professor, University of California and University of the Pacific Schools of Pharmacy; Adjunct Assistant Professor of Pharmacy Practice, University of Southern California School of Pharmacy.

The assistance of Ashley Vo, PharmD, in the preparation of the data for the CABG Clinical Pathway is acknowledged.

This manuscript is adapted from Saltiel E. Pharmacy's involvement in clinical paths: Cedars-Sinai Medical Center. *Am J Health-Syst Pharm* 1995;52(10) (accepted for publication).

At Cedars-Sinai Medical Center, pharmacy's involvement in clinical path meetings came about via at least three mechanisms: (1) prior involvement in patient focused-care implementation; (2) active communication with key members of clinical pathway planning teams (resource management, health services research, key physicians) to whom drug usage reports were provided; and (3) prior involvement in the development of practice guidelines for drug therapy and selected pharmacist-driven protocols through the Pharmacy and Therapeutics Committee (e.g., pharmacist-managed warfarin dosing protocol, antibiotic use review program) with clear implications for clinical pathway development.

Pharmacy's involvement in clinical paths can take many forms (**Table 26.1**). The Department of Pharmacy is involved at various stages of development with no less than twenty-four clinical paths at Cedars-Sinai Medical Center (**Table 26.2**). The following summaries describe specific pathways in which the Department of Pharmacy has participated. Each summary includes details on previous practices, drug utilization decisions, and anticipated or actual patient outcomes and cost data resulting from implementation of the clinical paths.

Table 26.1: ROLES FOR PHARMACY IN CLINICAL PATH DEVELOPMENT AND IMPLEMENTATION

- Developing a prioritization strategy regarding participation in specific clinical paths based on disease states or procedures with a prominent drug therapy component.
- Providing recommendations regarding drug selection, dose, route, and timing (initiation time, duration, timing of switch from parenteral to oral therapy, etc.), and monitoring of medications specific to the pathway.
- Performing drug use evaluation to examine variances in practice patterns.
- Reviewing the medical and pharmacy literature, focusing on outcomes.
- Benchmarking with similar institutions.
- Educating the medical staff, ideally in conjunction with physician representatives.
- Assisting with clinical pathway implementation by intervening to ensure optimal medication management.

Table 26.2: CLINICAL PATHWAYS AT CEDARS-SINAI MEDICAL CENTER IN WHICH PHARMACY IS ACTIVELY INVOLVED

- Mastectomy
- Urinary tract infections
- Diabetic foot ulcers
- Bone marrow transplantation
- Febrile neutropenia
- Pneumocystis carinii pneumonia
- Cytomegalovirus infection in AIDS
- Coronary artery bypass surgery
- Vaginal delivery
- Pediatric asthma
- Neonatal sepsis
- Total hip arthroplasty
- Total knee arthroplasty
- Hip fracture
- Community-acquired pneumonia
- Chronic obstructive pulmonary disease
- Deep venous thrombosis/Pulmonary embolism
- Acute renal failure
- Kidney transplantation
- Laminectomy
- Upper gastrointestinal bleed
- Unstable Angina
- Acute myocardial infarction
- Congestive heart failure

CABG Without Coronary Angiography

The initial meeting of the coronary artery bypass graft (CABG) without angiography clinical path committee was held in January 1994. Recent trends and figures indicated that length of stay (LOS) had been reduced from 13.2 days in 1990 to 8.9 days in 1993. Operating room costs were calculated at $10,853 per case. Total drug costs for a routine patient were approximately $900, based on the acquisition costs for the medications. Despite the small percentage of drug costs relative to total costs, the committee felt that important reductions could nonetheless be realized. Prior to the second meeting, pharmacy performed several drug use evaluations (DUEs) in a total of sixty-eight patients undergoing CABG. Fentanyl was used in 81% of cases (mean dose 2.18 mg, cost $11.12), and sufentanil was used in 29% (mean dose 256 mcg, cost $51.30). Pancuronium was used in 76% of cases (mean dose 15.9 mg, cost $2.54), and vecuronium was used in 38% (mean dose 24.5 mg, cost $43.86). For both of these drug classes, the anesthesiologist in the clinical pathway committee felt that the less expensive agent could be used as the standard and should be incorporated into the pathway. Also examined were colloids, sedatives and analgesics, and antibiotics. Albumin was used in 52% of the patients reviewed with a mean volume of 840mL. Hetastarch was used in 38% at a mean volume of 1035mL. The differences in postoperative use were more dramatic: 59% of the patients received albumin versus only 17% who received hetastarch. It was noted that the cost difference would be even more dramatic once hetastarch became generically available. The chairman of the committee suggested that hetastarch be the colloid of choice.

As discussions on blood use progressed, the committee asked about aprotinin. Pharmacy produced three studies on the use of aminocaproic acid or tranexamic acid, demonstrating that these agents were also associated with a favorable blood-sparing effect. [6-8] The committee felt that until patients undergoing CABG who were at high-risk of significant bleeding could be identified, there was no need to address the use of aprotinin in the pathway.

When prophylactic antibiotic use was examined in detail, some surprising patterns surfaced. Sixteen (35%) of forty-six patients reviewed received two doses of preoperative antibiotic within thirty minutes, and twenty-five (54%) received two doses within four hours pre- and intraoperatively. Duration of prophylaxis ranged from two to five days, with over 50% receiving five days. Pharmacy was asked to review the medical literature on antibiotic prophylaxis in patients undergoing CABG. Seven studies were reviewed, with the recommendation that a single dose of cefazolin or vancomycin prior to surgery would suffice for any CABG surgery lasting up to three hours.[9-15] Additionally, the committee felt that a twenty-four hour duration would be optimal. The potential use of cefazolin in patients with stated allergies to penicillin was also discussed.[16] In light of the recent Centers for Disease Control recommendations for curtailing vancomycin use due to increasing resistance, vancomycin was limited to patients with well-described immediate or accelerated reactions to penicillin or a derivative.[17]

Another issue discussed at the CABG clinical path meetings was the use of propofol versus midazolam versus lorazepam for postoperative sedation.[18-21] One trial demonstrated a more rapid recovery and earlier extubation with propofol than with midazolam.[18] Another study did not confirm this finding.[19] Another trial demonstrated that recovery times were at least as fast following diazepam than with midazolam, suggesting that plasma half-lives are less relevant than one might expect.[20] In patients requiring continuous sedation, a trial suggested that lorazepam is associated with a more rapid recovery than is midazolam, and requires less nursing time in dosage adjustments.[22]

In summary, the following medication-related aspects of care were incorporated into Cedars-Sinai's developing CABG clinical pathway: fentanyl is the short-acting opioid of choice; pancuronium is the neuromuscular blocking agent of choice; hetastarch is the colloid of choice for the first 1,000cc; a single dose of cefazolin will be given in the preoperative holding area, followed by a twenty-four hour postoperative course, vancomycin being reserved for patients with well-documented immediate or accelerated allergic reactions to ß-lactam antibiotics; and aminocaproic acid is to be used in patients deemed to be at high risk of bleeding, pending continued analysis of institutional data.

Low-Risk Community-Acquired Pneumonia

Community-acquired pneumonia is responsible for over one million hospital admissions per year in the United States. Contributing to the economic burden of this disease are wide variations in hospital admission rates and lengths of inpatient stay.[23] Based upon inhouse observations which appeared to mimic these variations, the Health Services Research Department at Cedars-Sinai Medical Center undertook a retrospective analysis of 503 patients admitted for community-acquired pneumonia. A total of 33% (n=166) of the patients were classified as low-risk at Day 3 of their hospitalization, utilizing several rating scales from the medical literature. The average length of stay for this subset of patients was 7.7 days. The authors concluded that this group could be safely switched to oral antimicrobial therapy on Day 3 and discharged on Day 4. Such a strategy would save 619 hospital bed-days per year.[23]

Following the analysis described above, the researchers met with members of the Divisions of Pulmonary Medicine and Infectious Diseases and the Department of Pharmacy to strategize gradual house-wide implementation of these guidelines. At present, clinical pharmacists are responsible for making recommendations on oral antimicrobial selection for all patients identified by utilization review as "low-risk" pneumonia. It should be emphasized that the pharmacy intervention is an integral part of the clinical pathway.

Based on the success of the low-risk pneumonia critical path, pharmacy was also consulted on a pathway for patients with chronic obstructive pulmonary disease. A total of 250 patients' charts were reviewed by Health Services Research Department, 232 patients satisfied criteria for being at low risk (the other 18 either had significant concurrent medical problems at admission or developed such problems during the first 72 hours of admission). The average length of stay for these 232 patients was 6.1 days. As was the case with pneumonia, a careful analysis demonstrated that discharge on Day 4 could be safely accomplished. One hundred eighty-five patients (79.7%) received parenteral antibiotics for a mean of 5.6 days. Oddly, only twenty-six patients had documented infections, and only two had a fever at some time during hospitalization. Two hundred nine patients (90.0%) received parenteral corticosteroids. Data supportive of corticosteroids was also found, but oral and parenteral administration appeared to be equiefficacious in the treatment of acute exacerbation of reversible airway disease.[24-26] In fact, a program at Kaiser Permanente was successful at increasing the percentage of patients switched from intravenous to oral corticosteroids from 28% to 71%.[27]

The pharmacists' role in the clinical pathway is to make recommendations on oral antibiotic selection and conversion to oral corticosteroids on Day 3 in patients admitted with COPD exacerbation, in preparation for discharge on Day 4.

Total Hip Replacement

A retrospective analysis of 230 patients at Cedars-Sinai Medical Center demonstrated that the mean length of stay was 8.3 days for patients undergoing total hip replacement and 10.7 days for those undergoing hip hemiarthroplasty. The analysis determined that discharge following a five-day length of stay would be safe in more than 90% of the patients.[28] As part of the clinical path development for total hip replacement, the Department of Pharmacy initially advocated the use of warfarin for prophylaxis of deep venous thrombosis and pulmonary embolism. This decision was based on a consensus review of the literature by the American College of Chest Physicians in 1992 and a cost-effectiveness analysis performed in 1991. [29, 30] Additionally, assuming equal efficacy rates, the Department of Pharmacy performed its own pharmacoeconomic analysis and determined that warfarin would be less costly than enoxaparin.[31] This latter analysis utilized benchmarking information on time spent for monitoring and adjusting warfarin therapy with the assumption that pharmacists would develop and run a warfarin-dosing protocol for orthopedic patients. As a result, a pharmacist-based warfarin dosing protocol was implemented. After 200 patients were dosed by the service, it became clear that pharmacist time involvement in the dosing service was markedly underestimated. A subsequent pharmacoeconomic analysis, utilizing actual times, demonstrated that enoxaparin was more cost-effective, if labor cost was included in the analysis. As a result, both options were allowed in the clinical path. Because of the demonstrated superiority of low molecular weight heparin relative to warfarin in total knee arthroplasty, enoxaparin was advocated for this latter procedure. [32, 33, 34]

Postoperative Pain Management Quality Action Team

In response to a number of concerns voiced at several surgical clinical path committees, the Department of Pharmacy assembled a Quality Action Team to address issues related to postoperative pain management with the goal of optimizing pain management in a number of surgical clinical pathways. Using the Acute Pain Management Guidelines from the Agency for Health Care Policy and Research (1992), the team has addressed no less than six issues pertinent to this area. Issues include the following: (1) the need for preadmission patient education on postoperative pain; (2) the need for regularly scheduled analgesics (not "PRN") for the first twenty-four hours or more following surgery (depending on the surgical procedure and thus the expected duration of pain); (3) the need for frequent assessment and reassessment of pain by nursing personnel; (4) the need for consistent use of a tool for patient self-assessment of pain (e.g., zero-to-ten verbal scale, or visual analogue scale); (5) the possibility of preemptive analgesic strategies to some or most patients scheduled for surgery; and (6) the specific analgesic strategies offered to patients.[32-34] Many of these issues have also been addressed as quality assurance standards by the American Pain Society.[35]

The Cedars-Sinai committee responsible for oversight of all the surgical clinical pathways has subsequently developed a preliminary template to incorporate specified postoperative pain management into the pathways being developed. (See **Figure 26.1**).

Figure 26.1: Postoperative Pain Management Template

CEDARS-SINAI MEDICAL CENTER
DEPARTMENT OF SURGERY

POST-OPERATIVE
PAIN MANAGEMENT

Note:
1. *All orders are to be completed, dated, timed, and signed by the physician and physician I.D. number is to be entered prior to transcription*
2. *Write in black ink only. Use a ball-point pen and press firmly.*
3. *The physician must check or circle all items that are to be ordered-items left unchecked will not be activated.*
4. *Orders are to be initiated, signed, dated, and timed when they are transcribed*
5. *Mark through all items that should not be ordered to avoid the inadvertent activation of an undesirable item*

PATIENT I.D.

PHYSICIANS ORDERS — INIT

Page 1 of 1

DATE:__________ TIME: __________

8. Pain Management:

[ ] PCA: See separate PCA Order sheet

[ ] Epidural Analgesia: See separate Order sheet

[ ] Injections:

[ ] Morphine _______ mg (usual doses: 7-10 mg) SQ every _______ hours (usual: 3 or 4 hrs)

[ ] around the clock

[ ] around the clock while awake

[ ] PRN for _________ hours, then ____________________

[ ] Hydromorphine (Dilaudid) ______ mg (usual doses: 1-2 mg) SQ every ______ hours (usual: 3 or 4 hrs)

[ ] around the clock

[ ] around the clock while awake

[ ] PRN for ________ hours, then ____________________

[ ] Other ______________________________

[ ] Oral Analgesics (if applicable) ________________________

[ ] For breakthrough pain, may give single dose of:

[ ] Morphine _________ mg (usual doses: 2-4 mg) IV push Q 2 hrs
May repeat x 1 in 30 minutes. Call MD for > 2 breakthrough doses given per 8 hr

[ ] Hydromorphine (Dilaudid) _________ mg (usual doses: 0.25 - 0.5 mg) IV push Q 2 hrs
May repeat x 1 in 30 minutes. Call MD for > 2 breakthrough doses given per 8 hr

[ ] Nursing: Patient Pain Assessment by verbal 0 - 10 scale Q 2 hours. If two consecutive scores are ≤ 3, reduce frequency to Q 6 hours. **For any report of pain score > 5:**

[ ] Call _______________ at _______________ for change in pain medication orders

[ ] Change pain medications as follows: ________________________
____

SIGNATURE OF PHYSICIAN					PHYSICIAN I.D. NUMBER	DATE	TIME
MD.							
SIGNATURE OF TRANSCRIBER	INIT	TITLE	DATE	TIME	SIGNATURE OF NURSE (NOTED)	DATE	TIME

DISTRIBUTION: White = Medical Record; Yellow = Pharmacy; Pink = Nursing

FORM S-PAINMGMT-MD 06/95

OPIOID EQUIANALGESIC DOSE CHART

DRUG NAME	PARENTERAL DOSE (mg)	ORAL DOSE (mg)[1]
Morphine	10	60[2]
Hydromorphone (Dilaudid)	1.5	7.5[3]
Meperidine (Demerol)	100	300
Methadone	10	20
Codeine	75	130
Pentazocine (Talwin)	60	180
Oxycodone tablets	NA	30 {6 tabs}
Oxycodone/acetaminophen (Percocet; Tylox)	NA	30 {6 tabs}
Hydrocodone/acetaminophen (Vicodin; Lortab)	NA	30 {6 tabs}
(Vicodin ES)	NA	30 {4 tabs}

NOTE: In switching from one agent to another or in changing from parenteral to oral therapy, all above doses are considered equianalgesic. For example, Vicodin 2 tabs q3h is equivalent in analgesic activity to Demerol 33mg or morphine 3.3mg IV or SQ q3h

1 Standard dosing regimens for all agents are q3-4h except: meperidine (Demerol): q2-3h; methadone: q6-8h.

2 The 60mg oral dose of morphine is equianalgesic to the 10mg injectable dose when oral morphine is given intermittently (or as a single dose). When given around the clock, the appropriate conversion is 30mg oral to 10mg parenteral.

Acute Myocardial Infarction

An analysis of 304 patients presenting to Cedars-Sinai Medical Center with acute myocardial infarction (AMI) demonstrated that 92 received a thrombolytic agent. Until the results of the Global Utilization of Streptokinase and Tissue Plasminogen Activator (TPA) for Occluded Coronary Arteries (GUSTO) trial, streptokinase was responsible for 62% to 89% of all thrombolytic use in the AMI setting at our institution.[36] The GUSTO trial demonstrated that front-loaded TPA with heparin provided an approximate 1% survival benefit over streptokinase combined with heparin. Subgroup analysis demonstrated that patients under seventy-five years of age, those with anterior AMIs, and those treated within four hours of the onset of chest pain had a significantly better survival than other patients. Although criticized for being open-labeled and affording more potentially life-saving emergency coronary artery bypass surgeries in TPA patients, GUSTO still made important inroads in many clinicians' perceptions of TPA's efficacy.[37, 38] The Division of Cardiology decided to recommend TPA in any patient with an AMI presenting with **any** of the three subsets in which TPA was shown to be more efficacious than streptokinase and reevaluate thrombolytic drug usage patterns in six months. At the time, the Division of Cardiology was participating in an investigational trial which provided free thrombolytic as part of the study. Therefore, the physicians felt that the impact of these recommendations on the drug budget would be minimal for the short term.

The pharmacy department's analysis demonstrated that if rigidly followed, these guidelines would result in the use of TPA in 86% of patients with AMI. The anticipated increase in costs associated with this shift in practice was estimated to be over $137,000 per year. In October 1994, a task force comprised of several leading cardiologists, the Pharmacy and Therapeutics Committee chairman, and members of the pharmacy department reviewed current usage and recent literature. TPA use had increased to 61% of all thrombolytic used in patients with AMI, representing an increase in $88,000 per year. The division of cardiology's assumption of a minimal impact on drug budget proved to be inaccurate, as only 28% of a forty-six-patient cohort reviewed were part of the investigational trial. The group discussed the relative values of TPA and streptokinase, reassessed the GUSTO trial and additional literature, and decided to designate streptokinase as the thrombolytic of choice except for patients who were under seventy-five years of age, have an anterior AMI location, **and** have received treatment within four hours of the onset of chest pain. Additionally, all patients with prior exposure to streptokinase or a derivative would receive TPA. This designation was closer to a literal reading of an editorial appearing in the same issue of the New England Journal of Medicine as the GUSTO trial.[39]

The recommendation of this task force was subsequently approved by the pharmacy and therapeutics committee and became a clinical guideline which, in turn, was approved by the clinical pathways committee. Other clinical guidelines for the AMI clinical pathway included: (a) use of angiotensin converting enzyme inhibitors; (b) use of ß-blockers; (c) use of heparin; and (d) use of aspirin. Pharmacy assisted in the development of each of these guidelines by providing supportive literature, and assuring that the most appropriate agent was used in each class, when possible.

Deep Venous Thrombosis (DVT) and Pulmonary Embolism (PE)

In October 1991, the Pharmacy and Therapeutics Committee approved a pharmacist-run heparin protocol for patients with DVT or PE. The protocol was derived as follows:

- Based on three studies demonstrating equivalent efficacy and equal or less toxicity, warfarin was automatically started on Day 1 of heparin.[40-42]
- The initial heparin infusion rate was based on gender, height, and weight, based on pharmacokinetic principles studied by Chenella et al, and evaluated in a retrospective study by Saya, et al. [43,44]
- The infusion rate changes were based on a protocol described by Hull, et al.[45]
- The rate changes were converted to weight-based figures, based on findings by Raschke, et al.[46]

In 1994, the pulmonary division initiated the development of a clinical pathway for DVT and PE. A representative of the pharmacy department met with members of the division in an effort to evaluate the literature on heparin dosing in patients with DVT and PE. The Cedars-Sinai's heparin protocol was also evaluated. Of twenty-one consecutive patients dosed per protocol over a six month period, twenty achieved a therapeutic APTT within twenty-four hours. The mean time to therapeutic APTT was less than ten hours. Following several meetings, the heparin protocol was formalized into the Cedars-Sinai's clinical pathway for DVT and PE. Additionally, the pathway requires that the pharmacist-run protocol be used, a service that was optional prior to the approval.

Conclusion

Rapid changes in the reimbursement for health care services are prompting institutions nationwide to rethink their approaches to providing care. As the evolution of health care towards managed care progresses, hospitals and physicians will become increasingly linked, the result being a more competitive entity from which to negotiate contracts with buyers of health care services. As managed care plans will increasingly profile hospitals' and physicians' performances and will continue to seek price concessions, it is incumbent upon health care professionals to develop optimal, cost-competitive plans towards management of patients.[1] Clinical paths provide an excellent tool to promote multidisciplinary efforts towards these ends. This article provides several examples of important roles the Department of Pharmacy can play in the development and implementation of clinical paths. In advocating optimal drug selection and monitoring, pharmacists can assist their institutions in reducing costs while maintaining or improving quality of care.

References

1. Shane R, B Vinson. "Use of Critical Pathways and Indicators in Pharmacy Practice." *Topics Hospital Pharmacy Management,* 1995 (in press).

2. Sox HC. "Practice Guidelines: 1994." *American Journal of Medicine* 97 1994: 205-7.

3. Woolf SH. "Practice Guidelines: A New Reality in Medicine. III. Impact on Health Care." *Archives of Internal Medicine* 153 1993: 2646-55.

4. Parmley WW. "Clinical Practice Guidelines. Does the Cookbook Have Enough Recipes?" *Journal of the American Medical Association* 1994; 272: 1374-5.

5. Shane R. "Development and Implementation Of Practice Guidelines (Part 1)." *Hospital Formulary* 29 1994: 711-9.

6. Yau MY, Carson S, Weisel RD, et al. "The Effect of Warm Heart Surgery on Postoperative Bleeding." *Journal of Thoracic and Cardiovascular Surgeon* 103 1992: 155-63.

7. Ovrum E, EA Holen, M Abdelnoor, et al. "Tranexamic Acid (Cyklokapron) Is Not Necessary To Reduce Blood Loss After Coronary Artery Bypass Operations. " *Journal of Thoracic and Cardiovascular Surgeon* 105 1993: 78-83.

8. Karski JM, SJ Teasdale, PH Norman, et al. "Prevention of Postbypass Bleeding With Tranexamic Acid and Epsilon-Aminocaproic Acid." *Journal of Cardiothoracic and Vascular Anesthesia* 7 1993: 431-5.

9. Klamerus KJ, KA Rodvold, NA Silverman, et al. "Effect of Cadiopulmonary Bypass on Vancomycin and Netilmicin Disposition." *Antimicrobial Agents and Chemotherapy* 32 1988: 631-5.

10. Van der Starre PJA, PH Trienekens, JE Harinck-de Weerd, et al. "Comparative study Between Two Prophylactic Antibiotic Regimens of Cefamandole During Coronary Artery Bypass Surgery." *Annals of Thoracic Surgery* 45 1988: 24-7.

11. Akl BF, G Richardson. "Serum Cefazolin Levels During Cardiopulmonary Bypass." *Annals of Thoracic Surgery* 29 1980: 109-12.

12. Austin TW, J Leake, JC Coles, et al. "Vancomycin Blood Levels During Cardiac Bypass Surgery." *Canadian Journal of Surgery* 24 1981:423-5.

13. Eigel P, A Tschirkov, P Satter, et al. "Assays of Cephalosporin Antibiotics Administered Prophylactically in Open Heart Surgery. Determination Of Serum Levels Before, During, And After Cardiopulmonary Bypass." *Infection* 6 1978:23-8.

14. Polk RE, GL Archer, R Lower. "Cefamandole Kinetics During Cardiopulmonary Bypass." *Clinical Pharmacology and Therapeutics* 23 1978: 473-80.

15. Miller KW, KH Chan, HG McCoy, et al. "Cephalothin Kinetics: Before, During, And After Cardiopulmonary Bypass Surgery." *Clinical Pharmacology and Therapeutics* 26 1979:54-62.

16. Rohr AS. Cephalosporins, pp. 209-10. In: Saxon A, moderator. " Immediate Hypersensitivity Reactions To Beta-Lactam Antibiotics." *Annals of Internal Medicine* 107 1987: 204-15.

17. Department of Health and Human Services, Center for Disease Control and Prevention. "Preventing the Spread of Vancomycin Resistance — A Report From the Hospital Infection Control Practices Advisory Committee." *Federal Register* (May 17) 591994: 25758-63.

18. Roekarts PM, FJ Huygen, S de Lange. "Infusion of Propofol Versus Midazolam for Sedation in the Intensive Care Unit Following Coronary Artery Surgery." *Journal of Cardiothorack and Vascular Anesthesia* 7 1993: 142-7.

19. Higgins TL, J-P Yared, FG Estafanous, et al. "Propofol Versus Midazolam for Intensive Care Unit Sedation After Coronary Artery Bypass Grafting." *Critical Care Medicine* 22 1994: 1415-23.

20. Wheeler AP. "Sedation, Analgesia, and Paralysis in the Intensive Care Unit." *Chest* 104 1993: 566-77.

21. Ariano RE, DA Kassum, KJ Aronson. "Comparison of Sedative Recovery Time After Midazolam Versus Diazepam Administration." *Critical Care Medicine* 22 1994: 1492-6.

22. Pohlman AS, KP Simpson, JB Hall. "Continuous Intravenous Infusions of Lorazepam Versus Midazolam For Sedation During Mechanical Ventilatory Support: A Prospective, Randomized Study." *Critical Care Medicine* 22 1994: 1241-7.

23. Weingarten SR, MS Riedinger, G Varis, et al. "Identification of Low-Risk Hospitalized Patients With Pneumonia. Implications for Early Conversion to Oral Antimicrobial Therapy." *Chest* 105 1994: 1109-15.

24. Rowe BH, JL Keller, AD Oxamn. "Effectiveness of Steroid Therapy in Acute Exacerbations Of Asthma: A Meta-Analysis." *Americal Journal of Emergency Medicine* 10 1992: 301-10.

25. Laurens RG, EG Honig. "Corticosteroids in the Treatment of Asthma." *Southern Medical Journal* 79 1986: 1544-52.

26. Webb JR. "Dose Response of Patients to Oral Corticosteroid Treatment During Exacerbations of Asthma." *British Medical Journal* 292 1986: 1045-7.

27. Tran A, S Litsey, M Cinnamond. "Implementation of the Use of Oral Corticosteroids Following Initial Dose of Intravenous Methylprednisolone for the Treatment of Airway Obstruction." Presented at the 1993 Western States Conference for Pharmacy Residents, Fellows, and Preceptors.

28. Weingarten S, M Riedenger, L Conner, et al. "Hip Replacement and Hip Hemiarthroplasty Surgery: Potential Opportunities to Shorten Lengths of Stay." *American Journal of Medicine* 97 1994: 208-13.

29. Clagett GP, EW Salzman, HB Wheeler, et al. "Prevention of Venous Thromboembolism." 102 (suppl) *Chest* 1992: 391S-407S.

30. Paiement GD, SJ Wessinger, WH Harris. "Cost-Effectiveness of Prophylaxis in Total Hip Replacement." *American Journal of Surgery* 161 1991: 519-24.

31. Saltiel E, L Nishimura, R Shane. "Pharmacoeconomic Analysis of Enoxaparin in Orthopedic Patients." Presented at the 51st annual meeting of the American Society of Hospital Pharmacists, Reno, NV, June, 1994.

32. Leclerc JR, WH Geerts, L Desjardins, et al. "Prevention of Venous Thromboembolism (VTE) After Knee Arthroplasty — A Randomized Double-Blind Trial, Comparing Enoxaparin to Warfarin Sodium (abstract)." *Chest* 106 1994: 48S.

33. Hull R, G Raskob, G Pineo, et al. "A Comparison of Subcutaneous Low-Molecular-Weight Heparin With Warfarin Sodium For Prophylaxis Against Deep-Vein Thrombosis After Hip or Knee Implantation." *New England Journal of Medicine* 329 1993: 1370-6.

34. The RD Heparin Arthroplasty Group. "RD Heparin Compared With Warfarin for Prevention of Venous Thromboembolic Disease Following Total Hip or Knee Arthroplasty." *Journal of Bone and Joint Surgery* 76A 1994: 1174-85.

35. Woolf CJ, M-S Chong. "Preemptive Analgesia — Treating Postoperative Pain by Preventing the Establishment of Central Sensitization." *Anesthesia and Analgesia* 77 1993: 362-79.

36. Ejlerson E, HB Andersen, K Eliasen, et al. "A Comparison Between Preincisional and Postincisional Lidocaine Infiltration and Postoperative Pain." *Anesthesia Analgesia* 74 1992: 495-8.

37. Richmond CE, LM Bromley, CJ Woolf. "Preoperative Morphine Pre-Empts Postoperative Pain." *Lancet* 342 1993: 73-5.

38. Committee on Quality Assurance Standards, American Pain Society. American Pain Society Quality Assurance Standards for Relief of Acute Pain and Cancer Pain. Proceedings of the VI th World Congress on Pain 1991, Chapter 21.

39. The GUSTO Investigators. "An International Randomized Trial Comparing Four Thrombolytic Strategies for Acute Myocardial Infarction." *New England Journal of Medicine* 329 1993: 673-82.

40. Ridker PM, C O'Donnell, VJ Marder, CH Hennekens. "Large-Scale Trials of Thrombolytic Therapy for Acute Myocardial Infarction: GISSI-2, ISIS-3, and GUSTO 1." *Annals of Internal Medicine* 119 1993: 530-2.

41. Ridker PM, C O'Donnell, VJ Marder, CH Hennekens. "A Response to 'Holding GUSTO Up to the Light.'" *Annals of Internal Medicine* 120 1994: 882-5.

42. Fuster V. "Coronary Thrombolysis — A Perspective for the Practicing Physician." *New England Journal of Medicine* 329 1993: 723-5.

43. Hull RD, GE Raskob, D Rosenbloom, et al. "Heparin for 5 Days as Compared to 10 Days in the Initial Treatment of Proximal Venous Thrombosis." *New England Journal of Medicine* 322 1990: 1260-4.

44. Gallus A, J Tillett, Jackaman, et al. "Safety and Efficacy of Warfarin Started Early After Submassive Venous Venous Thrombosis or Pulmonary Embolism." *Lancet* 2 1986: 1293-6.

45. Mohiuddin AM, DE Hillman, CJ Destache, et al. "Efficacy and Safety of Early vs Late Heparin Therapy in Acute Thromboembolism." *American Heart Journal* 123 1992: 729-32.

46. Chenella FC, MA Gill, JW Kern, et al. "Improved Method for Estimating Initial Heparin Heparin Infusion Rates." *American Journal of Hospital Pharmacy* 36 1979: 782-4.

47. Snyan FG, LT Coleman, JT Martinoff. " Pharmacist-Directed Heparin Therapy Using a Standard Dosing and Monitoring Protocol." *American Journal of Hospital Pharmacy* 421985: 1965-9.

48. Hull RD, GE Raskob, D Rosenbloom, et al. "Optimal Therapeutic Level of Heparin Therapy in Patients with Venous Thrombosis." *Archives of Internal Medicine* 152 1992: 1589-95.

49. Raschke RA, BM Reilly, JR Guidry, et al. "The Weight-Based Heparin Dosing Nomogram Compared With A 'Standard Care' Nomogram. A Randomized Controlled Trial." *Annals of Internal Medicine* 119 1993: 874-81.

Chapter 27

Analysis of Patient Care Monitoring Guidelines For Patients with Epidural or Intrathecal Morphine For Postoperative Pain: What is Appropriate?

Linda Burnes Bolton, DrPH, RN, FAAN
Carolyn E. Aydin, PhD
Peggy Kalowes, RN, MN
Susan Lewis-Colar, BA

The use of epidural and intrathecal administered morphine as an effective method for controlling patient pain has been well documented over the last two decades; however, patient responses to morphine administered under medical guidelines has varied, leading to the introduction of nursing monitoring guidelines to ensure patient safety. These monitoring guidelines have been widely used without an evaluation of their validity. This study evaluates nursing monitoring guidelines to determine if the demand for nursing care delimited in those guidelines is warranted based upon patient data.

In research on patients receiving epidural or intrathecal morphine for postoperative pain, investigators have documented a number of potential variations in physiologic response. The existing literature fails, however, to address the impact on postoperative nursing management of patients. Because of this lack of information, nursing clinical guidelines, policies, and procedures are based upon minimum patient care requirements to meet patient safety needs rather than upon data that delineates practical, efficient, and effective care.[1] Under these conditions, nurses may be required to assess patients more fre-

LINDA BURNES BOLTON, DRPH, RN, FAAN—Director, Nursing Research and Development and Director, Surgical Nursing, Cedars-Sinai Medical Center and Research Institute; Assistant Clinical Professor, University of California-Los Angeles, School of Nursing; Associate Professor, California State University, Los Angeles.

CAROLYN E. AYDIN, PHD—Assistant Administrator for Nursing Research, Cedars-Sinai Medical Center and Research Institute; Assistant Clinical Professor, University of California-Los Angeles, School of Nursing.

*PEGGY KALOWES, RN, MN—Clinical Nurse Specialist, Cedars-Sinai Medical Center.

*SUSAN LEWIS-COLAR, BA—Research Assistant, Cedars-Sinai Medical Center.

* The last two authors are no longer at Cedars-Sinai: these were their titles at the time of the project.

Acknowledgments: The Cedars-Sinai Medical Center Preoperative and Surgical Nursing Research Teams, consisting of Jan Berkowitz, RN, Paz Bon, RN, Janet Brewster, RN, Karyn Carneveli, RN, Rebecca Denny, RN, Diana Griffin, RN, Barbara Fields, RN, Josie Flores, RN, Elizabeth Garcia, RN, Peggy Giovinazzo, RN, Sandra Hardy, RN, Robin Hudson, RN, Chat Inducil, RN, DeeDee Klute, RN, Marci Langbaum, RN, Esther Mindoro, RN, Theresa Peterson, RN, Alie Resurrecion, RN, Naomi Tashman, RN, Betty Williams, RN, and Ann Mancini, RN, assisted in this research project.

quently than indicated by actual patient response to the analgesia. This need for close patient surveillance may require more nursing time than actually necessary for safe and effective patient care.[2]

In the present study a multidisciplinary team approach was used to develop guidelines for nursing management of patients with epidural or intrathecal morphine for postoperative pain. The research team focused on identifying variations in patient response among specific patient population subgroups (e.g., older patients, patients receiving redosage). The following research questions were addressed:

1. Is the incidence of variations in physiologic response among patients receiving epidural or intrathecal analgesia commensurate with findings in the literature?
2. What patient factors are associated with variation in physiological response?
3. What nursing assessment and monitoring guidelines should be adopted based on patient observations and a synthesis of literature findings?

The use of intraspinal narcotic analgesia and its appropriate medical management is well documented in the medical literature. Despite recent widespread use of intravenous (IV) patient-controlled analgesia (PCA), investigators comparing epidural to IV PCA morphine have shown epidural morphine to provide greater patient comfort for some groups of patients. [3,4,5] Investigators comparing epidural and parenteral opioid analgesia in adults undergoing thoracic and abdominal surgery also have suggested that epidural analgesia is superior for postoperative pain.[6, 7] Medical and nursing authors, however, have noted the need for a nursing management database from which appropriate parameters of care for patients with epidural or intrathecal morphine can be determined.

In prospective research studies, investigators have identified variations in physiologic response associated with intraspinal narcotic analgesia and investigated dosages, methods of administration, and the physiologic conditions associated with its use. Of particular importance for nursing, results indicate that patients may experience physiologic responses such as respiratory depression, pruritus, urinary retention, and nausea and/or vomiting, which may be dose dependent.[8] According to Cousins and Mather, urinary retention, pruritus, nausea, and vomiting have the same etiology for both epidural and intrathecal opioids, but the incidence is higher for intrathecal use.[9] Pruritus, nausea, and vomiting are generally reported as frequent, but they are easily treated.[10-17]

In research on the actual variations in patients' physiologic responses, however, investigators have shown conflicting results for different patient populations and doses.[18, 19, 20, 21] In peripheral vascular and orthopedic surgical patients, for example, Allen, et al. reported that nausea, vomiting, pruritus, and urinary retention were uncommon and did not appear to be dose related.[22] According to Stenseth, et al., postoperative nausea or vomiting were more frequent in women than in men.[23] Furthermore, although most variations in physiologic response are usually mild and easily treated, no data exist to document the nursing time involved in management of these patients.

In contrast to the less serious patient responses described above, respiratory depression often occurs after many hours, with potentially life threatening results. Etches, Sandler, and Lawson, for example, found that epidural morphine in postthoracotomy patients may be associated with "significant respiratory depression, which cannot be predicted on the basis of preoperative respiratory abnormalities, dose of drug, or hourly respiratory rate."[24] Blackman, et al., in a study of intrathecal morphine in patients aged eleven to sixteen undergoing spinal fusion, reported respiratory depression in five of their thirty-three patients.[25] Others note, however, that the actual incidence of late respiratory depression is probably low and depends upon a number of contributing factors, including advanced age.[26, 27, 28, 29] Allen, et al. reported late respiratory depression only in the highest (10-mg.) dose group.[30] Stenseth, et al. reported respiratory depression in only 10 (1%) of 1,085 patients.[31] Furthermore, in only two of the ten patients did it occur more than five hours after the last dose of epidural morphine. Stenseth, et al. also noted that the respiratory depression came on as a gradual declining respiratory rate that could be easily detected and treated. In fact, in a number of studies investigators have reported no occurrences of late respiratory depression at all.[32-38]

Method

Sample Selection

The study was conducted in the postoperative holding area, surgical intensive care units, and on the surgical floors of a 1,100 bed private teaching hospital in Los Angeles, California.

Inclusion criteria. One hundred ten patients scheduled to receive epidural or intrathecal morphine, fentanyl, or a combination were identified from the surgical schedule. The study included both patients scheduled to be admitted the day of surgery (37%) and patients admitted the night before (63%) in 1988. The sample was a convenience sample and the study was conducted over a three month time period.

Exclusion criteria. Obstetrical and pediatric patients, patients with chronic pain undergoing an operative procedure unrelated to the etiology of their pain, cancer patients whose pain was managed by epidural morphine, and patients who had received epidural morphine in the past were excluded. In addition, eleven of the original one hundred and ten patients were dropped from the study because of complicating diagnoses (e.g., preexisting cardiovascular and/or neurological conditions—seven patients) or abnormal vital signs prior to surgery (four patients), for a final sample of ninety-nine patients.

Sample Characteristics

Description. Background information was obtained to document demographic characteristics, the type of narcotic, and type of surgery for the ninety-nine patients eligible for the study. Of these ninety-nine patients, eighty-one (82%) were males and eighteen were females (18%). The mean age of patients in the sample was 66.2 years (SD=13.6). There were, however, age differences by type of narcotic, with a mean age of 64.4 years for patients receiving epidural morphine or epidural morphine combined with fentanyl and 71.1 years for patients receiving intrathecal morphine. Forty-one patients (41%) received epidural morphine, thirty-two patients (32%) received epidural morphine combined with fentanyl, and twenty-six patients (26%) received intrathecal morphine.

Type of surgery was coded in five categories: genitourinary/gastrointestinal (GU/GI), orthopedic, neurological/back, cardiovascular, and other surgeries. Seventy-five of the ninety-nine patients had GU/GI surgeries, with the most common procedure being transurethral prostate resection (TURP). Seventy-seven (78%) of the patients were transferred from postoperative holding directly to nursing floors, while twenty-two patients (22%) were transferred to intensive care units (ICUs). (Six of the ICU patients were subsequently transferred to nursing floors during the study period.) Eighteen percent of the ninety-nine patients were discharged during the study period.

Morphine dosage. Patients received epidural morphine dosages in the operating room ranging from 2 to 5 mg. Fentanyl dosages for those patients receiving morphine combined with fentanyl ranged from 40 to 200 mcg. Patients with intrathecal morphine received doses from 0.10 to 0.50 mg. Eleven patients were redosed after being transferred from the postoperative holding area to the ICU or patient care floor. Five of these patients received more than one redose during the study period.

To investigate whether physiologic variations were dosage related, patients were divided into three categories based on the initial morphine dosage they had received. About 79% of patients fell into the middle category, having received 3 to 4 mg. of epidural morphine or 0.2 to 0.3 mg. of intrathecal morphine. Only 4% (three patients) received lower dosages, while 17% (seventeen patients) received higher dosages. The lower dosage category had too few patients for separate analysis and was included with the patients in the middle category. The responses of the seventeen patients receiving higher dosages (4.5 to 5.0 mg. epidurally or 0.4 to 0.5 mg. intrathecally) were compared with the rest of the sample to isolate dosage related responses. Eleven of the ninety-nine patients also received morphine redoses in the intensive care unit or nursing floor. Effects of these redoses are detailed in the "Results" section.

Measures

Staff nurses used recording forms specifically designed for the research project to record patient data before and for seventy-two hours after the epidural/intrathecal narcotic was administered unless the patient was discharged sooner. Information recorded on each patient included age, sex, type of surgery, type of narcotic and dosage, postoperative vital signs, level of consciousness, and complaints of pain, nausea, vomiting, and pruritus. In addition, the medications administered to treat the observed variations in physiologic response were recorded by the nurse monitoring the patient. **Table 27.1** defines vital signs outside of normal parameters. The definition of abnormal level of consciousness included confused, agitated, sedated, and/or unresponsive. All complaints of pain, nausea, vomiting, and pruritus, regardless of severity, were recorded and included in the analysis.

Table 27.1: Vital Signs Outside Normal Parameters

Physiologic Measures
Systolic Blood Pressure - Greater than 150 or less than 90.
Diastolic Blood Pressure - Greater than 90 or less than 60.
Pulse - Greater than 100 or less than 40.
Respirations: Hyperventilation - Greater than 30.
Hypoventilation - Less than 10.

Validity and reliability. Content validity of the information to be collected was established by a panel of experts that included both nurses and anesthesiologists. All nursing staff in the units involved in the study received training in data collection. Reliability was established by comparing data collected by participating staff with data collected by members of the panel of experts on the same patients. The level of agreement for acceptable reliability was 0.85.

Procedures

The requirement for informed consent was waived by the institution's Human Subjects Review Committee. A research team consisting of a clinical nurse specialist, nurse managers, and staff nurses first conducted a pilot study on fifty-five patients receiving epidural morphine analgesia.[39] Following analysis of the pilot data, the team continued the research, observing the additional one hundred and ten patients described in the present paper for seventy-two hours postoperatively or up to the time of discharge if the patient was discharged earlier. As described above, eleven of the one hundred and ten patients were dropped from the study because a review of their medical records indicated complicating diagnoses or abnormal vital signs prior to surgery. The current analysis includes data collected on the final sample of ninety-nine patients during the first forty-eight hours after surgery.

Data were analyzed separately for the first and second twelve hours and the second twenty-four hours following release from the postoperative holding area. For each patient, the number of occurrences of each abnormal physiologic response in each time period, as well as nursing management data (e.g., the number of times medication was administered for that response during each time period), were coded for statistical analysis. The percentage of patients with at least one occurrence of each variation were then tabulated in three categories: (1) time period following surgery, (2) age, and (3) dosage. Patients receiving epidural and intrathecal morphine were combined because the number of patients receiving intrathecal morphine was too small for separate analysis. Also, because of the small number of females in the sample, separate analyses by gender were not conducted.

Statistical tests were conducted as appropriate to determine the statistical significance of findings. Because a small number of patients experienced many occurrences of some physiologic responses, the analysis used nonparametric tests to eliminate the effects of these outliers on the findings.

Results

Vital Signs

Table 27.2 shows the percentage of patients experiencing one or more occurrences of abnormal vital signs by time period after the patient was transferred to the ICU or nursing floor for the total sample and by age group. All of the observed variations constitute a change from preoperative status, since patients with abnormal vital signs, level of consciousness, and/or complicating diagnoses were excluded from the study.

Occurrence of physiological changes and patient age. Elevated systolic blood pressures occurred in 29% of the patients in the first twelve hours, dropping to 19% in later time periods. Age comparisons indicated significantly more occurrences in patients sixty-five years of age and older (X^2 [1, $\underline{N}$ = 99] = 14.53, $\underline{p}<0.001$). Abnormal diastolic blood pressures (both elevated and lowered) were observed throughout the forty-eight hour study, although the frequency decreased over time, with no significant differences by age. Pulses were accelerated in 14% of the patients during the first twelve hours, 13% in the second twelve hours, and 16% in the second twenty-four hours.

Initial dosage/redoses. There was no relationship between the initial morphine dose and occurrences of abnormal vital signs. Nine of the eleven patients (82%) receiving morphine redoses experienced abnormal blood pressures during the first twelve hours. Four of the six redosed patients (67%) still in the study during the second twenty-four hours also had abnormal blood pressure measures at that time.

Nursing monitoring. Nurses were required to monitor patient vital signs every fifteen minutes for the first two hours, then blood pressure and pulse every two hours for twenty-four hours. If a patient was redosed, the nurse observed the patient and obtained vital signs every fifteen minutes for two hours, followed by blood pressure and pulse every two hours for twenty-four hours.

Table 27.2

Percentage of Patients Experiencing Variations in Vital Signs Following Epidural or Intrathecal Analgesia for Total Sample and by Age Group[a]

Variations in Vital Signs	Time Period and Age Group[b]								
	First 12 Hours			Second 12 Hours			Second 24 Hours		
	Age Group			Age Group			Age Group		
	Total	20-64	65+	Total	20-64	65+	Total	20-64	65+
	(n=99)	(n=35)	(n=64)	(n=91)	(n=30)	(n=61)	(n=77)	(n=26)	(n=51)
Systolic B.P.	31%	6%	45%***	19%	10%	23%	19%	8%	26%
Elevated	29%	6%	42%***	19%	10%	23%	19%	8%	26%
Lowered	2%	0%	3%	0%	0%	0%	0%	0%	0%
Diastolic B.P.	32%	31%	33%	23%	20%	25%	18%	15%	20%
Elevated	14%	11%	16%	9%	7%	10%	6%	4%	8%
Lowered	21%	20%	22%	14%	10%	16%	13%	12%	14%
Pulse Heart Rate	14%	9%	17%	13%	10%	15%	16%	12%	18%
Accelerated	14%	9%	17%	13%	13%	15%	16%	12%	18%
Decelerated	1%	0%	2%	1%	3%	0%	0%	0%	0%
Respiratory Rate	3%	3%	3%	1%	0%	2%	3%	0%	4%
Elevated	3%	3%	3%	0%	0%	0%	2%	0%	4%
Depressed	2%	3%	2%	1%	0%	2%	1%	0%	2%

[a] *Percentage of patients with one or more occurrence.*

[b] *Sample includes only those patients observed for the entire time period indicated. Patients discharged during the time period are excluded. Total responses in each category may exceed the sum of the subcategories because one patient may have incidences of both high and low blood pressure, pulse, and/or respiration.*

* $p < 0.05$. ** $p < 0.01$. *** $p < 0.001$. *(Chi-square test for significant differences between age groups.)*

Respiratory Response

Incidence of respiratory depression, age, and redoses. Only two patients experienced the most significant complication, respiratory depression. Both had received morphine redoses. Both had respiratory depression during the first twelve hours; one also had respiratory depression in the second twelve hours and the second twenty-four hours (see **Table 27.2**). The lowest respiratory rate observed was charted at six respirations per minute. The patient observed with respiratory depression in all three time periods was seventy-three years old and received two redoses during the study period.

Nursing monitoring. Monitoring included vital signs (blood pressure, pulse, and respirations) every fifteen minutes for the first two hours, then respiratory rate every thirty minutes for twenty-four hours. Sedation (level of consciousness) was monitored every thirty minutes for twenty-four hours. If the respiratory rate was depressed, the patient was monitored every fifteen minutes until the respiratory status was stable for twenty-four hours. None of these patients was returned to the intensive care unit for invasive monitoring.

Postoperative Pain

Table 27.3 shows the incidence of postoperative pain, as well as pruritus, nausea, vomiting, and abnormal levels of consciousness, along with the percentage of patients receiving medication for relief, for the total sample and by age group.

Incidence and age. About 39% of the sample experienced pain during the first twelve hours, with the percentage increasing to 70% during the second twenty-four hours. Over half of the patients who complained of pain required pain medication. Patients age sixty-five years and older were significantly less likely to complain of pain (X^2 [1, $\underline{N}$ = 99] = 5.03, $\underline{p} < 0.05$), and receive pain medication (X^2 [1, $\underline{N}$ = 99] = 9.64, $\underline{p} < 0.01$) during the first twelve hours. There were similar differences between age groups in the second twenty-four hours.

Dosage and redoses. The incidence of postoperative pain was not related to the initial morphine dose. All of the patients receiving redoses experienced postoperative pain.

Nursing management. Nursing staff administered intramuscular analgesics every three to four hours as needed according to physician orders.

Pruritus

Incidence, age, and dosage. Records indicated that the incidence of pruritus dropped dramatically from 33% during the first twelve hours to 12% during the second twenty-four hours (see **Table 27.3**). Furthermore, many of the patients complaining of pruritus, especially during the second twenty-four hours, refused medication. Younger patients were significantly more likely than older patients to experience pruritus during the first twelve hours (X^2 [1, $\underline{N}$ = 99] = 5.67, $\underline{p} < 0.05$). The incidence of pruritus was not dose-related.

Table 27.3

Percentage of Patients Experiencing Variations in Physiologic Response Following Epidural or Intrathecal Analgesia for Total Sample and by Age Group[a]

Variations in Response	First 12 Hours			Second 12 Hours			Second 24 Hours		
	Time Period and Age Group[b]								
	Age Group			Age Group			Age Group		
	Total	20-64	65+	Total	20-64	65+	Total	20-64	65+
	(n=99)	(n=35)	(n=64)	(n=91)	(n=30)	(n=61)	(n=77)	(n=26)	(n=51)
Pain	39%	54%	31%*	43%	47%	41%	70%	89%	61%*
Pain Medication	20%	37%	11%**	37%	37%	38%	54%	73%	45%*
Morphine Redose	5%	6%	5%	7%	0%	10%	7%	4%	8%
Pruritus	33%	49%	25%*	20%	21%	9%	12%	12%	12%
Pruritus Medication	19%	37%	9%***	14%	17%	13%	3%	4%	2%
Nausea	29%	34%	27%	18%	23%	15%	5%	12%	2%
Vomiting	24%	26%	23%	13%	13%	13%	0%	0%	0%
Nausea/Vomiting Med.	24%	31%	20%	10%	10%	10%	6%	12%	4%
Abnormal Level of Consciousness[c]	7%	3%	9%	2%	3%	2%	6%	4%	8%

[a]*Percentage of patients with one or more occurrence.*

[b]*Sample includes only those patients observed for the entire time period indicated. Patients discharged during the time period are excluded.*

[c]*Includes confused, agitated, sedated, and/or unresponsive.*

*$p < 0.05$. **$p < 0.01$. ***$p < 0.001$. *(Chi-square test for significant differences between age groups.)*

Nursing management. Staff administered antipruritic treatments such as cooling measures as well as applying topical medications (Caladryl).

Nausea/Vomiting

Incidence, age, and dosage/redoses. Nausea decreased from 29% during the first twelve hours to 5% during the second twenty-four hours (see **Table 27.3**). There were no significant differences by age group. Nausea and vomiting were not dose-related. None of the patients receiving redoses experienced nausea during the first twelve hours.

Nursing management. Staff administered antiemetic drugs per protocol every three hours.

Level of Consciousness

Incidence, age, and dosage/redoses. As noted above, abnormal level of consciousness included patients who were confused, agitated, sedated, and/or unresponsive. During the first twelve hours, seven patients (7%) showed abnormal levels of consciousness (see **Table 27.3**). Only one of those patients had received a redose; five were sixty-five or older.

Five patients (6%) had abnormal levels of consciousness during the second twenty-four hours. Three were classified as confused, one agitated, and one had a petit mal seizure. Four of the five were sixty-five or older. Two of the patients had received redoses; three had not. None of the reactions was related to the initial morphine dosage.

Nursing management. Nurses observed patients and implemented safety precautions to prevent patient injury during periods of confusion, agitation, and sedation.

Discussion

Recommended Patient Management Guidelines

Since the first use of morphine in 1979, investigators have confirmed the efficacy of epidural analgesia.[40, 41, 42] Findings from the present study, as well as those reported in the literature, however, suggested that changes in the nursing management protocol could be implemented. The revised guidelines were based upon observed variations in physiologic response among patients in different subgroups. Given the sample size and study design, the findings are not generalizable; however, they suggest the need for database development across institutional settings on patient management for postoperative epidural morphine patients. The following sections detail findings for each of the three research questions.

Research Question 1: *Is the incidence of variations in physiologic response among patients receiving epidural or intrathecal analgesia commensurate with the literature?* The incidence of minor heart rate and blood pressure changes as well as nausea, vomiting, pruritus, and break through pain in our study was consistent with the literature (see **Table 27.4**).

Table 27.4

Incidence of Variations in Physiologic Response Compared to Expected Variation Based Upon Literature and Practice[52, 53, 54, 55, 56, 57]

Variation in Response	Expected	Observed
Elevated Blood Pressure	Less than 30% in first 12 hours	29% in first 12 hours
Decelerated Pulse Heart Rate	Less than 15% in first 12 hours	1% in first 12 hours
Respiratory Depression	0.1% in first 12 hours; <3% in 12 to 24 hours.	2% associated with redose in first 12 hours; 1% with redose and age >65 in 12-24 hours.
Breakthrough Pain	40% require additional opioids in first 12 hours; 50% in first 24 hours.	39% in first 12 hours; 43% in second 12 hours.
Pruritus	40-75% present 12 to 24 hours	12 to 33% over first 48 hours
Nausea/Vomiting	30-50% of patients	5-29% of patients
LOC	Less than 3% in 12-24 hour	2% in 12-24 hours

Research Question 2: *What patient factors are associated with variation in physiological response?* Patient age and redosing were the most significant factors associated with variations in physiologic response. Study findings showed significant differences between age groups, with patients age sixty-five and over more likely to experience variations in systolic blood pressure during the first twelve hours in particular. Patients under age sixty-five were more likely to experience both pain and pruritus during the same time period. Regardless of age, there was a potential for respiratory depression. Both of the patients experiencing respiratory depression, however, had received redoses.

Examination of the data indicated that two of the eleven patients receiving redoses experienced respiratory depression. Nine of the eleven patients (82%) experienced abnormal blood pressures during the first twelve hours. Four of the six redosed patients (67%) still in the study during the second twenty-four hours also had abnormal blood pressure measures at that time. Both of the patients with abnormal level of consciousness in the second twelve hours had received redoses; both were agitated.

Research Question 3: *What nursing assessment and monitoring guidelines should be adopted based on patient observations and a synthesis of literature findings?* Based upon these findings, recommendations were made to decrease respiratory rate monitoring from every thirty minutes for twenty-four hours to every sixty minutes for sixteen hours following the two hour post anesthesia care unit (PACU) monitoring phase. In addition to vital sign monitoring, the need to observe patients every thirty minutes for changes in level of consciousness was decreased (see **Table 27.5**). Together the data also suggest the need to develop specific nursing management guidelines for specific subgroups of patients. Nursing workload (demand for care) can be adjusted to meet patient needs.

Developing Guidelines

This study is an example of the multidisciplinary research required to develop appropriate guidelines that respond to the emergence of medical technology. The protocol in existence prior to the research study was developed by anesthesiologists based on reported medical experience, but with little input from nursing. The development of nursing management guidelines for any new technology requires that nurses observe variations in physiological response and develop monitoring modalities that address the anticipation and recognition of potential complications among specific patient population subgroups (e.g., older patients, patients receiving redosage). Findings from such studies provide a sound scientific basis for developing patient management guidelines and accompanying educational materials (e.g., Good Samaritan Hospital and Medical Center) that are generalizable to other institutions using the same technologies with comparable patient populations. [43]

Table 27.5

Nursing Assessment and Monitoring Guidelines
Nursing Management Protocols[a] Before and After Study and Rationale for Change

Response	Before Study	After Study	Rationale for Change
Initial Dose			
Blood Pressure	Every 2 hours for 24 hours.	Every 4 hours for 24 hours.	Literature and study indicate 70% show no change.
Pulse	Every 2 hours for 24 hours.	Every 4 hours for 24 hours.	Literature and study report 1% or less decelerated pulse.
Respiratory Rate	Every 30 mins. for 24 hours.	Every hour for 16 hours.	Literature and study report respiratory changes occur in first 16 hours. Only 3% (all age 65+) show later changes.
Level of Consciousness	Every 30 mins. for 24 hours.	Every 4 hours for 24 hours.	Literature and study report <=1% sedated and/or unresponsive.
Urinary Retention	Every 2 hours for 24 hours.	Every 4 hours for 24 hours.	Literature supports monitoring requirements.
Redose			
	Return patient to PACU or monitored bed.	Patient stays in general surgical unit.	Literature and study indicate it is not necessary to transfer patient higher level of care in absence of adverse physiologic parameters.
Vital Signs	Every 15 mins. for 2 hrs. Then respiratory rate every 30 minutes for 24 hours. Other vital signs every 2 hours for 24 hours.	Respiratory rate every 1 hour for 16 hours. All other vital signs every 4 hours for 24 hours.	

[a] *Following two-hour PACU monitoring phase.*

In the present case, patient variation and physician monitoring guidelines were first reported in the medical literature in 1979.[44, 45, 46] In each study, the authors suggested that nurses would need to closely monitor patients for extended periods, but did not support their recommendations with specific findings. Nursing investigators reported variations, but they did not suggest guideline development for monitoring until 1986.[47, 48, 49] The American Nurses' Association position statement for nursing management of patients receiving analgesia by catheter, endorsed by twenty-one other nursing specialty organizations, was issued ten years following the adoption of intraspinal narcotics for effective postoperative pain management.[50] As new technologies continue to emerge, nurses must pursue the development of patient care guidelines (e.g., Agency for Health Care Policy and Research) in collaboration with all members of the multidisciplinary clinical team.[51] Our findings also indicate the need for specific nursing care guidelines which delineate the amount of nursing time required to assure patient care quality.

References

1 Grinde JW, R Grina, T Gellaty. " Pain Management by Epidural Analgesia: The Challenge for Nursing." *Heart and Lung* 13 1984: 105-110.

2 Cramer C. "Morphine Epidural Anesthesia." *Journal of Post Anesthesia Nursing* 1 1986: 129-131.

3 Jiang C, C Liu, T Wu, et al. "Mini-Dose Intrathecal Morphine For Post-Cesarean Section Analgesia." *Acta Anaesthesiologica Sinica* 29 1991: 683-689.

4 Johnson RG, M Miller, M Murphy. "Intraspinal Narcotic Analgesia: A Comparison of Two Methods of Postoperative Pain Relief." *Spine* 14 1989: 363-366.

5 Loper KA, LB Ready, M Nessly, SE Rapp. "Epidural Morphine Provides Greater Pain Relief Than Patient—Controlled Intravenous Morphine Following Cholecystectomy." *Anesthesia and Analgesia* 69 1989: 826-828.

6 Simpson T, G Wahl, M DeTraglia, et al. "The Effects of Epidural Versus Parenteral Opioid Analgesia on Postoperative Pain and Pulmonary Function in Adults Who Have Undergone Thoracic and Abdominal Surgery: A Critique of Research." *Heart & Lung* 21 1992:125-140.

7 Simpson T, G Wahl, M DeTraglia, et al. "A Pilot Study of Pain, Analgesia Use, and Pulmonary Function After Colectomy With or Without a Preoperative Bolus of Epidural Morphine." *Heart & Lung* 22 1993: 316-327.

8 Bromage PR. "The Price of Intraspinal Narcotic Analgesia: Basic Constraints." *Anesthesia and Analgesia* 60 1981: 461-463.

9 Cousins MJ, LE Mather. "Intrathecal and Epidural Administration of Opioids." *Anesthesiology* 61 1984: 276-310.

10 Asantila R, P Eklund, PH Rosenberg. "Epidural Analgesia With 4 mg of Morphine Following Caesarean Section: Effect of Injected Volume." *Acta Anaesthesiologica* 37 1993: 764-7.

11 Blackman RG, J Reynolds, J Shively. "Intrathecal Morphine in Younger Patients for Postoperative Pain Following Spinal Fusion." *Today's O.R. Nurse* 13; 9 1991: 25-29.

12 Chestnut DH, WW Choi, TJ Isbell. "Epidural Hydromorphone for Postcesarean Analgesia." *Obstetrics and Gynecology* 68 1986: 65-69.

13 Jiang et al., 1991

14 Juneja MM, WE Ackerman III, K Bellinger. "Epidural Morphine Pruritus Reduction with Hydroxyzine in Parturients." *Journal of the Kentucky Medical Association* 89 1991: 319-321.

15 Kirson LE, JM Goldman, RB Slover. "Low-Dose Intrathecal Morphine for Postoperative Pain Control in Patients Undergoing Transurethral Resection of the Prostate." *Anesthesiology* 71 1989: 192-195.

16 Kotelko DM, PA Dailey, SM Shnider, et al. "Epidural Morphine Analgesia After Cesarean Delivery." *Obstetrics and Gynecology* 63 1984: 409-413.

17 Stenseth R, O Sellevold, H Breivik. "Epidural Morphine for Postoperative Pain: Experience with 1085 Patients." *Acta Anaesthesiologica Scandinavica* 29 1985: 148-156.

18 Cousins & Mather, 1984

19 Kirson et al., 1989

20 Stenseth et al., 1985

21 Yamaguchi H, S Watanabe, K Motokawa, Y Ishizawa. "Intrathecal Morphine Dose-Response Data for Pain Relief After Cholecystectomy." *Anesthesia and Analgesia* 70 1990: 168-71.

22 Allen PD, T Walman, M Concepcion, et al. "Epidural Morphine Provides Postoperative Pain Relief in Peripheral Vascular and Orthopedic Surgical Patients: A Dose-Response Study." *Anesthesia and Analgesia* 65 1986: 165-170.

23 Stenseth et al., 1985

24 Etches, RC, AN Sandler, SL Lawson. "A Comparison of the Analgesic and Respiratory Effects of Epidural Nalbuphine or Morphine in Postthoracotomy Patients." *Anesthesiology* 75 1991: 9-14.

25 Blackman et al., 1991.

26 Bromage 1981.

27 Brown DL. "Postoperative Analgesia Following Thoracotomy." *Chest* 88 1985: 779-780.

28 Corke CF & RG Wheatley. "Respiratory Depression Complicating Epidural Diamorphine. *Anaesthesia* 40 1985: 1203-1205.

29 Cousins & Mather, 1984

30 Allen et al., 1986

31 Stenseth et al., 1985

32 Chestnut et al., 1986

33 Gurel A, N Unal, M Elevli, A Eren. "Epidural Morphine for Postoperative Pain Relief in Anorectal Surgery." *Anesthesia and Analgesia* 65 1986: 499-502.

34 Johnson et al., 1989

35 Kirson et al., 1989

36 Kotelko et al., 1984

37 Loper et al., 1989

38 Yamaguchi, et al., 1990

39 Burnes Bolton, L, & P Kalowes. "A Clinical Study on Nursing Care Management of Patients Receiving Epidural Narcotics for Post Operative Pain." Paper presented at the 1988 Virginia Mason Medical Center Eighth Annual *Distinguished Nurse Lecture and Symposium*, Seattle, WA.

40 Baggerly J. "Epidural Catheters for Pain Management: The Nurses' Role." *Journal of Neuroscience Nursing* 5 1986: 290-299.

41 Samii K, M Chauvin, P Viars. "Postoperative Spinal Analgesia with Morphine." *British Journal of Anaesthesia* 53 1981: 817-820.

[42] Wang JK, LA Nauss, JE Thomas. "Pain Relief by Intrathecally Applied Morphine in Man." *Anesthesiology* 50 1979: 149-151.

[43] Good Samaritan Hospital & Medical Center. *Epidural Credentialing Workbook*. Portland, OR, 1990.

[44] Baggerly, 1986

[45] Samii et al., 1981

[46] Wang et al., 1979

[47] Baggerly, 1986

[48] Genge ML. "Epidural Analgesia in the Orthopaedic Patient." *Orthopedic Nursing* 7 1988: 11-19.

[49] Yeager M, D Glass, R Neff, T Brinck-Johnsen. "Epidural Anesthesia and Analgesia in High-Risk Surgical Patients." *Anesthesiology* 66 1987: 729-736.

[50] American Nurses' Association. *Nursing Management of Epidural Analgesia and Anesthesia.* Position Paper: Washington DC, 1991

[51] Agency for Health Care Policy and Research. *Acute Pain Management in Adults: Operative Procedures*. Department of Health and Human Services, Rockville, Maryland, 1992.

[52] Basu MS. "Intrathecal Buprenorphine for Postoperative Analgesia in Orthopaedic Surgery." *Journal of the Indian Medical Association* 90 1992: 5-6.

[53] Cousins & Mather, 1984.

[54] Cramer 1986

[55] Grass JA. "Fentanyl: Clinical Use as Postoperative Analgesic Epidural/Intrathecal Route." *Journal of Pain and Symptom Management* 7 1992: 419-430.

[56] Van der Auwera D, C Verborgh, F Camu. "Analgesic and cardiorespiratory effects of epidural sufentanil and morphine in humans." Anesthesia and Analgesia 66 1987: 999-1003.

[57] Whiting W, A Sandler, L Lau, et al. "Analgesic and respiratory effects of epidural sufentanil in patients following thoracotomy." *Anesthesiology* 69 1988: 36-43.

Chapter 28

Conclusion

Carolyn E. Aydin, PhD
Linda Burnes Bolton, DrPH, RN, FAAN
Scott Weingarten, MD, MPH

The health care system is undergoing significant change driven by market forces and societal needs. The health delivery whitewater period described five years ago as a tumultuous, storming, and ever-changing shifting force remains. States are struggling to pick up the ball on national health care reform, while the rapid rise of managed care is driving providers and payers to join forces in designing and implementing systems of care that are simultaneously efficient, effective, and valued. Policymakers, providers, and payers need time-sensitive data that can provide rapid and reliable information on the impacts of changes in organizations and their processes of care. This book explored the ways in which responsible providers and payers can evaluate the effects of these dramatic changes at the organizational and provider level on the health and health care of consumers. We conclude with a few summary comments on the case studies presented and a challenge to our colleagues on the next steps for improving health delivery system performance.

Restructuring Acute Care

We began by exploring several organizational concepts currently operating in the marketplace and presented data on the most popular organizational change effort in acute care delivery systems: patient-focused care. The goals of patient-focused care are to reduce the costs of providing acute clinical care services while improving the clinical and organizational outcomes associated with the care delivery process. This paradigm is being implemented in a national environment in which health care institutions are struggling with decreased inpatient volumes and shrinking revenue bases. The response to

CAROLYN E. AYDIN, PHD—Assistant Administrator for Nursing Research, Cedars-Sinai Medical Center and Research Institute; Assistant Clinical Professor, University of California-Los Angeles, School of Nursing.

LINDA BURNES BOLTON, DRPH, RN, FAAN—Director Nursing Research and Development, Cedars-Sinai Medical Center and Research Institute; Assistant Clinical Professor, University of California-Los Angeles, School of Nursing; Associate Professor, California State University-Los Angeles, School of Nursing.

SCOTT WEINGARTEN, MD, MPH—Director, Health Services Research, Cedars-Sinai Health System and Research Institute; Assistant Professor, University of California-Los Angeles, School of Medicine.

these external pressures has been a dramatic downsizing of acute care delivery systems and sharp increase in the number of integrated delivery networks. The popular belief is that, in order to finance health care delivery, provide expanded access to health care services, and meet the expectations of consumers, providers, and payers, the system as we know it today will evolve into five to eight integrated networks. Each network will consist of 600 to 800 community-based systems. The successful systems will employ strategies to deliver effective care that ensure quality outcomes at the lowest cost for large and diverse populations at both the acute and community care levels.[1] We provided several examples of structural and process changes that, if implemented, have the potential to influence the delivery of effective care and the monitoring of care processes at the organizational and clinical outcome level.

Delivering Appropriate and Effective Care

The implementation of evidence-based medicine and clinical guidelines is an important strategy for reducing variation in the delivery of appropriate and effective care. The exponential growth in the development of guidelines, practice parameters pathways, and algorithms stems from the interest of third party payers to have a reliable standard by which they can judge the performance of providers. According to D.M. Eddy, because guidelines are so pervasive and because they provide the fine tuning that touches the physician and patient most closely, they will probably be the visible and personal manifestations of the battle over evidence and cost of appropriate and effective care.[2]

Chapters 17-19 focused on methods to develop clinical guidelines and determine quality outcomes based on the best available scientific data and described the value of deploying interdisciplinary teams in this process. We believe in and highly recommend this organizational strategy. The development of pathways, which link clinical guidelines, protocols, and interdisciplinary planned interventions to expected patient outcomes, is another key organizational strategy. Chapter 19 detailed a template for pathway development while Chapter 23, among others, provided preliminary data on the effectiveness of the pathways and clinical guidelines developed by these interdisciplinary teams. The challenge remains to effectively link each of these measures into a system for ongoing organizational performance. We have initiated such an effort and have reported it here.

Measuring Quality Outcomes

Throughout the text we have illustrated the relationship between process and structural changes and the achievement of clinical and organizational outcomes. The chapters in Section I described the tools and methodology for patient-focused care. The ability to meet patient expectations, such as responsiveness, cleanliness, information and education, and access to clinical care (time spent with registered nurses and other clinicians), is vital to organizations seeking to attract key health care payers by demonstrating the presence of reengineering processes and systems. Chapters 15 and 16 detailed multiple methods to assess the outcomes of this effort, including both clinical outcomes and service outcomes that are valued by individual patients.

Clinical outcomes are valued by patients, payers, and providers. Whether they are attributed to patient-focused care or clinical guidelines and pathways, clinical outcomes must be tracked over time. The tools utilized to measure outcomes must also be reliable, valid, and subject to review by interdisciplinary groups. We provided several examples of clinical outcome monitoring by different health team members—medicine, nursing, physical therapy, pharmacy, pulmonary service, and medical social work. Each discipline described structural and process changes and the effects of those changes on patient outcomes. The pathway and guideline chapters synthesized the work of the interdisciplinary teams and delineated specific expected and observed clinical outcomes.

Reducing Costs

Delivering clinical care at the lowest cost requires an understanding of the factors contributing to the dollars expended. We recommend utilization of cost per discharge to evaluate organizational performance. Costs per discharge include all costs associated with the provision of care for large population groups. Patient-focused care seeks to reduce costs per discharge by restructuring the care team, removing barriers to effective team functioning, and identifying enablers to allow team members to provide care in an efficient manner. Clinical guidelines and pathways reduce costs per discharge by standardizing care processes and reducing variation in the consumption of resources to achieve desired clinical quality. Restructuring what care is provided, what resources are utilized to provide care, and who provides that care are effective organizational strategies to reduce the costs of delivering care for various clinical population groups.

Focusing on Effective Health Care Teams

The lessons learned from the various case studies presented in this book are illustrative of the various approaches to health system organizational restructuring. Taken together our findings indicate that, while we are usually successful in delivering the technical aspects of care, the interpersonal aspects of the quality of care require increased attention. Team function processes are more complex and require a longer period of transition and support to achieve expected care model outcomes. We recommend additional work at the interpersonal level on health care teams and the ways in which they are organized to achieve institutional outcomes. These recommendations stem from our collective experiences in organizational redesign. The relationship between effective team functioning and the ability to achieve desired organizational performance should be explored in greater detail. Self-directed teams that clearly understand their value-laden products are empowered to initiate structural and process changes to improve their ability to accomplish organizational goals. They also demonstrate a willingness to change for the better and are usually at the center of most successful organizations. These teams, whether in manufacturing or health care, are essential to our ability to address societal needs by organizing the work in a systematic manner that is responsive to reliable data on the effectiveness of the system's output. Teamwork among physicians, nurses, social services, and others has been shown to lead to cost-effective utilization of resources and tremendous, continuous improvement in the treatment of cancer.[3] We challenge readers to participate in the design of effective tools and processes to enable health care providers to evaluate the effect of continuous change on our collective ability to meet the health care needs of our society.

Next Steps

The quality improvement literature continue to cite the value of interdisciplinary work units to accomplish quality goals.[4, 5] Our next key steps are to develop and implement a systemwide approach to the creation and support of these work teams. Communication and commitment are critical to the success of any change initiative. People, who are motivated, empowered, and supported, are more likely to work together to improve processes and achieve outcomes. As simple as this sounds, it is difficult to accomplish.

We have embarked on a comprehensive program which includes the restructuring of our medical staff and administrative committee process. We will be deleting the departmentally-based quality improvement committees that promoted turfism. Typically, organizations have medical staff improvement committees, nursing improvement committees, and a variety of clinical ancillary improvement committees. We will have one interdisciplinary committee responsible for addressing the structural and process improvements necessary to sustain quality care at the lowest possible cost. The committee will function by launching continuous quality improvement teams to conduct the work of investigating and defining processes for improvement, delineating changes with the potential to affect outcomes, reporting on the best solutions, implementing and evaluating the solutions, and recommending ongoing monitoring efforts. We anticipate reducing the current committee structure of more than 100 medical staff and operational committees to possibly 25 or 30.

We are simultaneously launching a systemwide education effort for all employees on self-directed service teams. Self-directed service teams own the diverse processes of care. They are knowledgeable and communicate about how their work influences each other and ultimately patient outcomes. They are committed to eliminating steps that delay care or adversely affect patient outcomes. They are data driven and self managed. All employees will participate in customer simulation education to facilitate their understanding and empathy of the processes from the customer's perspective. Managers from diverse departments will continue their work on quality action teams designed to address system process improvement issues, such as patient education, turn around time, responsiveness, etc. We have identified core competencies for managers, which include their role as servant leaders. Managers, who are knowledgeable and committed to serving others by reducing barriers, providing enablers, and modeling the behaviors of customer-focused employees, are servant leaders. What effect will these managers have on process improvements and organizational and clinical outcomes? How will self-directed service teams enable health organizations to achieve their cost and quality objectives? What data and information about the health organization's system functions and outcomes are valued by consumers, providers, and payers? These challenges and question should be addressed by health researchers in collaborations with clinicians, administrators, consumers and payers. We look forward to working with the industry to meet the challenge.

References

1 Bergman R. "Getting the Goods on Guidelines." *Hospital and Health Networks*, Oct. 20, 1994:70-74

2 Eddy DM. "The Challenge of Producing Clinical Guidelines: Comparing the Benefits and the Harm." *Journal of the American Medical Association* 270(4) 1990:2493-2505.

3 Miles PV. "Use of Protocols for Effective Pediatric Oncology Treatment." *Journal of Quality Improvement* 21(1) 1995: 38.

4 Sneider D. "Healthcare Team Meetings: Sharing Responsibility for Cost and Quality Care." Definitions 4(2) 1989:1-3.

5 Berwick DM. *Organizational Dynamics-Quality Action Teams.* Burlington MA: 1990.